MIND-BODY UNITY

MIND-BODY UNITY

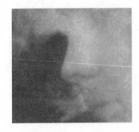

A New Vision

for Mind-Body

Science and

Medicine

——

HENRY DREHER

THE JOHNS HOPKINS UNIVERSITY PRESS

Baltimore and London

© 2003 The Johns Hopkins University Press
All rights reserved. Published 2003
Printed in the United States of America on acid-free paper
9 8 7 6 5 4 3 2 1

The Johns Hopkins University Press
2715 North Charles Street
Baltimore, Maryland 21218-4363
www.press.jhu.edu

Library of Congress Cataloging-in-Publication Data

Dreher, Henry.
Mind-body unity : a new vision for mind-body science and medicine /
Henry Dreher.
p. ; cm.
Includes bibliographical references and index.
ISBN 0-8018-7392-4 (hardcover : alk. paper)
1. Medicine, Psychosomatic. 2. Mind and body. 3. Mind and body therapies.
[DNLM: 1. Mind-Body Relations (Metaphysics)—physiology.
2. Psychophysiologic Disorders.
3. Psychosomatic Medicine. WB 880 D771m 2003] I. Title.
RC49 .D725 2003
616.08-dc21   2002152157

A catalog record for this book is available from the British Library.

For Harris Dienstfrey
and
Barbara Miller

Contents

Acknowledgments

I wish to thank Harris Dienstfrey, my editor at *Advances in Mind-Body Medicine*, for giving me my first chance in 1984 to write about mind-body science and medicine. Harris gave me open-ended opportunities to write for the journal, which I did regularly for the next seventeen years, and many chapters in this book are revised versions of articles that first appeared there. He has been a wonderful teacher and editor—patient and witty, blending constructive criticism with credible praise, a steadfast supporter and friend.

I am deeply grateful to the scientists and clinicians who have helped to shape my thinking, most importantly Lydia Temoshok, James Pennebaker, and the late George F. Solomon. Lydia opened my eyes to a deeper scientific and psychological sensibility about mind-body medicine, and we coauthored *The Type C Connection: The Behavioral Links to Cancer and Your Health* based on the research she conducted in the 1980s at the University of California at San Francisco. Her bold theoretical contributions have greatly influenced my writing of the chapters in this book on cancer and heart disease. I thank her for her wisdom and her friendship.

James Pennebaker's ever-changing repertoire of research methods has allowed him to sustain a freshness that makes his ever-broadening work on disclosure and health always relevant. Like Lydia, Jamie has moved beyond mind-body clichés to grasp how thoughts and feelings truly influence disease and health. We became friends the first time I went to Dallas to meet with and write about him, and I continue to enjoy his dry wit and penetrating insight.

My first assignment for *Advances* was a conference on psychosocial factors and AIDS. I knew little about the nascent mind-body field, and I was struck by the collective intellectual radiance of the conference participants, who included Lydia Temoshok, Michael Lerner, Rachel Naomi Remen, Joan Borysenko, and the late Bernard Fox. But the presentation made by George F. Solomon, the psychiatrist whose work in the early 1960s on the two-way communication between the brain and the immune system presaged the signal developments in mind-body science of the 1970s, 1980s, and 1990s, had a particular impact on me. George, who had used rigorous scientific methods to break down centuries-old Cartesian barriers, spoke eloquently about psychoneuroimmunology, the field he had helped to found.

George Solomon, an authentic visionary of modern mind-body science, died in 2001 at age seventy, far too young for a man of his vivacity whose lifework was not yet complete. I wrote about George's work, and I spent time with him and his wife, Susan. He was ornery, passionate, prescient, and gutsy enough to follow his nose and fight for his scientific beliefs. I feel honored to have known George and will always feel thankful for both his support of my work and his enormous contributions to the field of mind-body unity.

Many other leaders in this field have encouraged and helped me as I wrote about mind-body matters: Steven Locke, Candace Pert, Martin Rossman, Rachel Naomi Remen, Gary Schwartz, Belleruth Naparstek, Joan Borysenko, Michael Lerner, Steven Greer, Keith and Penny Block, David McClelland, Marilyn Schlitz, Jeanne Achterberg, Jon Kabat-Zinn, and the late Elizabeth Targ, whose brilliance, I am certain, continues to radiate wherever she may be in the cosmos. Jim Gordon, of the Center for Mind-Body Medicine in Washington, D.C., has given me wonderful opportunities to find my voice as a teacher and thinker, and physician Larry Dossey, who has brought so much integrity to integrative medicine, has been unwaveringly supportive and generous. I was honored to collaborate on two books with Alice Domar about mind-body medicine for women; she helped bring a plain-spoken, practical element into my writing. I also thank Larry LeShan, another farsighted mind-body pioneer, whose seminal work in cancer psychotherapy, as well as his friendship, have been especially meaningful.

Special gratitude goes to Candace Pert and Michael Ruff, my coauthors for chapter 1, "The Psychosomatic Network: Foundations of Mind-Body Medicine." The original version was published as an article in *Alternative Therapies in Health and Medicine*, and I was honored to work with them. Like Lydia and George, Candace Pert has helped move the mind-body paradigm from one of *linkages* to one of unity—roughly equivalent to the difference between occasional dating and lifelong marriage. I also thank my friends Jeanne Achterberg and Marilyn Schlitz for their help in steering that article from conception to completion.

Barbara Miller has not only guided my personal growth but also taught me the meaning of mind-body health on the deepest levels. I don't know that I could have written this book, an accumulation of more than a decade's work, without her grounded and loving support.

Jacqueline Wehmueller, executive editor at the Johns Hopkins University Press, has been a dream editor. Jackie was always available, her editing was meticulous and thoughtful, and in our conversations she was unfailingly positive, constructive, and generous. What more could a writer ask?

I am grateful to all those at the Johns Hopkins University Press who helped make the publication of this book possible, including those on the editorial and advisory boards; the copyeditor, Joanne Allen; Jackie Wehmueller's assistant, Susan Lantz; senior production editor Kim Johnson; Adam Glazer; and everyone involved in the book's production. I also thank my indexer, Alexa Selph. And a special salute goes to my dear friend Judy Nisenholt, who translated the concept of mind-body unity into the evocative image for the jacket and whose artistry never fails to inspire.

Finally, I thank my wife, Deborah Chiel, who, over the course of a decade, has seen me through the writing of every chapter in this book. She has put up with my odd hours and habits and my psychosomatic symptoms; she has been my constant, loving companion, and I could not have written this book without her input and guidance. Finally, I am thrilled to thank my daughter, Ava Rose, who exemplifies mind-body unity: her every gesture, giggle, smile, sob, raised eyebrow, new word, tight hug, and blown kiss is a whole mind, whole body experience. She lifts my spirit every day.

Introduction

We hear much today about the "mind-body connection." Physicians, biological scientists, mental health professionals, and the public at large discuss, debate, embrace, repudiate, criticize, and hold it up to scrutiny. Physicians and scientists are no longer wholly in the grip of Cartesian dualism, the nineteenth-century doctrine that separated mind (or soul) and body, but with rare exceptions they have not replaced the old dualism with a coherent, philosophically and scientifically rooted nondualism. A substantial portion of the public appears to believe in a mind-body connection, but the popular understanding of this phenomenon is a simplified dilution of an emergent body of knowledge, and the mind-body treatments widely available are too few and often superficial. Part of the reason for this lack of depth is the current conceptualization of the mind-body relationship. The popular belief, both in academia and among the public, is that we need only study and acknowledge how mind and body are "connected" to successfully set aside Cartesian dualism.

But the mind-body connection is itself a form of dualism. *Connection* implies two separate entities that are related via passageways—just as cities are connected by freeways, computers are connected by cables, oceans are connected by canals. Certainly there are brain-body connections: the brain is hard-wired to parts of the body, a point that has been self-evident since the birth of neuroscience. But the term *connection* can lose its validity when *mind* is brought into the equation.

The revelation of mind-body science has been that the brain regulates bodily systems (primarily but not exclusively the immune system) that were never thought to be commandeered by any systems other than themselves, let alone the material master of mind, the brain. This revelation has been a genuinely triumphant (if underrecognized) late-twentieth-century scientific achievement. Over the past three decades a group of pioneering investigators has used the technology of biomedical science to break through barriers of compartmentalization and specialization that were (and still are) being erected within biomedicine itself. The mind-body scientists followed every cellular and molecular trail that led from one system to another. They traced nerve fibers to the immune system's own teaching hospital, the thymus gland, trainer of immature T cells; tracked lines of innervation to other hubs of immunity, including the spleen, lymph nodes, and bone marrow; followed nerves as they thread alongside blood vessels through which lymphocytes pass on their defensive duties; detected receptors on immune cells for scores of different neuropeptides and neurotransmitters, more telltale evidence of nervous-immune interplay; searched out immune-cell products called cytokines in nooks and crannies of the brain, where they act as couriers in feedback loops of vital immunological and psychological information.

These explorers, leaders of such fields as psychoneuroimmunology, neuroimmunomodulation, and psychoneuroendocrinology, sneaked past the closed doors of biomedical compartmentalization with the fearlessness of cat burglars. Their work has been groundbreaking, yet the radical ramifications have hardly been understood, let alone fully integrated, by mainstream medicine. While their discoveries have spurred slight alterations in medicine's Cartesian paradigm, these breakthroughs have not overturned the paradigm, partly because of that lumbering word *connection*.

What is wrong with *connection?* It is a hard-edged, mechanistic term for describing the relational currency in an organism that is more flowing than fitted together, more thoroughly integrated than assembled like parts of an engine. Moreover, as the neuroscientist Candace Pert has argued, neuropeptides and their corresponding cellular receptors are substrates of human thought and feeling that act throughout the brain and body. Hence the mind cannot be completely defined by the brain any more than the body can be defined by bones and skin. Molecules once thought to belong to particular systems (e.g., the nervous, endocrine, and immune networks) turn out to speak a universal language of bodymind, and their signals carry information that is multileveled. For instance, a neurohormone that mediates fear can also activate natural killer cells roving the body in search of pathogens. There are countless examples of this blurring of boundaries between biological systems, so many, in fact, that it no longer makes much sense to talk about connections. Rather, as the molecular biologists Roger Booth and Kevin Ashbridge have argued, mind-body is an integral system of interacting elements governed less by sharply specialized functions than by a broader teleology—the preservation of the organism's integrity. That the "fear" molecule rouses the conscious mind when we are threatened and simultaneously stimulates natural killer cells reflects a teleological principle: it is a messenger warning both the brain and the immune system that injury may be imminent, and it prepares both for necessary actions. It is a "meaning" molecule, not a "mind" or "body" molecule.

Indeed, the very brain structures, cells, and molecules we associate with "mind"—the neuropeptides, neurohormones, and their receptors—are among the most versatile multitaskers in the human organism, dialoguing continuously with cells throughout the body, including immune cells. With the discoveries in the 1980s and 1990s that immune cells make nerve cell products and nerve cells make immune-cell products, old assumptions about biological specialization were turned upside down. Visionary mind-body scientists began to understand that connectivity was no longer the most useful or most accurate metaphor for understanding mind-body relationships. Mind and body are not connected; they are unified. The mind is not limited to the brain, the body is not limited to organs and tissues beneath the skull, and humans' endogenous healing network is not limited to the immune system; this network is a whole-organism entity.

The idea of mind-body unity opens up the field of mind-body science and medicine to limitless possibilities. Contrary to the therapeutic homilies of the 1970s and 1980s, when mind-body medicine was first popularized, love is not enough, and neither is relaxation. Love and relaxation may be necessary starting points for salutary mind-body interactions, but they are just starting points. Throughout this book I endeavor to show that mind-body unity runs as deep as the psyche itself, encompassing the full spectrum of our thoughts, feelings, memories, and personality traits, and its meshwork is as intricate as the molecular landscapes of the body. While I am certain that I fall prey to dualistic language from time to time, referring occasionally to "the mind's role in health," I offer this a priori corrective: our minds play a role in health the way our eyes play a role in sight.

The old model of mind-body, which still predominates in some academic and popular realms, focused mainly on stress, relaxation, and attitudes. The prevailing idea was that our health is influenced by our stress levels, our capacity to relax, and whether we confront stress, and illness itself, with a "positive attitude." While stress, relaxation, and attitudes matter, they represent only one level of mind-body unity. In fact, the popular health prescription of a positive attitude, a purported balm for all that ails us, was superficial and even harmful. It implied that harboring or expressing "negative" emotions—fear, anger, heartache—was bad for one's health, when the best evidence now suggests that acknowledging and working through negative emotions is adaptive and promotes health. If having a positive attitude means maintaining a façade of good cheer, it might do medical patients more harm than good, and it would not be salutary for healthy people either. The basic science of mind-body unity suggests that every shade of emotion and every facet of selfhood is curled together with bodily states relevant to health. And the most compelling mind-body studies suggest that how we feel, what we feel, and how we live in a relational world have as much bearing on our health as the pathogens we have been exposed to or the genes we were born with.

For the past nineteen years I have tried to delve beneath the surface of mind-body research and its popularization to uncover bedrock truths about mind-body unity. The interpenetration of systems once thought to belong solely to the psyche or soma calls upon researchers in the field, clinicians who apply the research findings, and people who wish to benefit from this knowledge to go deeper, to learn more about the mind and themselves, to discover whether and how unconscious as well as conscious intentions and emotions influence health. In various chapters of this book I have tried to integrate psychodynamic thinking with mind-body science because this integration has always seemed to me the farthest frontier of psychosomatic theory and practice. If mind and body are one, and if we want to promote our health and treat our diseases with psychological medicine, we need to plumb the psyche with the same skill and precision and openness we use to probe the mysteries of molecular messengers, cell receptors, and the human genome.

Part I is devoted to the scientific underpinnings of mind-body medicine, and Part II deals with the clinical applications of mind-body or behavioral medicine. Chapter 1, "The Psychosomatic Network: Foundations of Mind-Body Medicine," based on an article I coauthored with the neuroscientist Candace Pert, Ph.D., and the immunologist Michael Ruff, Ph.D., is an overview of basic scientific discoveries in psychoneuroimmunology and allied fields that represent the bedrock for the concept of mind-body unity. The chapter seeks to integrate biological research on mind-body unity with psychosocial research on emotions in human health, an approach that is consistent with Pert's vision of emotions as the common currency in the ceaseless interchange between systems we have long classified as belonging to either psyche or soma.

In chapter 2, "The Social Perspective in Mind-Body Studies," I write about the most neglected dimension in mind-body research, the social factor. The late George Engel, M.D., coined the tripartite term *biopsychosocial* to indicate that biology, the psyche, and the social fabric were inextricable aspects of health and therefore essential elements of a truly holistic medicine. Yet the social factor has been neglected, and in this chapter I use a report on a rare joint meeting of the American Psychosomatic Society and the Society of Behavioral Medicine as a launchpad for an exploration of social factors in mind-body health. I offer as a frame of reference an incisive critique of the mind-body movement's disregard of social factors written by the late medical sociologist Aaron Antonovsky, Ph.D.

Heart disease and cancer have been among the most pressing concerns of mind-body researchers and clinicians, both because they are the leading causes of mortality in the United States and because there is immense room for improvement in the prevention and treatment of both diseases. In chapter 3, "The Mindful Heart: Psychosocial Factors in Heart Disease," I present an overview of the astonishingly rich body of research on emotions, coping, and personality in coronary heart disease. I include both human studies and a section on basic research into mind-body mechanisms in coronary heart disease, which involves not only the nervous and cardiovascular systems but also the immune system. Finally, I offer what I call an "integrative process model," an effort to develop a coherent theoretical framework to help explain the sprawling, disparate research in this area. In presenting this model I integrate depth psychology into the mind-heart equation, hoping to bring more insight to an area that has too frequently relied on shallow psychological explanations. By taking into account psychodynamics, the unconscious (as difficult as it is to measure), and the ways in which people change and adapt over time, it is possible to weave seemingly contradictory bits of research into a whole that makes sense.

I offer a similar analysis in Chapter 4, "Cancer and the Mind: An Integrative Investigation," surveying mind-body-cancer research, while again presenting an integrative "process model," one first proposed by the mind-body researcher Lydia Temoshok, Ph.D. The chapter shows that contrary to conventional wisdom, there is a substantial body of research on psychosocial factors in cancer progression and survival and a modest but intriguing body of research on psychosocial contributors to cancer risk. While the findings suggest that the influence of the mind on both cancer recovery and the risk of developing the disease is modest, it may be clinically important, especially for cancer patients. In this chapter, I try to illuminate a thorny issue: whether mind-cancer findings blame the victim, a scientifically and philosophically complex question that dogs the field.

In Part II, "Clinical Applications of Mind-Body Medicine," I delve into the research on, and practice of, mind-body interventions for a range of medical conditions. I begin in chapter 5, "Behavioral Medicine's New Marketplace," using as a launchpad a report on a meeting, run by a nonacademic institute, that explored what was going on in the world of clinical mind-body medicine, often beyond the scrutiny or even the awareness of academicians. I describe presentations by such leading popularizers of mind-body medicine as Bernie Siegel, Deepak Chopra, and Joan Borysenko, as well as a host of relatively unknown practitioners working in clinics from California to Connecticut, exploring the cultural impact and medical value of widely employed clinical applications.

Chapters 6–9 delve into specific mind-body treatments for cancer, women's health conditions (including PMS, menopausal symptoms, and infertility), somatization disorder (which includes a vast variety of symptoms and illnesses), and surgery. In each chapter I describe the treatments and discuss the clinical research that supports their efficacy, with special emphasis on the work of particular investigators. I often characterize the social and political context of the research, taking a critical view of mainstream medicine's benign neglect of or outright disinterest in potentially effective mind-body therapies. I argue that the problem is manifold, being due to an information gap, in which doctors and scientists are typically unaware of clinical mind-body research; an institutional gap, in which the academic departments involved in mind-body studies are frequently walled off from other biomedical departments; a credibility gap, based on the differing paradigms underlying mind-body and mainstream medicine; and a funding gap, based on low prioritization by the National Institutes of Health (NIH) and the disinterest of private-sector investors, who have little profit motive for nonpharmacologic therapies. All too often the "more research is needed" pretext is unjustified; sound research has already been conducted, but few doctors and scientist know it. While I take an advocacy position when I feel it is warranted, I hope that the findings in these chapters will help stimulate broader implementation of mind-body interventions that have already been proven worthwhile.

Positive signs have recently appeared that the various gaps between mind-body and mainstream medicine are starting to shrink, if only modestly. In 1999 the NIH earmarked $50 million dollars for a new mind-body research initiative, and ten mind-body research centers have already been established around the country. The NIH's Integrative Neural Immune Program, which coordinates mind-body collaborations throughout the NIH, is directed by Esther M. Sternberg, M.D., who recently declared that "rigorous scientific evidence" has allowed the mainstream medical world "to welcome us with open arms" (Bunk 2001). Indeed, in 2001 the acting NIH director, Ruth Kirschstein, M.D., said, "It is now accepted as fact that the brain and the immune system communicate" (Bunk 2001). Kirschstein affirmed that this communication plays a role in disease and that mind-body research must cross disciplines, including the social sciences, psychology, neurobiology, neuroendocrinology, and immunology. In March 2001 fourteen NIH institutes, centers, and offices cosponsored the first in a series of meetings on the science of mind-body interactions. It was organized by the Integrative Neural Immune Program. "Frequently, we were greeted with skepticism and sometimes scorn," said Dr. Sternberg to the five hundred attendees at the fully subscribed event. "I think the packed house and the viewers on the internet are indications of the interest in this field" (Bunk 2001).

Considering the vast sums spent on other research domains, the funding level for mind-body research is minimal, but the ascendancy of the Integrative Neural Immune Program, the establishment of ten research centers, and the beginnings of cross-disciplinary collaboration bode well for the future. I would argue, however, that in some areas of clinical application we do not have to reinvent the wheel: the efficacy of certain mind-body treatments is sufficiently well established to be widely implemented now. That said, a groundswell of basic research opens doors to profound new understandings of mind-body unity and new, more effective mind-body therapies for chronic and life-threatening diseases.

I also detect a slight softening of the polarization between the mind-body and mainstream medical communities, in part as a result of advances in research and recognition. It has helped that reputable practitioners and advocates increasingly recognize that mind-body medicine is a *complementary* modality for most diseases, to be used alongside conventional treatments. These days, it is rarely promoted as an alternative panacea. Moreover, the mind-body research funded by the NIH's National Center for Complementary and Alternative Medicine highlights the increasing acceptance of mind-body as a form of complementary medicine.

As mind-body research evolves and deepens, it will continue to rub up against an age-old, seemingly insoluble problem: we still do not understand whether consciousness can be reduced to physical phenomena. Are our thoughts, dreams, and feelings attributable solely to their biological substrates—the neurons, neuropeptides, receptors, and twisty strands of DNA? Is consciousness an energetic or nonlocal realm that enlivens these biological bits? If so, are the unquantifiable dimensions of mind inseparable from the quantifiable dimensions of body? Can nondualism be rationally defended?

The transpersonal philosopher Ken Wilber has wrestled with this question as thoughtfully as any other contemporary thinker. Wilber uses a quadrant model to explicate reality: the left side is internal subjectivity (consciousness as we experience it); the right side is external objective reality. The upper quadrants represent the individual, the lower quadrants, the collective (fig. 1.1). With this model in mind, Wilber addresses the mind-body problem in *The Marriage of Sense and Soul:*

> The moment of truth of the scientific approach—a truth utterly lacking in premodern worldviews and among the Great Chain theorists— was that every Left-Hand event does indeed have a Right-Hand corre-

late. . . . The mind itself, far from being nothing but an otherworldly soul trapped in a material body, is intimately interwoven with the biomaterial brain (not reducible to it, but not drastically divorced from it either).

Science was bound to find this out sooner or later, and this shocking discovery—Left-Hand consciousness has a Right-Hand correlate—shook to its very foundations the entire "metaphysical'" approach to reality that had dominated every premodern worldview without exception. . . .

But as a confident modernity began to erase in earnest the entire Left-Hand dimensions . . . it failed to notice that this scientific endeavor was likewise erasing all sense and significance from the Kosmos itself. For there are no values, no intentions, no depths, and no meaning in any of the Right-Hand domains. The Left Hand is the home of *quality*, the Right Hand of *quantity*. The Left is the home of *intention* and *meaning;* the Right, of *extension* without purpose or plan. The Left has *levels of significance;* the Right has levels of magnitude. The Left has *better* and *worse,* the Right merely *bigger* or *smaller.*

For example . . . health is *better* than illness, but a mountain is not better than a river. Mutual respect is better than contempt, but an atom is not better than a photon. And thus, as you collapse Left to the Right, as you collapse compassion to serotonin, joy to dopamine . . . or contemplation to brain waves, you likewise collapse quality to quantity, value to veneer, interior to exterior, depth to surface, dignity to disaster. (Wilber 1998, 83–84)

Throughout this book I present the thesis, supported by evidence, that the *quantifiable* aspects of mind are no longer *classifiable* as they once were. Likewise, the *quantifiable* aspects of body are no longer *classifiable* as they once were. These realizations require a radical revision of the biomedical paradigm, one in which mind is no longer defined as brain, since cellular and molecular intelligence are operant throughout the organism. Wilber's point is that aspects of consciousness may be bound to physiological substrates but cannot be reduced to them, which suggests that mind transcends the brain and perhaps the body itself. It is a position that has been eloquently voiced by Larry Dossey, a physician, who argues in several of his books that prayer and distant healing are examples of transpersonal or nonlocal consciousness. While it is beyond the scope of this book to debate whether consciousness is nonlocal, the idea that mind is not ultimately reducible to its molecular or even atomic substrates means that mysteries will continue to abound in mind-body studies. Some aspects of

I	IT
Intentional	Behavioral
Subjective	Objective
Consciousness	Organism
"Mind"	"Brain"
WE	ITS
Intersubjective	Social
Cultural	Interobjective
	Environment

FIGURE 1.1 Ken Wilber's Four Quadrants
Adapted from figures in Wilber 2000.

consciousness (e.g., unconscious intention) may never be readily measurable, just as some physical substrates may never be revealed. But Wilber does not eschew the hard-science investigation of mind-body unity, the ongoing search for the right-hand correlates of left-hand states of being. He *does* eschew the effort to *purely* define compassion as serotonin, joy as dopamine, or contemplation as brain waves, for such efforts extinguish humanity, mystery, and spirit from the quest for scientific enlightenment. Wilber is saying that we must embrace visionary ways of knowing ("vision-logic," "transpersonal," "transrational") beyond the reductionism of modernity (even mind-body modernity), grasping the truth of subjective (emotional, spiritual, transcendent) experience both as it is tethered to and as it is distinct from physically measurable reality. We do not have to pit these kinds of knowledge against each other; we can encompass both, and in so doing we enrich our scientific understanding of mind-body health.

In human terms, a moving example of the tension between materialist science and vision-logic comes from a personal story told by David L. Felten, M.D., Ph.D., director of the Center for Neuroimmunology at the Loma Linda University School of Medicine. Felten is a neuroscientist who has conducted some of the most elegant mind-body research, tracing the innervation of immune tissues throughout the body and discovering the neural signaling of immune cells. In his essay at the end of the second edition of the classic text *Psychoneuroimmunology* (Ader et al. 1991) Felten pondered the mysteries of mind and immunity:

Although it is tempting for the basic scientist to ignore or deny that which cannot be explained on a mechanistic level, I am one such basic scientist who has been touched by the example of my mother, Jane Felten, a courageous woman who faced life crippled with polio and beset with medical problems, but whose determination and irrepressible spirit seemed to carry her through almost unbelievable medical adversity. Paralyzed at 8 years of age, she faced more than 10 orthopedic procedures to fuse bones of the lower extremities to allow her to stand with crutches. She never thought anyone would want to marry her, but she found a kind, gracious, and loving man, Harold Felten, whose example has been an inspiration to all who know him. She was told repeatedly by the medical establishment never to risk having children or trying to raise them but managed to have two sons at some risk to her own well-being. She spent many long and frustrating years learning to balance on crutches while gripping the tops with just her upper arms, to permit some use of her hands to care for her children, despite the inevitable damage to the brachial plexus this caused. Never once did I hear her complain about her affliction or her lot in life; rather, she took joy in her husband and children, her faith, and the kindness of others. She faced repeated cardiac problems with the attitude that it was a small price to pay for the good life she had been permitted. She faced repeated bouts of pneumonia and pulmonary problems with an astonishing determination to fight back and recover, which she managed to do for many years, beyond anyone's expectations. And when she faced ultimate deterioration, mental confusion, and death, in her more lucid moments she expressed gratitude to those who showed care and kindness to her.

Do we know the extent to which Jane Felten was able to assist herself to recover from illness, fight back from adversity, through some of the interactions described in this book? No. Do we understand how the support of a loving and caring husband contributed to neural signaling that helped her through overwhelming adversity, such as repeated bouts of pneumonia and cardiac failure? No. But does that mean that such factors are irrelevant just because we do not yet understand the mechanisms that underlie them? And does this mean that the example of Jane Felten and many others like her should be put aside, to be dismissed as mere anecdote or mythology? I think not. Rather, her example should serve as a constant reminder that healing involves far more than pharmacological mechanisms, and that the physician's role includes more than just the manipulation of currently understood physiological mechanisms. And her example should serve as an inspiration for us to explore further the scientific foundations and to unravel the mechanisms of in-

teraction of brain, behavior, and immunity, so that in the future we will xxiii
understand better how attitude, will, stressors, and "positive emotions"
are expressed in the periphery, including the immune system. (Ader et
al. 1991, 1120)

Felten's eloquent statement is a clarion call for a multidimensional
study of mind-body, one that simultaneously regards the psyche in its
depths, including both the measurable and the immeasurable, and the
molecular mechanisms of mind-body unity, holding both under the light
of scientific inquiry. It may be possible to take the search for physiological correlates down to infinitesimal levels—to genes, to atoms—and, with
no risk of logical contradiction, to also study the psyche and spirit in the
body, relying on the most penetrating schools of scientific psychology as
well as the wisdom traditions of East and West. Some might say that such
multileveled investigations deal with apples and oranges, but I believe that
this brand of mind-body science would go deeper, would be a genuinely
integral scientific endeavor. Felten is saying that his mother's perseverance
and kindness—something about her spirit—had much to do with her
physical resilience under impossibly challenging circumstances. The fields
of mind-body science and medicine must find ways to integrate a geography of the human spirit with a topology of mind-body unity.

REFERENCES

Ader R, Felten DL, Cohen N, eds. 1991. *Psychoneuroimmunology II*. New York:
    Academic Press.
Bunk S. 2001. Mind-body research matures. *Scientist*. 15(12):8.
Wilber K. 1998. *The Marriage of Sense and Soul*. New York: Academic Press.
Wilber K. 2000. *Integral Psychology*. Boston: Shambhala Press.

PART ONE

The Scientific
Basis of
Mind-Body
Medicine

Chapter 1

The Psychosomatic Network:
Foundations of Mind–Body Medicine

Mind-body medicine can help to heal diseases and promote health. In order to understand how, we need first to understand the unified mind-body dynamics that make it possible, on a molecular level, for these emerging new therapies to work. This chapter updates the concept of the human organism as a psychosomatic network, rooted in neuropeptides and their receptors; provides recent data on the clinical relevance of neuropeptide-receptor interactions for various human diseases; and offers new evidence that emotions are a bridge between mind and body, including data demonstrating that mind-body interventions that facilitate emotional expression can result in physiological healing. The broad view of the unified *body-mind* that emerges here is not only more complete; it is qualitatively different: a vision not only of mind-body interactions but also of dynamic mind-body unity. In this vision the integrity of the bodymind is protected and preserved by an internal healing system—a multidimensional entity guided by emotions and their biochemical substrates—vibrating with intelligence and purpose, with few, if any, functional boundaries inside the human organism.

Popular culture has enshrined the concept of a "mind-body connection," which has been promoted as the basis of clinical programs and popular books marketed to healthcare consumers hungry for a medicine that addresses the psychospiritual domain of their being. But the term reflects outdated ideas from the predecessor field of psychosomatic medicine, as

Reprinted by permission, with changes, from *Alternative Therapies in Health and Medicine* 4 (1998): 30–41, article co-authored with C. B. Pert and M. R. Ruff.

4 well as rather simplified concepts that stem from today's broader culture of alternative medicine, a culture that often peddles a one-dimensional "mind over matter" approach to mind-body medicine. (It is generally agreed among mind-body scientists that mind does not lord its putative powers over matter; rather, mind and matter are intertwined in a kind of dialectic dance.) As I argue in the introduction, the latest findings from the field of psychoneuroimmunology (PNI) and allied fields of psychosomatic understanding suggest that words like *connection* are misleading, since they conjure two separate entities attached via some biochemical, cellular, or other physiological pathway. A sort of "Panama Canal" metaphor has reigned, in which a limited passageway was thought to exist between these two vast oceanic entities known as *mind* and *body*.

While cells and substances we associate with mind and body are indeed connected by physical pathways, state-of-the-art investigations reveal that these very cells and substances can no longer be associated with just mind or just body. For instance, neurons make the same products that white blood cells do, and vice versa: the two groups of cells not only communicate with each other, they speak the same molecular language. Thus, the pathways "connecting" them do not join two otherwise unrelated entities. They are interlacing roadways within the geography of one vast, complex system of components that are frequently interchangeable with regard to functions we usually identify with mind or body.

The provable connections between the mind-brain, nervous, endocrine, gastrointestinal, cardiovascular, reproductive, and immune systems inform but no longer accurately reflect an emerging understanding of the human organism. In the form of neuropeptides and their corresponding cellular receptors, our biological systems (the body) are literally flooded by our cognitions and emotions (the mind). Furthermore, our minds are created anew on a moment-to-moment basis by the interplay of cellular messengers and growth factors, known collectively as *ligands,* and their corresponding cellular receptors, the whole system of which we have long associated only with the body. The cells and substances we used to view as connectors between biological subsystems, including those associated with mind, are really vibrant molecular packets of information swimming throughout a boundless sea, delivering messages to hosts of other cells and substances.

In illuminating the nature of mind (i.e., subjective experience, consciousness, feeling) the mind-body fields have contributed to a richer, more humanistic mind-body science. One sector of this science involves investigations of the very nature of consciousness in fields as disparate, yet overlapping, as physics, sociology, psychiatry, molecular biology, and bioenergetics. Such studies have set the stage for a profound integration in which disparate physical systems are no longer viewed as interconnected but are regarded as inseparable components of a dynamic mind-body unit. This vision is consistent with the concept of a "healing system," as characterized by the mind-body researcher Brendan O'Regan, of the Institute of Noetic Sciences. O'Regan and others have described this system as a unified body-mind network designed to foster homeostasis, the steady flow of information across biological systems with varying functional properties, and ultimately the capacity of the system for psychophysical regeneration, what we generally call *healing* (O'Regan 1987).

In the 1980s Candace Pert and Michael Ruff, who collaborated with me on this opening chapter, joined with their colleagues to elaborate the concept of a "psychosomatic network" composed of neuropeptides—short chains of amino acids present in the brain as well as in nonneural tissues— and their corresponding receptors (Pert 1986; Pert et al. 1985). This psychosomatic network, extending to every molecular corner of the body, functions as a living processor of information, a means of transmitting meaningful messages across organs, tissues, cells, and DNA. Moreover, the seventy to eighty neuropeptides identified to date can be viewed as the biochemical substrates of emotion.

In brain-mapping studies Pert and colleagues (1985) found that the paw-shaped hippocampus and the disc-shaped amygdala—structures in the brain's core that belong to the limbic system, long considered the emotional center of the brain—are infused with receptors for opioids, the painkilling class of neuropeptides. But their maps revealed much more: that these brain structures were rife with receptors for the majority of known neuropeptides. Their seminal work has been the very basis for a new concept of *mind-body unity*, which now ought to supplant the notion of psychosomatic or mind-body "connections." The paradigm of mind-body unity is one that suggests, in its imagery and actuality, an alive system characterized by *flow*, as opposed to more conventional paradigms that evoke a mechanical system of hard wiring between bits and pieces of molecular hardware.

Pert's concept broadened as it became clear that the biochemical substrates of emotion carry information across systems, from those traditionally associated with mind (i.e., the brain and autonomic nervous systems) to those traditionally associated with body (i.e., the endocrine, cardiovascular, digestive, and immune systems), and back again. Neuropeptide receptors are not limited to the brain; they are present on cells in tissues throughout the body. Emotions are therefore a veritable bridge between mind and body. Research from allied fields of behavioral medicine has verified that our state of disease or health is inextricable from our

6   emotional experience. The ubiquity of the neuropeptide-receptor network has provided the physiological basis for observations, from the age of Hippocrates to the modern age, that conscious and unconscious feelings are root factors in health and healing.

Despite these developments, the primacy of emotional experience in physical health and healing has yet to be recognized by mainstream medicine. Nor has it been fully integrated into studies in PNI, a still young field that sometimes contributes to compartmentalization by focusing on molecular substrates or physiological interactions to the exclusion of subjective experience, or vice versa. The challenge of today's mind-body science and medicine is to forge more deeply, to expand investigations of mind-body unity on the cellular level, while designing studies that simultaneously evaluate the psychospiritual domain, the feelings, thoughts, traits, and experiences that accompany molecular events.

The Psychosomatic Network Revisited

An early impetus for investigating mind-body communication was the recognition that for every mood-modifying synthetic drug there must be an endogenous (internal) neuropeptide ligand that binds to identical target receptor molecules. Put differently, if a psychoactive drug molecule can find a perfect lock-in-key fit in a specific cell receptor, there must be a highly comparable molecule made naturally by our own cells that hooks onto that same receptor and produces comparable effects in the brain and/or the body. During the 1970s Candace Pert and Solomon Snyder, at the Johns Hopkins University, identified the first brain drug receptor—the opiate receptor—a cell-surface molecule bound by both exogenous (external, synthetic) opiate drugs and their natural analogs in the body, the endogenous opioids, neuropeptides with powerful pain- and mood-modifying properties (Pert and Snyder 1973).

Herkenham and Pert (1982) developed sophisticated techniques (including autoradiography) for mapping neuropeptide-receptor distribution throughout the brain and body. Using these techniques, researchers in another study found that the amygdala, the hypothalamus, and other limbic structures of the emotional brain were highly enriched with opiate receptors (Lamotte et al. 1978). Later maps showing distribution of other neuropeptide receptors (e.g., substance P, bombesin, cholecystokinin, neurotensin, insulin, and transferrin) revealed the same pattern of enrichment in brain structures associated with emotional experience (Pert et al. 1985). It now appears that the emotional centers of the brain are flush with receptors for most neuropeptides.

Molecular neurobiology dictates that once bound in lock-and-key fashion by their corresponding ligands, cell-surface receptors undergo structural changes that trigger the sending of "messages" to the cell nucleus in a process known as *transduction*. Once these messages reach the nucleus, they stimulate a change in gene expression, which in turn yields a change in the production of cellular proteins that regulate one or another functional activity of the cell. Put simply, the presence of these receptors means that cells "receive" messages from matching neuropeptide carriers of biochemical "information." And these messages are ultimately transduced to the cell's genetic core in ways that are biologically meaningful. For instance, an immune cell may be primed for action or restrained by a message from a neuropeptide such as endorphin.

Pert and her colleagues found that other anatomical locations, both inside and outside the brain, were "nodal points" of neuropeptide receptor distribution. The dorsal horn of the mammalian spinal cord, where neurons transmitting information from glands, skin, and other peripheral organs first make synaptic contact with the central nervous system (CNS), is enriched with virtually all neuropeptide receptors (Lewis et al. 1981; Pert et al. 1985). Thus, the entry point within the CNS for filtering the body's sensory information is replete with neuropeptide receptors, and similar nodal points were found in virtually all locations in the brain where sensory information enters the nervous system. Another receptor-rich locus is the periaqueductal gray region of the brain stem, which is hardwired to the limbic brain—the seat of emotions often referred to as the "emotional brain"—by neuronal pathways. The periaqueductal gray region has also been shown to modulate pain thresholds (Pert et al. 1985).

The boundaries of the classical CNS were vastly expanded with the discovery of nodal points rich in neuropeptide receptors throughout the body. The entire gastrointestinal tract, from the esophagus to the large intestine, is lined with cells that contain neuropeptides and their receptors. The phrase *gut feeling*, referring to instinct or intuition, is much more than a metaphor; it describes a biological reality (Pert et al. 1986). We probably experience emotions in our gut precisely because of the richness of its receptors for brain and nervous-system chemicals. Specific neuropeptides and their receptors have also been found in the kidney, the testis, and the pancreas, as well as in immune system organs and cells, a point to which we will return shortly.

These and other related findings spurred a reevaluation of traditional notions of neurotransmission. Until recently, every aspect of mental activity, including perception, integration, and performance, was thought to be determined solely by the action of the classical neurotransmitter mol-

8 ecules—brain chemicals such as serotonin, norepinephrine, dopamine, GABA, and acetylcholine—in the busy space between neurons known as the *synapse*. The neurotransmitters ferry information across these neuronal junctures in bursts of electrochemical discharge. The whole of biological psychiatry has been rooted in an understanding and a biochemical manipulation of neurotransmitters in the synapse. Moods, emotions, and cognitions were—and to some extent still are—believed to be determined solely by the amount of certain neurotransmitters present in the synapse and their actions within that space: Do they linger? Do they degrade? Do they return from the neuron from which they came? Or do they cross that electrochemical bridge and connect to receptors on the neighboring *(post-synaptic)* neuron? Our states of mind have been thought to depend, on the most fundamental level, on the strength of neurotransmitter-receptor connections, which hinge on the nature of the frenzied molecular traffic in that tiny synaptic space.

But research by Pert and others on the neuropeptide-receptor network revealed that these linear channels of neurotransmission were not the only meaningful pathways for biochemical substrates of thought and emotion. Certainly these channels represent an essential "mechanism" of mental processes and mind-body interactions. But in ways quite different from the classical neurotransmitters, neuropeptides flow throughout brain and body, finding their respective receptors and altering cell function through transduction of messages to the cell nucleus (Pert 1986). Thus, neuropeptides can act at great distances from their cellular targets, without synaptic or linear connections, and it is the specificity of the receptors that allows for such far-flung mind-body communication. Returning to the gut, there are neurotransmitter actions in the brain that mediate an emotion such as fear, but neuropeptide actions in the gut that have nothing to do with synapses in the brain may also, simultaneously, mediate that queasy feeling that one gets in the abdomen when something frightening happens. One neuropeptide, cholecystokinin (CCK), stimulates structures in the brain stem when we experience fear, but it is also highly active in the gut, regulating its motility and probably causing a whole range of so-called gut feelings.

Work by the recent Nobel Prize winner Eric Kandel of Columbia University suggests that biochemical change at the receptor level is the molecular basis for memory and learning (Kandel et al. 1986). Modulation of receptors at nodal points by various neuropeptides determines which memories, perceptions, and sensations readily percolate across synapses and up the neuroaxis to emerge as conscious thought, as well as which are "repressed" in the unconscious mind. These findings have important ramifications for the psychosomatic network because memory storage must extend beyond the brain to the entire body—particularly to receptor-rich areas between nerves and ganglia—distributing not only in proximal structures of the spinal cord but out along pathways to internal organs and the surface of the skin (Pert 1997). In other words, the unconscious mind is located not only in anterior brain structures but throughout the network of peptide interconnections spanning the autonomic nerves known as ganglia, various internal organs, the immune system, and even the skin. The notion that we store memories and repressed emotions in the body—not just in the brain—should no longer be considered a psychoanalytic flight of fancy.

The purposes and functional abilities of the neuropeptide-receptor network are manifold, but one overriding function is the transmission of information. The neuroscientist Francis O. Schmitt first suggested that the vast variety of neuropeptides, neurohormones (most of which are peptides), steroid hormones, neurotransmitters, growth factors, cytokines, and protein ligands communicate across the alleged barriers between biological systems and that they all transmit information (Schmitt 1984). (For example, growth factors such as the epidermal growth factor, insulin-like growth factors I and II, and immune-cell products such as interleukin-1 [IL-1] all have feedback loops and receptors in emotion-mediating brain structures [Pert and Dienstfrey 1988].) Schmitt therefore termed these molecules *informational substances.* He proposed the existence of a parasynaptic (parallel) system in which these information-bearing substances circulate throughout extracellular fluids to reach specific target-cell receptors.

If Schmitt's model has been largely accepted, its ramifications have been just as widely neglected. Understood from the perspective of the emerging field of information theory, the idea that ligands are informational substances that transmit messages to cells through membrane receptors calls for a whole new mind-body paradigm. The bodymind can no longer be wholly characterized as a hierarchical system of hard-wired connections that descend down from a putative ruling station (the brain); rather it must be seen as an expansive network of free-flowing information transmitted by molecules that enter at any nodal point and move rapidly to any other point (Pert 1997; Pert et al. 1985). Moreover, the fact that many of these molecular messengers are biochemical substrates of emotion underscores the role of mind—both conscious and unconscious—in linking and coordinating the major systems and their organs.

With regard to the healing system, two-way communication between neuropeptides and the immune system holds a key to the influence of mind on healing processes. Michael Ruff and his colleagues (Pert et al. 1985; Ruff, Schiffman, et al. 1985; Ruff, Wahl, et al. 1985) realized that they

10   could learn which ligands could hook onto immune-cell receptors (and therefore regulate the cells' actions) by studying patterns of *chemotaxis*, the process by which messenger molecules sway the movement patterns of various cell populations. (Ruff's assumption, based on a known biochemical and immunological principle, was that any cell type that can be swayed in its movements by a specific molecule must have receptors with which that molecule can interact.) He therefore used chemotaxis assays to find out what kind of receptors were present on monocytes, roving immune cells that recognize and digest foreign invaders and promote tissue repair.

Ruff found that this vital class of immune cells possess receptors for a wide range of neuropeptides and psychoactive drugs, including opioids, benzodiazepines (e.g., Valium), and bombesin. His chemotaxis investigations therefore confirmed that specific neuropeptides help regulate the routing and migration of monocytes.* Think of the peptides as tiny magnets that drag along iron filings, in this case the immune cells, wherever they roam. And monocytes play vital roles in the immune system, presenting foreign antigens to B- and T-lymphocytes, the respective kingpins of the humoral and cellular arms of the immune system. The fact that neuropeptides are traffic managers for monocytes means that they influence systemwide immune responses to pathogens in the body.

Perhaps the strongest support for the notion of informational substances was research by Daniel Carr and Ed Blalock, at the University of Texas, showing that immune cells also synthesize, store, and secrete neuropeptides (Carr and Blaylock 1991). In other words, the cellular agents of healing produce the same chemical messengers that regulate mood and emotion. Because these cells also receive input from neuropeptides, there can be no doubt that there is two-way communication (scientists term it *bidirectional*) between brain and body. Moreover, we now know that nerve cells can produce immune-cell products, such as interleukin-1, and that in the brain they exhibit receptors for CD4 (a protein found on immune T cells) as well as many peptides associated with the immune system (Farrar et al. 1987; Pert et al. 1986).

During the 1980s the now burgeoning field of psychoneuroimmunology yielded copious findings regarding brain-body interactions that were relevant to healing. As investigators came to understand the pathway running from the hypothalamus to the pituitary gland and downward to the

---

* The existence of distinct neuropeptide receptors on human monocytes was further suggested by the finding that chemotaxis can only be blocked with the precise antagonist for a given neuropeptide receptor class. For example, chemotaxis via the fMet-Leu-Phe receptor, though antagonized by specific fMet-Leu-Phe antagonists, is not affected by the opiate-receptor antagonist naloxone'4 or by benzodiazepine PK-11195 (Ruff, Pert, et al. 1985).

adrenal glands—the hypothalamic-pituitary-adrenal (HPA) axis—various research teams found that stress and emotional responses could influence levels of corticosteroid hormones; these in turn were shown to modulate immune-cell functions, most notably inflammation (Sternberg et al. 1992; Sternberg and Gold 1997). This is now a fairly well understood and widely accepted hierarchy, one that regulates immune responses through feed-back loops involving neuropeptide messengers (e.g., corticotropin-releasing factor, or CRH) that either stimulate immunity when pathogens invade or tamp it down when the battle has been won and an accelerating immune response would only cause excessive inflammation, leading to chronic pain or even autoimmune disease. At the same time, acting in a parallel fashion to the hierarchical HPA axis, our circulating network of informational substances interacts with cell-surface receptors throughout the body. This parallel network, less hierarchical and more freely flowing, also regulates immune cells as they travel our interior landscape performing tasks associated with host resistance and healing.

The Psychosomatic Network: Recent Findings

Since the 1980s, PNI and its allied fields (e.g., neuroimmunomodulation, psychoneuroendocrinology, behavioral medicine) have produced reams of published findings that, taken together, dismantle previously erected barriers between biological subsystems. These fields have lent legitimacy to efforts dating back to the 1960s to bring mental and emotional processes into the healing equation by showing their influence over immune functions. Often classified as part of this endeavor, research on neuropeptides as informational substances is at the core of the emerging picture of the mind-body system as an integrative psychosomatic network.

In the early days of PNI research it became apparent that neurotransmitters involved in the stress response (namely, the catecholamines adrenaline and noradrenaline), as well as the messenger molecules of the HPA axis, can lock onto receptors on the surface of immune cells and influence their actions. In other words, when we experience "fight or flight" during stress, the flood of hormones and transmitters produce concomitant changes in the immune system. A major leap came when Pert and others found that those circulating neuropeptides, such as the opioids, also have corresponding receptors on immune cells, which enables them to have potent effects on the cells' actions in the body. Today, the number and types of messenger molecules that influence immune cells have expanded rapidly and surprisingly: the list now includes hormones such as insulin, melatonin, and prolactin; sex hormones, including both estrogens and an-

12   drogens; thymic hormones; human growth hormone (Ader et al. 1991); and a vast variety of neuropeptides, including beta-endorphin, enkephalins, substance P, bombesin, corticotropin (ACTH), gastrin-releasing peptide, vasoactive intestinal polypeptide (VIP), somatostatin, calcitonin gene-related peptide, peptide histidine isoleucine, and peptide histidine methionine (Geoetzl et al. 1991).

Consider the immunological influence of one such peptide, VIP. First described as a vasodilator, VIP is present in both the central and the peripheral nervous systems, where it functions as a classical neurotransmitter. But VIP-secreting cells and receptors also line the entire gastrointestinal tract, suggesting that they are mediators of those "gut feelings." Scores of recent investigations (e.g., Wiedermann et al. 1988; and Ottoway 1991) further confirm that VIP is "a potent immunoregulatory signal which can influence a variety of lymphoid cells around which immune responses pivot" (Ruff et al. 1987). The interplay of emotional and immune responses is arguably typified by the protean properties of VIP, a multitasking molecule that speaks the biochemical language of many biological subsystems, including the nervous, gastrointestinal, endocrine, and immune systems.

VIP is far from alone among neuropeptides in its widespread influence on immunity. VIP, substance P, and calcitonin gene-related peptide are clearly involved in the movement patterns of key immune cells, the lymphocytes and monocytes (Ruff et al. 1987; Schratzberger et al. 1997). Substance P also manages the traffic of neutrophils, eosinophils, and monocytes (Carolan and Casale 1993; Ruff, Wahl, and Pert 1985; Wiedermann et al. 1993). And a newly discovered neuropeptide, secretoneurin, which is widely distributed throughout the central and peripheral nervous systems, was recently shown to direct monocyte traffic, reduce the movement of neutrophils, and regulate the migration of cells called fibroblasts (Schratzberger et al. 1997). In short, biochemical substrates of emotion are like the air traffic controllers of immune cells hurtling through the field of the body, modulating the duration and intensity of immune responses to the foreign entities they encounter in inner space.

Such findings have radically altered the landscape of basic immunology research, which as recently as ten years ago trained its search for immune-regulating agents exclusively on substances belonging to the immune system itself—cytokines, lymphokines, chemokines, and growth factors. Put another way, immunologists had always believed that immune behavior was tightly controlled within the family of immune cells and signalers, that no outsider from another "system" had any regulatory power. But it is now clear that nerve-cell products are pivotal regulators of immunity. Moreover, many immune-cell products that govern the action of immune cells—all of which were once believed to belong exclusively to the immune family—are now recognized as global citizens of the body. They have business in many subsystems and are essentially "multilingual" when it comes to the molecular language of these other systems.

The discovery of receptors for a wide array of neuropeptides on monocytes has been matched in studies of lymphocytes, key effector cells of the immune system. Among the neuropeptide receptors identified and characterized on human lymphocytes are those for B-endorphins, enkephalins, somatostatin, substance P, VIP (Geoetzl et al. 1991), and ACTH (Bost et al. 1987). Radiographic techniques have been used to map the distribution of neuropeptide receptors, including VIP, CCK, substance P, and bombesin, embedded in tissues associated with immunity—lymph nodes, glands, and other lymphoid tissues (Sacerdote et al. 1988; Wiedermann et al. 1988). This analysis reveals that particular neuropeptide receptors are located on particular types of immune cells, suggesting that these immune-cell populations have specific jobs that depend on the specific neuropeptides that regulate them. In many cases, immunobiologists have yet to pinpoint these specialized functions or to determine how brain chemicals control them. Still, the presence of neuropeptide receptors on lymphocytes and monocytes is irrefutable evidence that the nervous and immune systems are involved in intimate communication. So intimate, in fact, that hard-and-fast distinctions between the two systems are beginning to melt away.

Equally strong evidence comes from ongoing research demonstrating that immune cells actually produce neuropeptide molecules. This line of inquiry began with the observation by E. M. Smith and J. Edwin Blalock (1981) that an insult to the immune system, such as a viral or bacterial invasion, causes white blood cells to produce the pituitary neurohormone ACTH, as well as endorphin-like molecules. (Only a few years ago the idea that white cells could make brain chemicals would have been considered heresy.) After further study these molecules were shown to be more than just similar to ACTH and endorphin—they were identical to them. Accumulating research would finally turn classical neurobiology and immunology on their respective heads, with findings that immune cells contain and probably synthesize the neuropeptides VIP, somatostatin, substance P, oxytocin, and neurophysin. They also make thyrotropin, a glycoprotein secreted by thyrotropes of the anterior lobe of the pituitary gland; chorionic gonadotropin; and human growth hormone (Carr and Blalock 1991).

Finally, completing the reversal of old theoretical constructs about the

14   separateness of the nervous and immune systems, we have come to recognize that nerve cells make immune-cell products as surely as immune
cells synthesize brain chemicals. For instance, purified and enriched cultures of astrocytes and microglia—brain cells—secrete key immune-cell
products (known as cytokines), including interleukin-1, interleukin-6, and
tumor necrosis factor (TNF) (Benveniste et al. 1995; Farrar 1988). Microglia also secrete IL-10 (Williams et al. 1996), and Schwann cells found
in the brain produce TNF-alpha (Wagner and Myers 1996). Such discoveries were the rough equivalent of finding out that a seemingly invio-
lable law of physics is not only inaccurate but the polar opposite of what
new experiments reveal as truth.

A recent, barrier-breaking pair of mouse studies, published together
in the journal *Science,* suggest that blood cells can even transmogrify into
brain cells. In the first experiment, researchers in the Laboratory of Developmental Neurogenetics of the National Institute of Neurological Disorders and Stroke (NINDS) transplanted bone marrow stem cells into a
strain of mice incapable of making their own myeloid and lymphoid blood
cells (Mezey et al. 2000). These stem cells, which give rise to a variety of
blood cell types and which repopulate blood throughout adult life, were
found to migrate into the brains of the mice, where they differentiated into
cells expressing neuronal antigens. In short, the blood cells turned into
brain cells. In the second study, investigators at Stanford University delivered genetically marked adult mouse bone marrow into normal mice
whose own bone marrow had been destroyed by radiation (Brazelton et al.
2000). They later found hundreds of marrow cells in the mouse brains,
and as in the first study, the blood cells now expressed gene products typical of nerve cells. The researchers commented that the "generation of
neuronal phenotypes 1 to 6 months after an adult bone marrow transplant
demonstrates a remarkable plasticity of adult tissues with potential clinical applications." (Bone marrow cells may thus be used as an alternative
source of neurons in patients with degenerative nerve diseases or brain and
spinal cord injuries.) In light of these studies, Candace Pert's comment in
the mid-1980s that immune cells were "bits of brain floating around the
body" (Pert 1989) now seems even more starkly factual than metaphoric.

Certainly, biologists have known for over a decade that immune-cell
products, cytokines, communicate directly and indirectly with the brain.
They can signal the brain via direct nerve routes, such as the vagus nerve.
In some instances, as during inflammation or illness, they can be carried
across the blood-brain barrier with nutrients from the blood (Ader et al.
1991). Interleukin-1 is a cytokine secreted by immune cells when we are
challenged by a pathogen, such as a rheovirus, and it mediates the fever

response that occurs during any infectious illness. IL-1 also participates in an immune-modulating feedback loop, first by signaling the brain cells in the hypothalamus to start making CRH, which then triggers a relay of messages leading ultimately to the release of corticosteroids from the adrenal glands (Sternberg et al. 1992). And what do these steroids do? They tamp down the very inflammation that IL-1 helped to produce, the inflammation that fights infection but can also get out of control unless checked by the counterregulation of steroids. It is a perfect feedback loop that requires the so-called immune agent (in this case IL-1) to work its way through the nervous system (Sternberg et al. 1992).

But the story does not stop there. Interleukin-1 mediates not only immune responses but behavioral responses as well. The activation of the brain by IL-1 and perhaps other cytokines can induce mild anxiety and cautious avoidance, emotional states that prompt us to stay "out of harm's way" until an illness has run its course. The sleepiness and lethargy characteristically experienced during, say, a bad case of the flu are direct results of the neuropsychological effects of IL-1 (Sternberg and Gold 1997). It is another example of molecular multitasking: beyond its immune function, IL-1 serves our well-being by making us so weary with fatigue that we stay in bed, where we avoid the elements and get the rest we need to recover. (Another example of the neuropsychological effects of an immune cytokine is that people taking interferon for diseases ranging from chronic leukemia to multiple sclerosis may be subject to depression or to other psychiatric conditions resulting from the brain effects of this immune cytokine.)

When challenged by antigens, immune cells produce neuropeptides, whereas nerve cells produce immune-associated cytokines, suggesting that the dynamic interplay among systems occurs in response to pathogens and other foreign entities. The informational substances are couriers engaged in continuous feedback loops among these systems whose purpose is ongoing self-regulation of defensive responses to external challenges. Because it has been shown that neuroimmune communications are clearly sensitive to stress and emotional factors, there is no question that psychological traits and states influence immunity, and vice versa—that immune activity can influence mental and emotional states and their physical manifestations.

From an evolutionary, psychobiological perspective, it makes sense that social and environmental conditions and concurrent emotional states—fear, anxiety, sadness, anger, joy—should impact immunity since events and emotions necessitate a more or less vigorous defense of the integrity of the self. (For instance, when one is mugged, one's body may go into spasms of fear; the body's immune system must also be instantly prepared

16   to heal any wounds or fight any foes that enter through injured tissues.) Our emotions provide a way to prioritize the competing information to which the bodymind must pay attention. Events with higher emotional charge compel our attention as well as the physical and mental resources of our bodies (i.e., whether to run to "escape the tiger" or to lie down and rest to allow healing). Because we cannot attend to all external and internal stimuli at once, some demands necessarily suffer at the expense of others. It is this interplay of our conscious as well as our unconscious emotions and thought processes that lies at the border between health and disease.

Emotions, Neuropeptides, and the Healing System

The interconnectedness of the nervous, endocrine, and immune systems surely suggests a unified healing system. But what of the emotions? That biochemical substrates of emotion are intimately involved in immune regulation does not, in itself, help us to understand how and why states of mind are integral aspects of the healing system or what kind of treatments will strengthen that system.

Researchers at the forefront of mind-body science are tackling these questions with multileveled investigations. For instance, William Gerritsen and colleagues (1996) developed an experimental situation designed to induce social fear: a difficult public-speaking task. Seventy-nine healthy subjects were required to prepare and give an oral presentation in front of an audience; a control group comprised thirty healthy persons subjected to a nondemanding task of the same duration. Compared with the control group, those subjects who gave an oral presentation experienced tension accompanied by increases in blood pressure, elevated levels of various hormones (e.g., cortisol, prolactin, and β-endorphin), and immune changes consistent with short-term stress: a rise in natural killer (NK) cells, a drop in helper T cells (CD4 cells), and a reduction in the responsiveness of T cells to challenges by foreign antigens (Gerritsen et al. 1996). Gerritsen's research showed how informational substances (neuroendocrines and neuropeptides) that "carry" emotion also influence the cardiovascular and immune systems when people are in the midst of stress.

What function does it serve for the immune system to be modified when we experience stress or certain emotions? The answer is far from clear, in part because the immunological fluctuations reported in these studies are enormously complex. Generally speaking, however, when we experience acute stress—such as when dodging a car hurtling through an intersection or after receiving a serious diagnosis from a doctor—the sympathetic nervous system, which governs the "fight or flight" response, kicks into gear, and the result is a rapid increase in the activity of natural killer cells (Naliboff et al. 1991). (Natural killer [NK] cells are like free-lance assassins that destroy viruses, cancer cells, and other pathogens without receiving signals from other immune components. Some mind-body theorists suggest that acute stress heralds an increase in NK cells because we need swift elimination of pathogens during this period of threat.) At the same time, other immune responses may be down-regulated, perhaps to prevent excessive or prolonged inflammatory reactions, which can result in autoimmune disorder. Chronic stress, on the other hand, often results in down-regulation of NK cells and other indicators of immunity, a long-term, low-level immune suppression that may leave us vulnerable to disease.

Based on these findings, mind-body research teams pursued the possibility that chronic stress was the more significant causal factor in diseases of immune suppression or imbalance. The most revealing body of evidence regarding such stress and its effect on immunity comes from the work of Yehuda Shavit and his colleagues. Shavit and colleagues showed that certain forms of shock administered to the feet of rats during experimental procedures resulted in suppression of NK cell activity (Shavit et al. 1984; Shavit et al. 1985). Specifically, suppression of NK cells resulted from exposure to prolonged intermittent (unpredictable) shocks but not from a brief continuous footshock. Similar suppression of NK cell activity occurred when rats were exposed to inescapable as opposed to escapable shocks (Shavit, Ryan, et al. 1983). This model, in which pairs of rats are yoked to one another—one rat able to "control" the administration of shocks (escapable stress) and the other unable to control them (inescapable stress)—was also used in studies that found that rats in the "inescapable" situation had suppressed T-cell responses to challenge by substances called mitogens (Laudenslager et al. 1983) as well as enhanced growth of injected tumor cells (Sklar and Anisman 1979; Visintainer, Volpicelli, and Seligman 1982). These studies suggest that "learned helplessness," induced by unpredictable or inescapable stress, has pronounced suppressive effects on several important classes of immune cells.

Shavit called these forms of stress "opioid" because unlike other predictable or controllable stressors, they were associated with analgesia (pain reduction) and could be reversed by an opioid antagonist called naloxone (Shavit 1991). These findings suggested that the NK cell deficits were caused, at least in part, by chronic increases in levels of endogenous opioid peptides. Subsequently, Shavit and colleagues (1986) injected morphine (20 and 40 mg) into the lateral ventricle of the brain, which caused suppression of NK cell activity to the same degree as a systemic dose a

18   thousand times as great; this effect was blocked by naltrexone. The mimicking of the NK cell–suppressing effect by an exogenous opiate drug confirmed Shavit's theory that opioids—the natural kind in the body or drug sources—can dampen immunity. (The well-known susceptibility of morphine and heroin addicts to infectious disease may be an example of opiate-mediated immune suppression, though nutrition and other environmental factors must be taken into account.)

In an elegant series of follow-up studies rats subjected to the opioid forms of stress were subsequently injected with rat breast-cancer cells. In contrast to rats exposed to non-opioid stress, as well as to controls, rats exposed to opioid stress before tumor injection were later shown to have reduced median survival time and reduced survival, having succumbed more quickly to malignant tumors (Shavit, Lewis, et al. 1983). In support of the hypothesis that chronically high levels of endogenous opioids played a role in the swift decline of these animals, subsequent experiments showed that the tumor-enhancing effect of opioid footshock had been entirely blocked by naltrexone. This same tumor enhancement also was mimicked by morphine administered four days before the tumors were implanted (Shavit 1991). Shavit later theorized that the NK cell deficits shown in prior studies of opioid-type inescapable stress had probably been the reason for the animals' inability to slow the growth of tumors.

A consistent equation was emerging from Shavit's research: when animals, probably including humans, are exposed to stress that yields a sense of helplessness, they experience chronic elevations of natural opioids, which in turn depress NK cells, leaving them vulnerable to the progression of tumors. (The relationship between opioids and NK cells is complex, but Shavit and others repeatedly have confirmed the link between chronic and/or inescapable stress and elevated levels of opioid peptides.) Thus, chronic, inescapable, or unpredictable stress appears to be the more significant factor contributing to cancer and other diseases involving an imbalanced immune system.

These layered studies penetrate to the heart of the concept of a unified bodymind: social and physical conditions, emotional states, neuropeptide interactions, and surveillance capabilities of the immune system are inseparable aspects of a seamless response by an organism. Shavit's work also supports clinical observations of human patients, as well as many psychosocial studies, suggesting that people who respond to life stresses with helplessness or hopelessness, who view their circumstances as "inescapable" and therefore become emotionally withdrawn, may be at increased risk for the development or progression of cancer (Temoshok 1987). (Compelling recent evidence for this thesis comes from research by

Margaret Watson and her colleagues in London, who followed 578 breast cancer patients for five years. Women who scored high on an established measure of helplessness or hopelessness as an initial reaction to their diagnosis were significantly more likely to relapse or die from their disease [Watson et al. 1999]. This finding held true after the researchers controlled for all established prognostic risk factors, including the number of metastatic lymph nodes.)

Studies directly comparable to those of Shavit are more difficult to perform on human beings, but several lines of inquiry have produced parallel results. One small but intriguing study of the effects of physical trauma compared levels of opioid neuropeptides in twenty-one patients severely traumatized at the scene of an accident. The opioid levels were measured from the first blood sample drawn at the scene, within an average of thirty-two minutes after injury, and for eight days after the trauma. Compared with five control subjects tested immediately after elective surgery, the traumatized persons had markedly elevated levels of beta-endorphin and, on the third day after trauma, significantly suppressed reactivity of polymorphonuclear neutrophils (a class of infection-fighting white blood cells) (Nerlich et al. 1994). (On the third day after trauma the reactivity of neutrophils to low opioid concentrations was suppressed to 80% of the baseline value.) In other words, people who experienced the shock of a serious accident and the attendant sense of loss of control had marked increases in levels of endogenous opiates, resulting in weakened immunity, whereas those who experienced physical trauma for which they had been emotionally prepared—indeed, trauma they had chosen—showed no such deleterious physiological changes.

The human analogs of helplessness are even more complex. One analog may be repression, or the nonexpression of emotions. Larry Jamner and Gary Schwartz (Jamner et al. 1988) conducted psychological evaluations of 312 patients seen at their medical clinic and found that those who exhibited repressive or "defensive high anxious" coping styles had significantly reduced numbers of monocytes, a sign of relative immunological weakness. ("Defensive high anxious" persons have been theorized by Schwartz and others to be repressors whose defenses have become ineffective, leaving them in a state of chronic distress [Jamner et al. 1988].) These individuals also had high serum glucose, which coincides with studies showing that hyperglycemia occurs when beta-endorphin is injected directly into the cerebrum (Van Loon and Appel 1981) and that opioid antagonists, by contrast, can reverse stress-induced hyperglycemia (Amir and Bernstein 1982; Amir and Harel 1983). The investigators concluded that their behavioral, immunological, and endocrine profile was consistent

20   with the "opioid peptide hypothesis of repression" (Jamner et al. 1988). The theory implies that habitual repression of strong emotions results in chronically high levels of endogenous opioids, which in turn cause immune deficits that reduce the person's resistance to infectious and malignant disease. It is a thesis that perfectly parallels the findings of Shavit in his studies with mice, although in mice the more complex construct of *repression* is replaced by the simpler animal analog, *helplessness.*

Although Jamner and associates did not link their patients' immune decrements to disease, other studies have correlated repression, immune dysfunction, and poor health. A longitudinal study of one hundred HIV-positive patients showed that patients who developed symptoms over the course of one year were significantly more likely to exhibit psychological defenses of repression or denial, whereas those who remained asymptomatic evidenced fighting spirit (Solano et al. 1993). In research with fifty-eight melanoma patients Lydia Temoshok (1985) demonstrated that repressors—persons who evidenced nonexpression of emotions in videotaped structured interviews coded by independent raters—had thicker and more aggressive lesions and fewer lymphocytes infiltrating the site of the tumor to stem the tide of malignant growth. In a related series of studies, Temoshok found that melanoma patients who did not express emotions exhibited other related coping characteristics, including appeasement, extreme self-sacrifice, and a pleasant facade, a constellation she and others referred to as "type C behavior" (Temoshok and Dreher 1992).

From a psychological perspective, the "learned helplessness" animal studies, which show similar relationships between a psychosocial factor, elevations in opioid peptides, and suppression of immunity, may indeed be comparable to the work of Jamner and Temoshok on repression in human beings. The helplessness induced in experimental animals is a state of resignation that occurs when no active response seems possible or purposeful. Human beings experience helplessness under circumstances of chronic stress; they often believe that no expression of emotion or active behavioral response will change inescapably unpleasant conditions or alleviate the pain of loss or separation. In time, the helpless human may become the repressed human, worn down by relentlessly bad experiences to believe that expressive action is simply no use.

Indeed, in many social settings (e.g., family, school, work) we get the message that expression of strong emotion—anger, fear, grief—will exacerbate interpersonal tensions and hasten rejection or opprobrium. Our response is often helplessness, and our long-term coping strategy may be repression. (Genetic and early environmental factors may also play a role in the evolution of habitual coping styles.) From a psychobiological perspective, the release of opioid peptides is our organismic attempt to quell pain or at least to establish the bliss or bonding associated with interpersonal closeness. If emotional pain or loss is repressed and never resolved, the continuing synthesis and release of endogenous opiates may result, with unintended injurious consequences for our own health and well-being.

Put differently, we banish socially unacceptable or exceedingly painful emotions from consciousness when we feel powerless to change conditions that cause ongoing stress, anguish, rejection, abandonment, hunger, or physical discomfort. This repressive defense, often useful for a period of time, can eventually carry a substantial psychobiological price. A long-term incapacity to express emotion is maladaptive because it disables people from protecting themselves in relationships, meeting their needs, and experiencing the full spectrum of feelings. If we are emotionally "locked" in a certain psychobiological state, we preclude expression of a fuller range of emotional adaptive responses. Homeostasis and host resistance mechanisms are thus disrupted, creating the conditions for ill health.

Is it possible that the symptoms or diseases of a compromised mind-body system—the infections, chronic pains, autoimmune disorders, even the cancers—are, in part, messages to the chronic repressor that his or her defense no longer protects his or her well-being? Can illness be a macro-cosmic variant of the microscopic molecular feedback loops that govern the workings of the internal healing system? Is it simply another signifier in the language of mind-body distress?

If so, illness is a signifier that must be properly interpreted. Disease is never a punishment. The etiology of most illnesses involves complex biological, psychological, and social factors (as in the "biopsychosocial model of health and illness" first developed by Dr. George Engel), and the psychological components, including both affective states and personality traits, are unconscious, unintentional contributors to host vulnerability (Temoshok and Dreher 1992). "Blaming the victim" should be expunged from any scientifically and ethically sound model of mind-body medicine. Although disease is no indicator of character flaws, many one-time medical patients insist that it can be a wake-up call. From their perspective, illness signifies that imbalance—psychosocial, emotional, nutritional, physiological—reigns in the mind-body system and that efforts made to restore balance will yield benefits in both the psychospiritual and physical realms even when a "cure" is not a likely or possible outcome.

Emotional Expression: Flow in the Psychosomatic Network

What are the clinical ramifications of research on the biochemical substrates of emotion, the psychosomatic network, and the healing system? In some quarters the simplistic answer is to promote "positive" emotions while discouraging "negative" feelings. But refined research in the mind-body field suggests that the variety of emotions, though associated with different biochemical substrates and unique correlates in the immune system, are not intrinsically maladaptive, immune suppressive, or bad for our health. Primary emotions such as anger, sadness, grief, fear, and joy are essential elements of the repertoire of human experience, and each emotion serves adaptive psychobiological and evolutionary functions (Temoshok 1983). Emotions carry information, and we benefit by paying attention to their messages. By contrast, long-term states of distress (e.g., helplessness, hopelessness, depression, despair) often result from inescapable or overwhelming stress, rigidly repressive psychic defenses, anger turned against the self, unresolved grief, and ineffective coping styles. These states of chronic distress are frequently present in people with documented disturbances in their healing systems—depressed immunity, autoimmune disorder, and hormone imbalances with worrisome consequences in terms of disease susceptibility.

Schwartz (1990) and Temoshok and Dreher (1992) have tried to clarify the linkages between repressive defenses, chronic helplessness or hopelessness, and dysfunction of the healing system. Over time, the inability to express emotion reinforces unconscious hopelessness because the person who is unable to experience or communicate emotions may be unable to alter stressful social conditions or assert legitimate needs or rights. He or she may also lack contact with inner sources of creative energy and relatedness to other people in their families and social networks. Viewed from an existential perspective, the repressive coper is out of touch with some essential components for an authentic selfhood, having unconsciously sacrificed access to emotions that form the foundation of a mature identity. The sacrifice is usually made in childhood for a protective, even noble purpose—to maintain self-integrity. But much later, in adolescence and adulthood, this sacrifice may become an unconscious impediment to self-realization and fulfillment.

This line of reasoning leads inevitably to the hypothesis that emotional expression, disinhibition, and self-realization strengthen the healing system. We now have experimental, longitudinal, and clinical evidence to support this hypothesis. Steve Cole and his colleagues at the University of California, Los Angeles, analyzed data from a longitudinal psychosocial study of eighty HIV-positive gay men who were otherwise healthy from the outset (Cole, Kemeny, Taylor, et al. 1996). The subjects were examined at six-month intervals for nine years. The investigators sought to evaluate whether the extent to which these gay men were "closeted" influenced the course of their disease. The men were asked to rate themselves as being "definitely in the closet," "in the closet most of the time," "half in and half out," "out most of the time," or "completely out of the closet." HIV progression was measured in terms of the time from entry to the study to a critically low CD4 lymphocyte count (15% of total peripheral blood lymphocytes), AIDS diagnosis, and AIDS mortality. On all measures, the rate at which HIV infection advanced was in direct proportion to the extent to which participants concealed their gay identity (Cole, Kemeny, Taylor, et al. 1996). The investigators successfully ruled out explanations based on demographic characteristics, health practices, sexual behavior, or the use of antiretroviral therapy.

Relative to participants who reported being "mostly" or "completely" out of the closet, those who reported being "half" or more "in the closet" experienced a 40 percent reduction in time to reach a critically low CD4 count, a 38 percent reduction in time to AIDS diagnosis, and a 21 percent reduction in time to death—statistically significant differences in each instance (Cole, Kemeny, Taylor, et al. 1996). Viewed from another angle, the HIV-positive men who were relatively more "out of the closet" did not experience the rapid disease progression experienced by their counterparts. These results were consistent with data from a study of 222 HIV-negative gay men showing that men who concealed their gay identity experienced a significantly higher incidence of cancer and several infectious diseases (pneumonia, bronchitis, sinusitis, and tuberculosis) during a five-year follow-up period (Cole, Kemeny, Taylor, and Visscher 1996). In this study as well the researchers could not attribute these effects to health behaviors, socioeconomic factors, anxiety, depression, or reporting biases.

The findings of Cole et al. (Cole, Kemeny, Taylor, and Visscher 1996; Cole, Kemeny, Taylor, et al. 1996) are consistent with prior research linking psychological inhibition to physical illness, and these results suggest that concealing one's identity, which certainly encompasses a whole gamut of emotions, personality traits, and proclivities (e.g., insight, humor, self-expression, honest communication with others) can compromise the healing system. (Although concealing homosexual identity may not be completely consonant with repressive coping, these constructs may overlap to some extent, and Cole's finding may be consistent with the opioid peptide hypothesis of repression.) By contrast, being able to fully accept and acknowledge one's identity may be interpreted to mean that one is freed

24   from the physiological "work" of inhibition, which has been shown to have negative effects on immunity and health, primarily in the work of James Pennebaker.

Pennebaker's extensive body of research (Pennebaker 1989) has shown that disinhibition—emotional expression and processing—has a salutary influence on immune functions and resistance to illness. In experimental studies, subjects who wrote down their deepest thoughts and feelings about past traumas experienced greater T-cell responsiveness (Pennebaker et al. 1988) and better overall health (Pennebaker 1989; Pennebaker and Beall 1986) than did control subjects, who wrote about trivial events. Pennebaker has shown that in order for disinhibition to foster health or healing, previously blocked emotions must be not only expressed but also cognitively processed—understood and resolved over the course of three or four twenty-minute writing sessions on successive days. Moreover, the degree to which subjects disclosed previously inhibited painful memories and emotions was associated with better health outcomes (Pennebaker and Beall 1986).

Drawing from the Pennebaker model, researchers at the University of Miami explored the immunological effects of both repression and disinhibition. One measure of cellular immune responses is the capacity to control latent viruses, specifically the ubiquitous herpes and Epstein-Barr viruses. The investigators administered a personality inventory to eighty students and had them write about stressful or traumatic events in their lives, after which blood was drawn. Essays were scored based on the degree of emotional disclosure according to an analysis of the ratio of so-called emotion words used (e.g., *I feel. . . , angry, upset, afraid*). A lesser degree of emotional disclosure was found to be associated with impaired control of latent Epstein-Barr virus (EBV) as measured by high antibody titers to EBV capsid antigen (Esterling et al. 1990). (High antibody titers to EBV viral capsid antigen have been shown to indicate poor T-cell-mediated immune control of the latent virus.) Furthermore, participants who scored high on a test of emotional repression also demonstrated poorer immunological control of the latent virus.

The data linking emotional disclosure, disinhibition, or expression with a more efficient immune system, whether the subjects are compared with other, more inhibited subjects or with themselves prior to an experimental procedure involving disclosure, continue to build. The relevance of these findings to disease and health has been questioned because it is not certain that the observed immune fluctuations are clinically meaningful. The question asked repeatedly is, do these immune changes really matter to health? A handful of studies have indeed shown that, contrary to prevailing medical opinion, various immune improvements are clinically relevant.

Temoshok's study showing links between emotional expression and levels of tumor-infiltrating lymphocytes in melanoma is clinically relevant because these infiltrates can block tumor progression. (In several reports, patients with this potentially life-threatening skin cancer who had relatively more tumor-infiltrating lymphocytes had a better prognosis [Temoshok 1985].) Also, in Temoshok's study patients with fewer infiltrating lymphocytes had generally thicker tumors made up of melanoma cells with a higher growth rate, both of which indicate a poor prognosis (McGovern et al. 1981; Thompson 1973). (Further support for the role of emotional expression in cancer survival comes from a joint study by investigators from Freiburg, Germany, and the University of South Florida. After tracking seventy-nine breast cancer patients for a median of 8.4 years, researchers found that emotional defensiveness and anger suppression were independent predictors of recurrence, while somatic symptoms of depression and habitual suppression of anger were independent predictors of mortality [Kuderer et al. 1998].)

Although the clinical relevance of a wide array of immune measures has yet to be established, psychoneuroimmunological researchers have begun to show associations between psychological factors and health that are arguably determined, at least in part, by the intervening role of the immune system. For instance, in a classic study Sheldon Cohen and colleagues (1991) demonstrated that in volunteers inoculated with rhinoviruses the risk of contracting a cold or a respiratory infection was directly proportional to the amount of stress the subjects reported experiencing in the preceding year. In a study of 116 postsurgical breast cancer patients, Andersen and colleagues (1998) found that women with higher stress levels had NK cells with a significantly reduced capacity to destroy human tumor cells in test tubes or to respond to the activating effects of interferon. Compared with less stressed patients, they also had less robust proliferation of peripheral blood lymphocytes to challenge by plant lectins. These patients continue to be observed by Andersen for long-term outcomes. In a separate study (Levy et al. 1991) NK cell activity was shown to be a strong predictor of recurrence of early-stage breast cancer. Thus, among breast cancer patients stress modulates immune factors that involve NK cell activity, a measure with clear clinical importance in this particular disease.

Cole's research on concealing gay identity among HIV-positive patients provides evidence that not only are emotional factors clinically *relevant* to disease outcomes but they may also be *predictive*. Although the study did not examine whether a drop-off in immune measures was linked to

26 concealment of gay identity or to progressive disease, as noted, the investigators did rule out a vast range of alternative hypotheses (Cole, Kemeny, Taylor, et al. 1996). Based on the existing literature of psychological inhibition, one compelling theoretical construct for these findings is the mediating role of neuroimmunomodulation. The role of emotional factors in viral disease generally could also be explained, in part, by the fact that viruses bind to the same receptors as neuropeptides, and the ability of viruses to enter the cell may therefore depend on the relative availability of neuropeptides with an affinity for these receptors.

One of the most intriguing lines of inquiry involves the long-term health effects of early physical and sexual abuse, traumas that are typically suppressed or repressed. The best studies of the long-term pathological effects of early abuse involves gastrointestinal diseases, most notably irritable bowel syndrome (IBS) and inflammatory bowel disease (Drossman et al. 1990; Drossman et al. 1995; Leserman et al. 1996). The prevalence of early sexual and physical abuse in patients with IBS has been documented by one of the country's leading gastroenterologists, Douglas Drossman. From his work, considered alongside research on the biology of the gastrointestinal (GI) tract, we can reasonably hypothesize that biochemical substrates of repressed emotion may play a central role in some GI disorders. Neuropeptide receptors line the entire GI tract, and research has shown that three of these neuropeptides—VIP, somatostatin, and substance P—have profound stimulatory (and occasionally inhibitory) effects on T cells, which reside throughout the mucosal lining of our intestines (Nio et al. 1993). One hypothesis worth investigating is whether the inhibition of emotions and memories of early abuse causes an overactivation of immune-regulating intestinal peptides, resulting in chronic inflammatory bowel disease. In language that better suits a memoir than a medical text, early abuse is a kick in the gut, and the psychophysical repercussions may be felt for decades.

The experimental studies of disinhibition are building blocks for clinical research on whether a psychosocial treatment that systematically encourages emotional expression and proactive coping sufficiently strengthens our host defenses to promote healing of disease. Several of these studies have been conducted, and the results have been well documented and publicized. In a decade-long study of eighty-six women with metastatic breast cancer the psychiatrist David Spiegel and colleagues (1989) found that patients who participated in "supportive/expressive therapy," a group psychosocial intervention, lived twice as long (mean of 36.6 months) as control subjects, who did not participate (mean of 18.9 months). Spiegel has emphasized that the intervention was designed to

encourage emotional expression—sharing and processing the most difficult emotional states associated with a life-threatening condition. We await
results from his current replications, which also address whether neuroendocrine and immune factors act as mediators between psychological
states and disease progression—or survival.

The psychiatrist Fawzy I. Fawzy and his colleagues (1993), who conducted a similar, randomized, controlled trial with sixty-eight patients
with melanoma, found that participation in a six-week, structured psychosocial intervention was associated with a reduction in the risk of recurrence and a statistically significant, threefold reduction in the risk of
mortality over six years. Although emotional expression was not an explicit
goal of his cognitive-behavioral intervention, Fawzy's participants did
share their ordeals with others, learned and adopted methods of active
coping, and practiced relaxation techniques. Although it has received little
attention, the study also found that patients who expressed more distress
at the outset of the study, and who evidenced an increase in active-
behavioral coping, were significantly less likely to experience a recurrence
or to die of their disease. In an earlier study, Fawzy et al. (1990) demonstrated that participants in his treatment program experienced a significant increase in NK cells, large granular lymphocytes, and the ability of
interferon to augment NK cell activity.

These intervention studies support our contention that the healing system, in all its multilayered complexity, is strengthened and balanced, not
simply by "good" emotions, but by the experience, expression, and cognitive resolution of all emotions. Indeed, we propose that emotional expression and resolution is a psychodynamic process that correlates with a
properly balanced flow of neuropeptides throughout the mind-body system. Put differently, flow in one system is both responsive to and genera-
tive of flow in the other system. This appropriately balanced flow within
and between both systems generates a functional healing system, which
also involves a balanced flow of endocrine secretions, a vigorous but finely
tuned immune system, perhaps even the minimization or control of cellular abnormalities caused by inappropriate gene expression.

Mind-Body Medicine and the Healing System

Research on the biochemical substrates of emotion emphasizing the pivotal role of neuropeptides and receptors in the psychosomatic network has
enhanced our understanding of the healing system. Consciousness studies, as well as continuing investigations in psychodynamics and transpersonal psychology, which have shed light on the unified fields of mind, body,

and spirit, have further broadened our understanding of the healing system. Although the immune system is clearly central to the body's healing endeavor, the healing system is larger than one subset of organs, tissues, and cells: it encompasses the integral activities of virtually all the biological subsystems, including those associated with mind and emotion.

Research on the nature of the healing system should now also focus on what Ernest Rossi (1993) calls "the mind-gene connection." Our state of health or disease cannot simply be measured by immune increments or decrements; dysfunction at the cellular level must also be the result of altered gene expression. Moreover, informational substances, especially neuropeptides, that interact with receptors can modify gene expression through the transduction of messages from the cell's surface to its nuclear core. A remarkable series of studies by the immunovirologist Ronald Glaser, the psychologist Janice Kiecolt-Glaser, and their colleagues have shown the influence of stress and emotional factors on gene expression. In one study seventeen first-year medical students were tested for levels of messenger RNA expression of the genes *c-myc* and *c-myb* in peripheral blood leukocytes at the time of academic examinations and at a baseline period approximately one month before the examinations. *C-myc* and *c-myb* are proto-oncogenes; that is, they play a normal role in regulating cell growth patterns, but when inappropriately activated, they can trigger malignant cell growth, thus becoming full-fledged cancer genes, known as oncogenes. Glaser and Kiecolt-Glaser found higher levels of messenger RNA expression of *c-myc* and *c-myb* in the white blood cells of these subjects only during the stressful examination period (Glaser et al. 1993). The increased expression of *c-myc* and *c-myb* was consistent with previous data demonstrating down-regulation of these immune cells during stress.

In other words, gene expression is altered during stress, and this alteration changes cellular functions, with consequences for the health of the individual. What does this finding augur for research on the link between emotional factors and the oncogenes that represent a pivotal "mechanism" in most human cancers? If stress can increase expression of proto-oncogenes, presumably through the intermediary effect of stress-related neuropeptides interacting with receptors and causing transduction of messages to cellular DNA, can it transform benign proto-oncogenes into active cancer genes?

Janice Kiecolt-Glaser and Ronald Glaser have also shown that stress can hamper DNA repair mechanisms (Kiecolt-Glaser et al. 1985), so malignantly transformed cells may be more likely to develop into full-blown tumors. Our healing systems must now be broadened to include the dialectic relationships between emotions, neuropeptides, endocrine glands and secretions, immune system components, and the influence of this entire cascade on gene expression and the regulation of gene products within the cell.

Working together, two creative scientists have grappled with the question why psychological traits and states should be so fully intertwined with biological systems of defense and healing. In seeking answers to this perplexing problem, the molecular biologists Roger Booth and Kevin Ashbridge developed an encompassing model of the psychoneuroimmune system (Booth and Ashbridge 1993). They proposed that the immune system, commonly viewed as a defense network, is engaged in a broader process of self-determination. In their view, the psychological, neurological, and immmunological subsystems share a common goal: establishing and maintaining self-identity. They refer to this unifying principle as "teleological coherence," and they argue that biological subsystems overlap so closely because of their common purposes, which is to maintain harmony within and without the organism and to uphold the integrity of the organism by distinguishing "self" from "nonself."

Booth and Ashbridge's model is reinforced by the many conspicuous metaphors between the mind-brain and immune-healing systems, many of which were postulated in the 1960s by the psychoimmunology pioneer George F. Solomon (Dreher 1995). Both systems have the capacity for memory, the mind/brain through short- and long-term memory storage at the level of the neuron, the immune system through T- and B-cell memory of encounters with foreign agents. Both are designed for adaptation to environmental stressors, the mind/brain honing its coping mechanisms through cognitive and behavioral shifts, while the immune system acts swiftly to identify and vanquish interlopers that "stress" the organism. Both act as defenders, the mind/brain employing sophisticated gating systems to block overwhelming bits of cognitive and emotional information, such as traumas, while the immune system is fully armed to defend against any pathogenic assault. Both are harmed by inadequate defenses, the mind/brain when it cannot endure or integrate painful stimuli, the immune system when it fails to destroy microbes and cancer cells. Both are harmed by excessive defenses, the mind/brain when it relies so rigidly on repression or denial that it leaves the person unable to deal with reality, the immune system when it zealously and indiscriminately reacts against the body's own tissues, resulting in autoimmune disease. And both develop either tolerance or sensitivity to "noxious" agents, the mind/brain by responding with too little or too much anxiety to stressful challenges in the environment, the immune system by ignoring or overreacting to antigenic challenges.

As we have argued, not only are these systems analogous but they are

30   wholly intertwined. The critical questions regarding this integrative model include: At what level in the mind–body "system" can we interpolate our own awareness? Are these overlapping and intertwined processes, as purposeful and coherent as they may be, susceptible to conscious intervention? To what extent do we consciously participate in self-determination at the psychological, the immunological, or even the genetic level?

One speculative approach that is consistent with Booth and Ashbridge's ideas suggests that the mind is a nonphysical substrate that holds together the flowing psychosomatic network of informational substances and cells, linking and coordinating the major systems and their molecular constituents in an intelligently orchestrated symphony of life processes. Although the operation of this network occurs below the level of consciousness, it is impinged upon by biochemical substrates of unconscious mental processes. Moreover, various therapies can bring unconscious mental processes into awareness, and we can make psychosocial and behavioral changes that transduce down through the mind–body network, resulting in concomitant physical changes. Therapies that encourage emotional expression are prime examples of the interpolation of consciousness into otherwise autonomic (unconscious) psychobiological processes, resulting in health benefits for the person. Other examples are the use of conscious breathing techniques, imagery, or meditation to ameliorate pain. A major nodal point of pain transmission is the periaqueductal gray region of the midbrain, which is filled with opiate receptors, making it a control area for pain (Pert 1980). Yogis and other practitioners of Eastern meditative and breathing disciplines have demonstrated their ability to vastly alter pain perception. It is conceivable, even likely, that these individuals gain access to the periaqueductal gray region, consciously resetting their pain thresholds.

Psychological treatments that encourage us to consciously engage in identity formation, self-assertion, and self-expression may indeed generate comparable qualities in our healing systems. Teleological coherence is an organismic reality, but in the human animal consciousness may indeed intervene in seemingly involuntary processes of the bodymind. Without simplifying too much, it seems that when we stand up for ourselves, we provide fuel for elements in our biological healing system that "stand up" for our organism's integrity. When we actively reshape and solidify our identity in the world, we also strengthen our biological "selfhood," more ably resisting attacks by external invaders and our own misguided immune sentries. The findings cited above by such clinical investigators as Cole, Spiegel, Fawzy, Solomon, and Pennebaker, among others, suggest that the psychological quest for physical health is more than just a metaphorical metaphysic: it is a testable hypothesis that is already bearing fruit.

Deeper questions concern the nature of the mind—that presumably nonmaterial, nonphysical substrate of observable processes characterized by a flow of information centered in, but not limited to, the brain. The word *soul* is still assiduously avoided by academic scientists. But what animates the neuropeptides in their flow patterns through the body? What animates the receptors? These flexible cell-surface molecules vibrate, shimmy, and even hum as they change shapes, awaiting arrival of their matching ligands. The entire healing system is propelled by chemical energies, but to reverse the usual question, What is the immaterial substrate of these ceaseless biochemical reactions? Rachel Naomi Remen refers to the "life force," the heretical psychoanalyst Wilhelm Reich spoke of "life energy," and poets and theologians conjure an élan vital and "spirit."

These questions may be largely unanswerable by the current methods of mainstream science, though researchers have sought to explain how varieties of energy medicine (Rubik 1995), prayer (Dossey 1993), and other spiritual practices (Levin 1994) support the healing system. But research on healing energies, whether delineated in Western terms (bioelectromagnetism, nonlocal consciousness) or in Eastern spiritual or medical terms (e.g., qi, *kundalini,* prana), may shed light on the immaterial substrates of the molecules of emotion. The epidemiologist Jeffrey Levin (1994), who has uncovered more than 250 published empirical studies on the largely beneficial health effects of religious or spiritual practice, has developed a series of hypotheses for these effects, including behavioral and social factors as well as the psychodynamics of belief systems and religious rites. He also includes as an alternative hypothesis the role of a "superempirical force," an energetic phenomenon that is accessed through spiritual or religious practice, a pantheistic, discarnate force or power (Levin 1994). Levin emphasizes that in the near future this force may be considered empirical rather than superempirical; some scientists are claiming success in measuring bioenergy fields (Motoyama 1991; Rubik 1995).

A point of intersection between efforts to explain the psychosomatic network and efforts to explain biological energies is the concept of information. We noted that in the biomedical realm the neuroscientist Francis O. Schmidt used this model when he described molecular messengers as "informational substances." Likewise, in studies of bioelectromagnetic fields, which are relevant to energy-medicine treatments such as acupuncture, homeopathy, and healer interventions, the biophysicist Beverly Rubik has endeavored to shift the emphasis from a strictly energetic model to an information-based paradigm. In her view, energy-medicine applications may involve bioinformation that interacts with internal electromagnetic biofields or at the level of membrane receptors in the organism (Rubik

32   1995). Thus, information can be viewed as a unifying concept that spans many levels of organization of living systems, including emotional, energetic, biochemical, molecular, and genetic levels.

Using the principle of information as a guide, it may be possible to develop a hybrid of an energy-based model (one variation of which is the foundation of ancient healing arts, including traditional Chinese medicine) and a neuropeptide-receptor model. It may be possible to ground such a model in Western science, particularly if it encompasses both state-of-the-art quantum physics and psychobiology. The unifying idea is that information is passed among the components of living systems in concurrent streams of biologically active molecules and biophysical energy.

But the unification of these seemingly disparate realms through an information-based model brings us into another domain. As Larry Dossey (1991) has argued, we must consider the possibility that *meaning* is translated on both energetic and molecular levels. For instance, psychological states of "hopelessness" or "joy" have specific energetic and molecular correlates—our experience of such states cannot be reduced to either level but appears to be translated on both—simultaneously and indivisibly. One can best "read" such meanings and their multileveled correlates by evaluating the whole person, combining the clinician's art with the biologist's technological probes. Perhaps that is why we have emphasized the pivotal role of emotional expression in the healing system: it may be the best marker for activation of a life force, however one defines such an uncertain phenomenon. The forms of mind-body medicine that awaken our healing potential are those that rouse emotion and generate spirit, which could be defined in terms once used by Rollo May (1981): "Spirit is that which gives vivacity, energy, liveliness, courage, and ardor to life."

REFERENCES

Ader R, Felten DL, Cohen N, eds. 1991. *Psychoneuroimmunology II*. New York: Academic Press.

Amir S, Bernstein M. 1982. Endogenous opioids interact with stress-induced hyperglycemia in mice. *Physiol Behav*. 28:575–577.

Amir S, Harel M. 1983. Role of endorphins in endotoxin-induced hyperglycemia in mice. *Neuropharmacology*. 22:1117–1119.

Andersen BL, Farrar WB, Golden-Kreutz D, et al. 1998. Stress and immune responses after surgical treatment for regional breast cancer. *J Natl Cancer Inst*. 90:30–36.

Benveniste EN, Huneycutt BS, Shrikant P, Ballestas ME. 1995. Second messenger systems in the regulation of cytokines and adhesion molecules in the central nervous system. *Brain Behav Immun.* 9:304–314.

Booth RJ, Ashbridge KR. 1993. A fresh look at the relationship between the *psyche* and immune system: teleological coherence and harmony of purpose. *Advances.* 9:4–23.

Bost KL, Smith EM, Wear LB, Blalock JE. 1987. Presence of ACTH and its receptor on a B-lymphocyte cell line: a possible autocrine function for a neuroendocrine hormone. *J Biol Regul Homeost Agents.* 1:23–27.

Brazelton TR, Rossi FM, Keshet GI, Blau HM. 2000. From marrow to brain: expression of neuronal phenotypes in adult mice. *Science.* 290:1775–1779.

Carolan EJ, Casale TB. 1993. Effects of neuropeptides on neutrophil migration through non-cellular and endothelial barriers. *J Allergy Clin Immunol.* 92:589.

Carr DJ, Blalock JE. 1991. Neuropeptide hormones and receptors common to the immune and neuroendocrine systems: bidirectional pathway of intersystem communication. In: Ader R, Felten DL, Cohen N, eds. *Psychoneuroimmunology II.* New York: Academic Press.

Cohen S, Tyrrell DAJ, Smith AP. 1991. Psychological stress and susceptibility to the common cold. *New Engl J Med.* 325:606–612.

Cole SW, Kemeny ME, Taylor SE, Visscher BR. 1996. Elevated physical health risk among gay men who conceal their homosexual identity. *Health Psychol.* 15:243–251.

Cole SW, Kemeny ME, Taylor SE, et al. 1996. Accelerated course of human immunodeficiency virus infection in gay men who conceal their homosexual identity. *Psychosom Med.* 58:219–231.

Dossey L. 1991. *Meaning and Medicine.* New York: Bantam.

Dossey L. 1993. *Healing Words: The Power of Prayer and the Practice of Medicine.* New York: HarperCollins.

Dreher H. 1995. *The Immune Power Personality: Seven Traits You Can Develop to Stay Healthy.* New York: Dutton.

Drossman DA, Leserman J, Nachman G, et al. 1990. Sexual and physical abuse in women with functional or organic gastrointestinal disorders. *Ann Intern Med.* 113:828–833.

Drossman DA, Talley NJ, Leserman J, et al. 1995. Sexual and physical abuse in gastrointestinal illness: review and recommendations. *Ann Intern Med.* 123:782–794.

Esterling BA, Antoni MH, Kumar M, Schneiderman N. 1990. Emotional repression, stress disclosure responses, and Epstein-Barr viral capsid antigen titers. *Psychosom Med.* 52:397–410.

Farrar WL. 1988. Hemopoietic cytokines in brain. *Prog Neuroendocrinimmunol.* 1:18–19.

Farrar WL, Hill JM, Ruff MR, Pert CB. 1987. Autoradiographic distribution of IL-1 receptors in rat brain. *J Immunol.* 139:459–463.

Fawzy FI, Fawzy NW, Hyun CS, et al. 1993. Malignant melanoma: effects of an early structured psychiatric intervention, coping, and affective state on recurrence and survival six years later. *Arch Gen Psychiatry.* 50:681–689.

Fawzy FI, Kemeny ME, Fawzy NW, et al. 1990. A structured psychiatric interven-

34   tion for cancer patients. II. Changes over time in immunological measures. *Arch Gen Psychiatry.* 47:729–735.

Geoetzl EJ, Turck CW, Sreedharan SP. 1991. Production and recognition of neuropeptides by cells of the immune system. In: Ader R, Felten DL, Cohen N, eds. *Psychoneuroimmunology II.* New York: Academic Press.

Gerritsen W, Heijnen CJ, Wiegant VM, et al. 1996. Experimental social fear: immunological, hormonal, and autonomic concomitants. *Psychosom Med.* 58:273–286.

Glaser R, Lafuse WP, Bonneau RH, et al. 1993. Stress-associated modulation of proto-oncogene expression in human peripheral blood leukocytes. *Behav Neurosci.* 107:525–529.

Herkenham M, Pert CB. 1982. Light microscopic localization of brain opiate receptors: general autoradiographic method which preserves tissue quality. *J Neurosci.* 2:1129–1149.

Jamner L, Schwartz CE, Leigh H. 1988. The relationship between repressive and defensive coping styles and monocyte, eosinophil, and serum glucose levels: support for the opioid peptide hypothesis of repression. *Psychosom Med.* 50:567–575.

Kandel ER, Klein M, Castellucci VF, et al. 1986. Some principles emerging from the study of short- and long-term memory. *Neurosci Res.* 3:498–520.

Kiecolt-Glaser JK, Stephens RE, Liepetz PD, et al. 1985. Distress and DNA repair in human lymphocytes. *J Behav Med.* 8:311–320.

Kuderer NM, Krasner S, Spielberger CD, Lyman GH. 1998. Psychological measures and breast cancer survival. *Proceedings of the American Society of Clinical Oncology.* Vol 17. Alexandria, Va: American Society for Clinical Oncology. Abstract 238.

Lamotte CC, Snowman A, Pert CB, Snyder SH. 1978. Opiate receptor binding in rhesus monkey brain: association with limbic structures. *Brain Res.* 155:374.

Laudenslager ML, Ryan SM, Drugan RC, et al. 1983. Coping and immunosuppression: inescapable but not escapable shock suppresses lymphocyte proliferation. *Science.* 221:568–570.

Leserman J, Drossman DA, Li Z, et al. 1996. Sexual and physical abuse history in gastroenterology practice: how types of abuse impact health status. *Psychosom Med.* 58:4–15.

Levin JS. 1994. Religion and health: is there an association, is it valid, and is it causal? *Soc Sci Med.* 38:1475–1482.

Levy SM, Herberman RB, Lippman M, D'Angelo T, Lee J. 1991. Immunological and psychosocial predictors of disease recurrence in patients with early-stage breast cancer. *Behav Med.* 17:67–75.

Lewis ME, Mishkin M, Bragin E, et al. 1981. Opiate receptor gradients in monkey cerebral cortex: correspondence with sensory processing hierarchies. *Science.* 211:1166.

May R. 1981. *Freedom and Destiny.* New York: Delta Books; 220.

McGovern VJ, Shaw HM, Milton GW, et al. 1981. Lymphocytic infiltration and survival in malignant melanoma. In: Ackerman AB, ed. *Pathology of Malignant Melanoma.* New York: Masson; 341–344.

Mezey E, Chandross KJ, Harta G, Maki RA, McKercher SR. 2000. Turning blood into brain: cells bearing neuronal antigens generated in vivo from bone marrow. *Science.* 290:1779–1782.

Motoyama H. 1991. *The Correlation between Psi Energy and Ki: Unification of Religion and Science.* Tokyo: Human Science Press.

Naliboff BD, Senton D, Solomon GF, et al. 1991. Psychological, psychophysiological, and immunological changes in young and old subjects during brief laboratory stress. *Psychosom Med.* 53:121–132.

Nerlich ML, Holch M, Stalp M, et al. 1994. Neuropeptide levels early after trauma: immunomodulatory effects. *J Trauma.* 37:759–768.

Nio DA, Moylan RN, Roche JK. 1993. Modulation of T lymphocyte function by neuro-peptides: evidence for their role as local immunoregulatory elements. *J Immunol.* 150:5281–5288.

O'Regan B. 1987. Healing, remission, and miracle cures. *Inst Noetic Sci Spec Rep.* 3–14.

Ottoway CA. 1991. Vasoactive intestinal peptide and immune function. In: Ader R, Felten DL, Cohen N, eds. *Psychoneuroimmunology II.* New York: Academic Press.

Pennebaker JW. 1989. Confession, inhibition, and disease. *Adv Exp Soc Psychol.* 22:212–244.

Pennebaker JW, Beall S. 1986. Confronting a traumatic event: toward an understanding of inhibition and disease. *J Abnorm Psychol.* 95:274–281.

Pennebaker JW, Kiecolt-Glaser JK, Glaser R. 1988. Disclosure of traumas and immune function: health implications for psychotherapy. *J Consult Clin Psychol.* 56:239–245.

Pert A. 1980. Psychopharmacology of analgesia and pain. In: Ng L, Bonica JJ, eds. *Discomfort and Humanitarian Care.* New York: Elsevier.

Pert CB. 1986. The wisdom of the receptors: neuropeptides, the emotions, and bodymind. *Advances.* 3:8–16.

Pert CB. 1989. Untitled presentation at Elmwood Symposium, "Healing Ourselves and Our Society," Dec 9, Boston, Mass.

Pert CB. 1997. *The Molecules of Emotion: Why We Feel the Way We Feel.* New York: Scribner.

Pert CB, Dienstfrey H. 1988. The neuropeptide network. *Ann NY Acad Sci.* 521:189–194.

Pert CB, Hill JM, Ruff MR, et al. 1986. Octapeptides deduced from the neuropeptide receptor-like pattern of antigen T4 in brain potently inhibit human immunodeficiency virus receptor binding and T-cell infectivity. *Proc Natl Acad Sci U S A.* 83:9254–9258.

Pert CB, Ruff MR, Weber RJ, Herkenham M. 1985. Neuropeptides and their receptors: a psychosomatic network. *J Immunol.* 35:820s–826s.

Pert CB, Snyder SA. 1973. Opiate receptor: demonstration in nervous tissue. *Science.* 179:1011–1014.

Rossi EL. 1993. *The Psychobiology of Mind-Body Healing: New Concepts of Therapeutic Hypnosis.* New York: W. W. Norton.

36   Rubik B. 1995. Energy medicine and the unifying concept of information. *Altern Ther Health Med.* 1:34–39.

Ruff MR, Martin BM, Ginns EI, Farrar WL, Wahl SM, Pert CB. 1987. CD4 receptor binding peptides that block HIV infectivity cause human monocyte chemotaxis: relationship to vasoactive intestinal polypeptide. *FEBS Lett.* 211:17–22.

Ruff MR, Pert CB, Weber RJ, et al. 1985. Benzodiazepine receptor-mediated chemotaxis of human monocytes. *Science.* 229:1281–1283.

Ruff MR, Schiffman V, Terranova V, Pert CB. 1985. Neuropeptides are chemoattractants for human tumor cells and monocytes: a possible mechanism for metastasis. *Clin Immunol Immunopathol.* 37:387–396.

Ruff MR, Wahl SM, Mergenhagen S, Pert CB. 1985. Opiate receptor-mediated chemotaxis of human monocytes. *Neuropeptides.* 5:363.

Ruff MR, Wahl SM, Pert CB. 1985. Substance P receptor-mediated chemotaxis of human monocytes. *Peptides.* 6(suppl 2):107–111.

Sacerdote P, Ruff MR, Pert CB. 1988. Cholecystokinin and the immune system: receptor-mediated chemotaxis of human and rat monocytes. *Peptides.* 9:29–34.

Schmitt FD. 1984. Molecular regulation of brain function: a new view. *Neuroscience.* 13:991.

Schratzberger P, Reinisch N, Prodinger WM, et al. 1997. Differential chemotactic activities of sensory neuropeptides for human peripheral blood mononuclear cells. *J Immunol.* 158:3895–3901.

Schwartz GE. 1990. Psychobiology of repression and health: a systems approach. In: Singer JL, ed. *Repression and Dissociation: Implications for Personality Theory, Psychopathology, and Health.* Chicago: University of Chicago Press.

Shavit Y. 1991. Stress-induced immune modulation in animals: opiates and endogenous opioid peptides. In: Ader R, Felten DL, Cohen N, eds. *Psychoneuroimmunology II.* New York: Academic Press.

Shavit Y, Depaulis A, Martin FC, et al. 1986. Involvement of brain opiate receptors in the immune-suppressive effect of morphine. *Proc Natl Acad Sci U S A.* 83:7114–7117.

Shavit Y, Lewis JW, Terman GW, Gale RP, Lieberskind JC. 1984. Opioid peptides mediate the suppressive effect of stress on natural killer cell cytotoxicity. *Science.* 223:188–190.

Shavit Y, Lewis JW, Terman GW, et al. 1983. Endogenous opioids may mediate the effects of stress on tumor growth and immune function. *Proc West Pharmacol Soc.* 26:53–56.

Shavit Y, Ryan SM, Lewis JW, et al. 1983. Inescapable but not escapable stress alters immune function. *Physiologist.* 26:A64.

Shavit Y, Terman GW, Martin FC, et al. 1985. Stress, opioid peptides, the immune system, and cancer. *J Immunol.* 135:834s–837s.

Sklar LS, Anisman H. 1979. Stress and coping factors influence tumor growth. *Science.* 205:513–515.

Smith EM, Blalock JE. 1981. Human lymphocyte production of ACTH and endorphin-like substances: association with leukocyte interferon. *Proc Natl Acad Sci U S A.* 78:7530–7534.

Solano L, Costa M, Salvat S, et al. 1993. Psychosocial factors and clinical evolution in HIV-1 infection: a longitudinal study. *J Psychosom Res.* 37:39–51.

Spiegel D, Bloom J, Kraemer HC, Gottheil E. 1989. Effect of psychosocial treatment on survival of patients with metastatic breast cancer. *Lancet.* 2:888–891.

Sternberg EM, Chrousos GP, Wilder RL, Gold PW. 1992. The stress response and the regulation of inflammatory disease. *Ann Intern Med.* 117:854–866.

Sternberg EM, Gold PW. 1997. The mind body interaction in disease. *SciAm.* 7:8–15.

Temoshok L. 1983. Emotion, adaptation, and disease: a multidimensional theory. In: Temoshok L, Van Dyke C, Zegans LS, eds. *Emotions in Health and Illness: Theoretical and Research Foundations.* Orlando, Fla: Grune & Stratton.

Temoshok L. 1985. Biopsychosocial studies on cutaneous malignant melanoma: psychosocial factors associated with prognostic indicators, progression, psychophysiology, and tumor-host response. *Soc Sci Med.* 20:833–840.

Temoshok L. 1987. Personality, coping style, emotion, and cancer: towards an integrative model. *Cancer Surv.* 6:545–567.

Temoshok L, Dreher H. 1992. *The Type C Connection: The Behavioral Links to Cancer and Your Health.* New York: Random House.

Thompson PG. 1973. Relationship of lymphocytic infiltration to prognosis in primary malignant melanoma of the skin. *Pigment Cell Res.* 1:285.

Van Loon GR, Appel NM. 1981. B-endorphin-induced hyperglycemia is mediated by increased central sympathetic outflow to adrenal medulla. *Brain Res.* 204:236–241.

Visintainer MA, Volpicelli JR, Seligman MEP. 1982. Tumor rejection in rats after inescapable or escapable shock. *Science.* 216:437–439.

Wagner R, Myers R. 1996. Schwann cells produce tumor necrosis factor: expression in injured and non-injured tissues. *Neuroscience.* 73:625–629.

Watson M, Haviland JS, Greer S, Davidson J, Bliss JM. 1999. Influence of psychological response on survival in breast cancer: a population-based cohort study. *Lancet.* 354:1331–1336.

Wiedermann CJ, Sertl K, Zipser B, Hill JM, Pert CB. 1988. Vasoactive intestinal peptide receptors in rat spleen and brain: a shared communication network. *Peptides.* 9:21–28.

Wiedermann FJ, Kahler CM, Reinisch N, Wiedermann CJ. 1993. Induction of normal human eosinophil migration in vitro by substance P. *Acta Haematol.* 89:213.

Williams KC, Dooley N, Ulvestad E, et al. 1996. IL-10 production by adult human derived microglial cells. *Neurochem Inl.* 29:55–64.

Chapter 2

The Social Perspective in Mind-Body Studies

In an arresting article published in 1994 the late Israeli medical sociologist Aaron Antonovsky concluded that the "well-being" movement—what we in the United States variously refer to as mind-body health, holistic medicine, or complementary/alternative medicine (CAM)—has largely neglected the fundamental importance of social factors in generating the conditions that favor disease or health (Antonovsky 1994). Antonovsky was a galvanizing figure in this movement, a researcher and theorist on matters of health who bucked convention with a passionate insistence. When psychosomatic investigators were seeking to identify the dysfunctional coping styles and maladaptive personality traits linked to poor mind-body health, Antonovsky was searching for the *positive* styles and traits linked to robust mind-body health. Referring to psychological tendencies that generate good health, he coined the term *salutogenesis* (meaning "generating that which is salutary"). He conducted studies on the human coping capacity he found to be most salutary, which he dubbed a *sense of coherence,* and found that this capacity was possessed by people who believed that in a stressful world they could still operate effectively, with agency and meaning. Antonovsky's most important statement was his 1979 book *Health, Stress, and Coping,* a substantive work on salutogenesis.

Antonovsky's salutogenic strengths, which include a sense of coherence, control, self-efficacy, and other health-promoting psychological states and traits, would seem to be intrapsychic capacities that a person possesses *apart* from the stressful world he or she presently inhabits. Conventional

Reprinted by permission, with changes, from *Advances in Mind-Body Medicine* 11 (1995): 39–54.

mind-body wisdom holds that such gifts (or their lack) are traceable to one's genetic endowment and learning experiences from early life. But in his 1994 critique Antonovsky argued forcefully that one's ability to develop a sense of coherence, or indeed any psychological strength in the face of stress, depends greatly on one's social network, one's social environment, and one's economic resources. He ridiculed mind-body theorists who pay lip service to a *systems* approach to health, often referred to as the *biopsychosocial* model, yet drop the question of social influences in their theories and clinical applications. In his article Antonovsky repeatedly referred to the "structural sources of salutogenic strengths." He was suggesting that our "innate" psychological abilities are not so innate, that they depend almost completely on nurturance from social networks. And they depend on whether we have enough food and resources to live decently; whether we have opportunities for creative work; whether we are free from the constant fear of violence in our communities. In other words, we gain much of our capacity for coherence, control, and self-efficacy from our social and economic support systems.

Antonovsky believed that the well-being movement had simply ignored the structural—societal—sources of salutogenic strengths and, further, that it had neglected social factors in every important equation involving health. Antonovsky's article was based on a paper he had delivered at the Second International Dead Sea Conference on the Anatomy of Well-Being in 1993. Speaking to a community of mind-body-oriented clinicians and theorists, he said:

> Most of us are, in theory, committed to systems theory. And yet the voluminous writing of—shall we call it the holistic approach to health?—as far as I can tell shows a near-total absence of reference to or awareness of the larger social system in which the mind-body relationship operates. History, social structure, and even culture do not seem to exist. Let me quote almost at random from this writing to convey the flavor of what I mean. The source does not matter; "We must search for health within ourselves. If we don't have balance within ourselves, then we cannot expect the world to stay in balance . . . we must begin within the borders of our own skin."
>
> From a scientific point of view, I submit, this new version of Freudianism, of looking within the skin, prevents understanding the social burdens that pressure people to behave in pathogenic fashion, and that block them from behaving salutogenically. From a moral point of view, the focus on the "health within" is at the very least a passive and unconscious approval of the social status quo. If I prove to be wrong, I will be

delighted to apologize. I add quickly, so that I am not misunderstood: the world of techno-biomedicine is no better. This comforts me not at all.

Antonovsky went on, not simply to toss ideological brickbats, but to set forth social conditions that favor the development of salutogenic strengths: solid social networks; social structures (political, corporate, community-based, familial) that provide us with clear informational input rather than confusing, brutalizing noise; a socialization process that grants us tools of language and information processing; the availability of resources—money, time, friends, and freedom; and our embeddedness in social systems that are flexible and responsive to our communications.

Here again he faulted the well-being movement for failing to consider these factors in a meaningful way. (It should be said that what Antonovsky called the well-being movement is as heterogeneous as the biomedical establishment, including institutions and individuals with countless underlying philosophies and therapeutic strategies.) Taken broadly, his provocative arguments raise a valid question for the mind-body establishment: Does it pay enough attention to society? Or does it, as Antonovsky implied, pay too much attention to the self?

In April 1994 the American Psychosomatic Society and the Society of Behavioral Medicine, the two most prestigious groups organizing, promoting, and sponsoring mind-body medicine, held a joint annual meeting. Many leading lights of the mind-body establishment came together to share recent data and discoveries, to generate new hypotheses and research possibilities, and to discuss the health policy ramifications of developments in their respective fields. The first full day's event was a joint symposium called "Superhighways of Disease: Shared Determinants of Health Outcomes." This unusual joint symposium, an event unlike any occurring before or since, seemed a made-to-order opportunity to test Aaron Antonovsky's contention that in studying the conditions favoring disease and health, the mind-body and holistic movements largely neglect social factors.

I attended the event, and I shall report and interpret my experiences and observations through the lens of Antonovsky's critical perspective. I should say from the outset that I largely accept Antonovsky's propositions. I believe, as he did, that economic and social factors in health are rarely given their due by the mind-body and CAM movements. Yet I take issue with Antonovsky's derisive attitude toward the relative contribution of psychospiritual factors to health. (He seems to view any focus on these factors as a form of narcissistic navel gazing.) I consider these variables independent contributors to well-being (or disease), and I hue to a systems philosophy in my belief that psychospiritual factors intertwine with the social factors that contribute to health. In his article Antonovsky did briefly refer to "autopoiesis," which he described as "the capacity of human systems for self-reorganization." Beyond this nod to the power of autonomous action, Antonovsky flirted dangerously with social determinism.

My own two-year experience as a reading teacher in an after-school day-care program in New York City's Hell's Kitchen area informs my wariness about any philosophy bordering on social determinism. Most of my students lived in terrible neighborhoods, rife with poverty, drugs, and demoralization. An astonishing majority of the children were from broken families, no fathers in sight. Some kids suffered more than others, of course, both emotionally and physically. But I was struck by the children who came from the worst imaginable homes and neighborhoods and yet possessed a maturity and resilience that I could not explain. I knew their makeshift families (many with no parents), I went to their homes, and I spent hours with some of the children in and out of school. I did not know why their wounds did not cut deeper than the wounds of some children whose social conditions were slightly better or, put another way, why they were able to heal so much more readily. I never thought they were inherently superior to any other children, yet, in my understanding of them, they had psychospiritual qualities—whether from genes, early experiences, or unknown influences—that enabled them to thrive. Their external "stressors" did not cause the same degree of internal distress—the helplessness, hopelessness, and hostility we associate with physical illness and continued economic deprivation—as they generated in others.

Although Antonovsky's thesis is trenchant, my experience with the kids in Hell's Kitchen leads me to believe that researchers or practitioners who focus on psychological or spiritual factors should not have to apologize at every turn for omitting social influences. Their piece of the health-promotion pie is legitimate unto itself because there is a dimension of coping that is indeed independent of the external conditions that challenge people. Clearly, therapies designed to facilitate coping should take social conditions into account, and they can encourage individuals to shape their own environments. But at times they must deal with people who, in a social sense, *are* helpless because no sociopolitical revolution is about to save them and no imaginable personal actions can substantially reorder their brutal environments. That is when pure psychological medicine has its place, respecting and shepherding the process whereby a person turns within for sources of energy, hope, and meaning.

That said, the balance in mind-body studies has been weighted decidedly toward pure psychological medicine, with far too little consideration given to social environments, no discussion of economic factors, and a one-

42   sided preoccupation with getting people to change their inner lives as a cure for every ailment of mind and body. (I stand accused myself, having written two books on the role of personality and health with nary a mention of macrosocial influences, although in my first book, which was about cancer prevention, I set forth critiques of the tobacco and meat industries.)

As if to underscore the validity of Antonovsky's thesis, on the first day of the meetings, 12 April 1994, a front-page story in the *New York Times* entitled "Study Confirms Some Fears of U.S. Children" reported findings from a wide-ranging study concluding that "millions of infants and toddlers are so deprived of medical care, loving supervision, and intellectual stimulation that their growth into healthy and responsible adults is threatened." These children were vulnerable, the story said, because their parents (if they had parents) were overwhelmed by poverty, teenage pregnancy, divorce, or work.

These findings came as no great surprise. What was astonishing was the portion of the story devoted to the effect such social conditions had on brain development. "The quality of these young lives is deteriorating even as mounting scientific evidence indicates that children's environment, from birth to age three, helps determine their brain structure and ability to learn." The article went on to state that "advances in molecular biology and neurology have shown that children's experiences in these early years can influence how many brain cells, or neurons, they develop, and how many connections, or synapses, are formed between them. Activating these synapses allows learning to take place." (Of course, this report must be read cautiously. It deals with statistical trends, not with a "hard-wired" cause-and-effect relationship. It leaves room for adaptive responses to even the most injurious environments. But such studies underscore what people deprived of supportive early environments are up against and how the damage can extend to the physical realm.)

If a harsh environment can influence brain and nervous-system development at the primordial level, there is no telling how profound the effects of such environments are on the cardiovascular and immune systems (which are regulated by the nervous system) and, thus, on lifelong patterns of physical health.

In this chapter the presentations at the joint meeting of the American Psychosomatic Society and the Society of Behavioral Medicine provide a launchpad for deeper exploration of the balance between self and society in the mind-body and CAM movements. While I discuss a number of the talks and sessions from the four-day meeting, I focus primarily on the "Superhighways of Disease" joint symposium, which sought to map the converging roads to disease and health.

Shared Risk Factors on the Superhighways of Disease . . . and Health

The symposium "Superhighways of Disease: Shared Determinants of Health Outcomes" comprised nine addresses delivered under four topic headings: "Shared Risk Factors," "Shared Mechanisms," "Interventions," and "Health Policy Implications." (All of the addresses were published in a special issue of *Psychosomatic Medicine*, volume 57 [1995].) Norman B. Anderson, Ph.D., an associate professor in the Departments of Psychiatry and Psychology at Duke University, opened the section on "Shared Risk Factors" by examining social class. In a talk titled "The Ubiquity of Social Class as a Determinant of Health Outcomes: A New Challenge for the Biopsychosocial Approach," Anderson cited research that underscored Antonovsky's concern with the effects of social conditions: many long-term, population-based epidemiological studies have associated socioeconomic status (SES) with morbidity and mortality (Adler et al. 1993; Adler et al. 1994; Fox et al. 1985; Haan et al. 1989). Anderson covered all possible answers to the question, How does the objective phenomenon of socioeconomic status "get under the skin" to contribute to disease? His list of factors included access to healthcare; health-promoting or health-damaging behaviors (including smoking, drug use, and alcohol); residential setting; stressful life events; degree of social support; and socially determined differences in personality. But Anderson interpreted the data as showing that no single factor accounts for the influence of socioeconomic status on health. For instance, countries with universal access to healthcare still show the same steep gradient in the relationship between socioeconomic status and health: despite universal access, the lower a person's socioeconomic status, the worse, on average, his or her health (Adler et al. 1993).

Moreover, while income is a strong factor in health outcomes, other aspects of class and ethnicity appear to be equally important. Anderson pointed out that low-income African Americans report considerably more psychological distress (see Kessler and Neighbors 1985) and higher mortality rates (see Pappas et al. 1993) than white counterparts with the same incomes. Racism is a health issue, apart from and alongside social class and income.

Anderson asked, If socioeconomic status is a causal factor in illness, shouldn't we explore ways to move people out of poverty? This question raises a larger issue: Should behavioral medicine, which purportedly accounts for all relevant factors in health and illness, begin to move beyond its traditional borders of individualized and even community-based inter-

44 ventions? Should it join new initiatives against poverty, all in the name of disease prevention and physical health promotion? On the basis of Anderson's evidence, the answer is yes. But mounting such an initiative seems almost too utopian and far-fetched. This is especially true in a political climate in which antipoverty movements are still branded as hopelessly liberal anachronisms, even when they differ in spirit and structure from the Great Society programs of the 1960s.

The next examination of shared risk factors turned away from the macrolevel of society to the microlevel of the individual. Michael F. Scheier, Ph.D., of Carnegie-Mellon University, in a talk called "Person Variables and Health" presented an overview of the current state of research on the role of personality in health and disease (Scheier and Bridges 1995). Scheier emphasized "person variables," as he called them, in contrast to "personality predispositions," since, in his view, person variables included acute psychological states as well as stable character traits.

Scheier cited correlations between person variables, on the one hand, and heart disease, cancer, and other causes of mortality, on the other, distinguishing areas where the evidence was substantial from those where the evidence was spotty. He identified three broad streams of person variables—anger/hostility, depressed affect, and pessimism/fatalism. He cited the associations between anger/hostility and coronary heart disease as perhaps the strongest and clearest in the entire field of personality and disease.

Scheier's address focused on how various disease entities "share" personality patterns as contributing risk factors. For example, an attitude of fatalism has been linked to mortality among HIV-positive patients (Reed et al. 1994) as well as among younger cancer patients (Schulz et al. 1996). But he did not address the factors that contribute to such personality tendencies as fatalism, depression, and hostility. Here, of course, the admonishing finger of Antonovsky would have pointed again at social conditions. Is it not true, he might have said, that being unemployed, poor, disenfranchised, or consistently discriminated against is enough to drive any sane person toward fatalism, depression, or hostility? Or, on another socioeconomic level, isn't being stuck in a reasonably well paying but alienating job in an authoritarian corporate structure enough to make some people feel continually helpless or angry?

Scheier went on to present a disease model that pivoted on people's capacity to remain engaged rather than become disengaged. Whether and how people struggle to cope with their circumstances, he argued, will determine their emotional states and behaviors, which in turn influence illness. He cited clinical studies—mainly in the area of cognitive psychotherapy—in which patients who became more optimistic and proactive had better outcomes in their struggles with serious illness (Fawzy et al. 1993; Greer et al. 1990). His emphasis, then, is on the individual, who needs to bolster his or her commitment and coping skills to prevent the lapses into fatalism, depression, or hostility that cause or worsen illness via mind-body pathways.

The model is compelling, but the onus is exclusively on the person to change person variables. What if these variables developed and are reinforced in response to social conditions? Can a woman who is angry primarily because she works in an environment in which she is ill-treated and poorly paid use mind-body treatments to eradicate her hostility? Can an HIV-positive gay man who has no support from his family and no health insurance and is constantly exposed to negative cultural feedback about what it means to be infected with the AIDS virus avoid feeling fatalistic?

In answer to such questions Scheier might say that most cancer, heart disease, or AIDS patients cannot transform their social environment overnight or join political movements that will succeed in their lifetime, so they do well to seek social support and psychological reorientation as a means toward wellness. He would be right, of course. But Antonovsky would have been right, too, in pointing to the larger sociocultural context that makes such a psychological reorientation so difficult and so necessary.

In his stinging critique Antonovsky accused the mind-body movement of engaging in the same sort of mechanistic thinking on a macrosocial level that biomedicine applies to the microlevel of the person. Indeed, mind-body adherents blame biomedical scientists for mechanistic thinking, not recognizing that their implicit view of the person disconnected from his or her social environment is just as mechanistic. In his prescient 1974 book *Earthwalk* the sociologist Philip Slater summed up the contradiction:

> It has taken more than a century for Western medicine to rediscover what witch doctors and shamans have known all along: (1) that a disease occurs in a whole organism, not, as in a machine, in one defective part; and (2) that every organism is organically related to others, and to the total environment, and hence any "cure" that does not take account of these relationships is likely to be ephemeral. What we stigmatize as magic is scientific inasmuch as it teaches the wholeness and interconnectedness of living forms. Scientific medicine, on the other hand, is irrational in that it treats the organism as if it were a machine, disconnected from its surroundings and internally disconnectable.

Western medicine gets both points wrong; it recognizes neither the wholeness *within* the organism nor the wholeness of the organism in its organic relationships, its social context. Meanwhile, mind-body medicine

46   gets the first part right—recognizing wholeness within—but neglects the second part, "the interconnectedness of living forms." When people are treated with cognitive therapy to bolster their optimism, their inner wholeness is honored, but their wholeness in a family, community, culture, nation, and planet is often set aside. To be fair, mind-body clinicians frequently emphasize the need for loving support from family and friends, but they rarely address economic questions (How does your financial status influence your state of mind and body?), issues of workplace politics (Is your sense of self being cultivated or crushed on the job?), the soul-sickening impact of racism (Is your self-esteem wounded by experiences of bigotry?), or the affect of culture (What cultural messages make you feel worthless, helpless, or hopeless?).

Next, Lisa Berkman, a professor of epidemiology at Yale University, made a presentation titled "The Influence of Social Networks and Social Support on Health." Berkman is renowned for her work with S. Leonard Syme at the University of California, Berkeley, particularly the Alameda prospective study of about seven thousand adults, which demonstrated that social isolation caused a twofold increase in mortality rates among men and a threefold increase among women. Berkman reviewed these findings and reported data from her recent study of 194 patients who had suffered heart attacks. Thirty-nine of the patients died within six months of their heart attack. Fifty-three percent of these people had no one they could count on for emotional support, 36 percent had one such person, and 11 percent had two or more individuals they could rely on. Compared with patients with at least one support person, those with no supporters were about three times more likely to die within six months (Berkman et al. 1992).

Berkman indicated that there are numerous pathways linking support and outcome after a heart attack. The presence of emotional and practical help may influence health behaviors such as smoking and diet, access to medical care, compliance with doctor's orders, and, of course, the internal pathways of psychophysiology, this last implying that the succor of support calms the cardiovascular system through neuroendocrine channels. Based on these and other findings, Berkman called for preventive interventions facilitating healthy forms of social support, harnessing family and community strengths.

With Antonovsky on my shoulder, I could not resist taking the inquiry one level deeper. What determines whether a person who has had a heart attack has enough people in his or her life to offer support? For many, socioeconomic factors are likely to be crucial. Consider the divorced man who moonlights two jobs to make ends meet and has so little time left over that his social life is impoverished. Or a woman whose husband died because he had inadequate access to healthcare, so that she is left to fend for herself with several children. When such individuals suffer a heart attack, their sources of support are tragically limited.

Community interventions that help ailing people to recognize their emotional and practical needs for support and find ways to meet them may certainly be healing. Such interventions do little to rectify suprastructural causes, but they can set in motion a collective awareness and responsibility that offsets some of the damage caused by the social isolation associated with poverty, poor education, and fractured communities.

SHARED MECHANISMS: PATHWAYS BETWEEN SOCIETY AND THE BODY

By what "mechanisms" do social and psychological factors influence the pathogenesis of disease or the promotion of health? Two speakers addressed this question. The first, Stephen B. Manuck, Ph.D., of the University of Pittsburgh, described the activation of the sympathetic nervous system as a common pathway for both a wide range of cardiovascular diseases and diseases associated with immune dysfunction. Manuck, who called his talk "Sympatho-adrenal Activation, Stress and Disease," focused mainly on heart disease, pointing out that stress, inadequate support, and maladaptive personality traits can harm the cardiovascular system through a variety of mechanisms that probably overlap: atherosclerosis, activation of blood platelets and resulting thrombus formulation over arterial plaque, ischemia, vasomotor spasm, cardiac arrhythmias, and myocardial infarction resulting from one or many of these pathologies.

Manuck detailed his fascinating work with his colleagues, including Jay Kaplan at the Bowman-Gray School of Medicine at Wake Forest University in North Carolina. The scientists administered a high-fat diet to groups of macaque monkeys, placed the monkeys in unstable social settings (e.g., frequently changing their cages and compatriots), and then watched their behavior. They found that the level of atherosclerosis in monkeys who tended toward dominant social behavior was twice as high as that in monkeys who were subordinate.

When such dominant animals received adrenergic inhibitors—which block the effects of the stress hormone adrenaline—their levels of atherosclerosis dropped. Manuck's discovery suggests that adrenaline, which is secreted during activation of the sympathetic nervous system, plays a mediating role in the pathogenesis of blocked arteries (Manuck et al. 1988a, 1988b). Manuck reported that social dominance in unstable environments promoted atherosclerosis even *without* high-fat diets.

48   Manuck's findings provided more evidence to support the biobehavioral models of heart disease that identify aggressive Type A behavior and
hostility as factors in pathogenesis of the disease. At the end of his talk
Manuck briefly suggested that a low socioeconomic level could increase
sympathetic activation by setting in motion stressful events leading inevitably to the human responses of aggression and hostility. This was his
only reference to the social dimension of health, which Antonovsky in-
sisted should claim more of our attention. Can more be said about the
social context of heart disease? It seems possible to recast the entire literature of Type A behavior and hostility in sociological terms. Chronic activation of the sympathetic nervous system is, at least in part, a learned
response to chronically stressful conditions. It is also a learned coping style
that Freudians would argue originates in childhood. Even if one accepts
the psychoanalytic proposition of early origins, Type A behavior and hostility are certainly reinforced in cultural settings, and they are driven by
economic conditions and social cues.

For instance, an African American man raised in an inner-city environment of desolation, with few educational and job opportunities, may
enlist in an economic subculture of drug dealing while unleashing his hostility in acts of violence, behavior sanctioned by the subculture as appropriate expressions of the rage born of hopelessness. At the other end of the
socioeconomic spectrum, the Type A business executive may learn the
corporate message (driven by profit motives) that his worth to the company—and hence to himself—depends on barracuda-like deal-making behavior. Paul Ekman of the University of California, San Francisco, has
shown that people who willfully contort their facial muscles into expressions of happiness, fear, or anger will soon come to *feel* happiness, fear, or
anger (Ekman 1984). For the Type A executive, conditioned dog-eat-dog
behavior and underlying hostility may begin to spiral in self-reinforcing
fashion. Meanwhile, the cardiovascular system becomes vulnerable to the
damage wrought by an overheated sympathetic nervous system.

The work of Redford Williams, M.D., a recognized leader in research
linking hostility and cardiovascular disease, is relevant here. His studies
have solidified connections not only between hostility and heart disease
but also between hostility and the psychophysiological mechanisms (many
addressed by Manuck) that cause heart disease. Williams chaired the symposium's first section, on shared risk factors, and the following day he
chaired a workshop entitled "Controlling Hostility: A Workshop for Use
in Cardiac Rehabilitation Programs and Stress Management Programs in
a 'Wellness' Context." The purpose of the workshop was to teach strategies for controlling hostility and stress control that practitioners could

adapt in their work with patients. These strategies were derived from Williams's book *Anger Kills: Seventeen Strategies to Control the Hostility That Can Harm Your Health,* which he coauthored with his wife and collaborator, Virginia Williams, Ph.D. Williams's approach seems eminently wise and applicable, and it has been proven successful in clinical settings (Williams and Williams 1993). But an Antonovskian would say that it falls short of the whole story.

The Williamses' seventeen strategies for controlling hostility are as follows: "reason with yourself"; "stop hostile thoughts, feelings, and urges"; "distract yourself"; "meditate"; "avoid overstimulation"; "assert yourself"; "care for a pet"; "listen"; "practice trusting others"; "take on community service"; "increase your empathy"; "be tolerant"; "forgive"; "have a confidant"; "laugh at yourself"; "become more religious"; and "pretend today is your last." This list of practical strategies is reasonable and helpful when considered from the point of view of a middle- or upper-class person experiencing a "normal" range of difficulties in work and family life. Your boss is driving you nuts; your kids are having trouble in school; you go crazy whenever you get behind the wheel of a car. What if you consider them from the point of view of a homeless person? Or a lesbian fired from her job by a homophobic employer? Or a poverty-stricken woman suffering from post-traumatic stress syndrome after being raped as she walked home in her dangerous neighborhood? Suddenly suggestions such as "distract yourself," "care for a pet," "forgive," "be tolerant," and even "assert yourself" seem the psychosocial equivalents of puffballs.

My point is not to critique Redford Williams, whose work I greatly admire, but simply to suggest its practical limit—or, as Antonovsky might have said, its sociopolitical context. Williams's psychological medicine may be empowering, but probably not always and not for everyone. In many instances individual efforts to control hostility caused by macrosocial factors may be only stopgap measures. If a person's social conditions are horrific and, for the time being, inescapable, he or she may benefit by practicing psychological techniques such as relaxation and stress management. But when the conditions never change, the person's reservoir of hostility can never be depleted. All a person can do is turn off the spigot, again and again. Turning off the spigot may be better than letting the water spill over onto the floor, but pressure will build up nonetheless—pressure that is still harmful to one's health.

A person in a supportive social environment with adequate food, shelter, healthcare, and amenities may drain his or her sources of hostility in dynamic psychotherapy or control them comfortably with cognitive strategies. But the person in an ongoing environment of scarcity or brutality has

50   a more difficult task. The fact remains that in the lives of many people
structural societal changes are necessary to reverse the root causes of heart-
damaging hostility. For instance, Norman Anderson's studies of African
Americans showed that racism and poverty are associated with cardiovascular disorders in general and hypertension in particular. And he ruled out
access to healthcare as the exclusive cause of this epidemiological relationship. The evidence strongly suggests that racism and poverty cause
heart-damaging hostility. Thus, programs promoting economic justice, job
training, and civil rights may not only protect people's rights, they may
protect their hearts.

THE SOCIAL CONTEXT OF PSYCHOLOGICAL STRESS

The second talk on shared mechanisms was delivered by Janice Kiecolt-
Glaser, Ph.D., of Ohio State University, whose address was titled "Social
Support, Chronic Stress, and Immune Function." Professor Kiecolt-
Glaser has long collaborated with her husband, the immunovirologist
Ronald Glaser, M.D., to produce an impressive body of data on psychoneuroimmunological interactions. After reviewing the burgeoning
body of research on stress, social support, psychosocial interventions, immunity, and health outcomes, she then focused on her own recent investigations into the effect of psychosocial stress on immunity and health
among caregivers for patients with Alzheimer's disease (Kiecolt-Glaser
and Glaser 1995).

     According to Kiecolt-Glaser, most such caregivers are spouses, adult
children, or other close relatives for whom the experience is a form of "living bereavement." Their loved ones gradually slip away from them
through loss of cognitive abilities, memory, independence, and familiar facets
of their personalities. The stresses on these (mostly elderly) caregivers are
financial, emotional, and physical; they must provide for every need of the
patient, all the while experiencing that painfully drawn-out bereavement.

     In 1987 Kiecolt-Glaser began comparing caretakers of persons suffer-
ing from Alzheimer's disease with matched control groups. She documented declines in cellular immune functions in 32 percent of the caretakers as compared with only 1 percent of the controls. In a novel study,
she and Ronald Glaser evaluated the caregivers' responses to an influenza
vaccine. Previous studies had shown that the development of antibodies
after such vaccinations is diminished by stress and anxiety. As the Glasers
had hypothesized, measures at two weeks after vaccination showed that
the development of antibodies was greater in the controls than in the caregivers. Three months later the control group again had a considerably

more vigorous T-cell response. The study also had clinical relevance since influenza vaccines are often necessary to prevent the flu among elderly caretakers. A weak response to the vaccine could keep people from developing protective antibodies.

Kiecolt-Glaser stressed that as the immune system ages, a normal decline in function occurs but a certain resilience remains. However, that resilience is compromised when an elderly person is subjected to chronic stress, such as that experienced by the caregivers of Alzheimer's patients. Her work is testimony to the powerful interconnections between stress, coping, social roles, grieving, immunity, and health.

A sociological critique would also seek to unearth the social dimension of Kiecolt-Glaser's findings. The immune-compromised caregivers had been exposed to a form of stress with two dimensions, one largely social, the other largely psychological. The social dimension, which Kiecolt-Glaser did not fully address, encompasses finances, access to healthcare, and social support. The caregiver who has enough money, a spacious home, complete health coverage, home care, and supportive friends and family members with time on their hands will probably suffer less in mind and body than a caregiver who lacks these vital buffers. Social class and economics must play a crucial role in the caregiver's capacity to cope with his or her travails and maintain immunological vigor. By the same token, a caregiver's psychological suffering will not be entirely ameliorated by even the best social circumstances because all the buffers in the world cannot extinguish the pain of "living bereavement." Psychosocial treatments for caregivers must therefore address both dimensions.

Psychoneuroimmunology (PNI) studies span several levels of interaction, usually involving the psyche, the central nervous system, the endocrine system, and the immune system. Often, the "psyche" level is summed up by the enduringly imprecise term *stress*. From the perspective of a sociological critique, PNI studies can expand their sphere of reference by taking a harder look at sources of stress. Hans Selye's definition of stress—life circumstances that exceed an organism's capacity to cope— suggests that two dimensions, external circumstances and an individual's coping capacity, come together to create it. The Antonovsky model would take this further: The individual's coping capacity may *itself* depend partly on socioeconomic realities unfolding over time rather than solely on genes or early-childhood conditioning.

Thus, PNI studies that evaluate stresses in a person's life and their effects on neuroendocrine-mediated immune disturbances ought to identify the causes and nature of these stressors. Since mind–body interventions aimed at preventing or treating diseases of imbalanced immunity will be

52   guided by basic PNI research, the stressors to be alleviated must be clearly defined, and socioeconomic status should be considered whenever it is relevant. In general, there needs to be more communication between PNI researchers, on the one hand, and social epidemiologists and sociologists, on the other. When a person's stress involves economic privation, poor educational and occupational opportunities, and racism, these issues can hardly be ignored by experts designing therapeutic fixes.

INTERVENTIONS: HEALING ON THE SUPERHIGHWAYS

The portion of the symposium on interventions began with a talk on community-based prevention by David G. Altman, Ph.D., a senior research scientist at the Stanford Center for Research in Disease Prevention. In his talk, titled "Community Intervention on the Superhighway: Promise, Paradoxes, Pitfalls," Altman spoke to Antonovsky's thesis. He hammered home the need to get to the bottom of the shared determinants of disease, which for him lead down a chain of causality to socioeconomic status. His own community interventions in poor neighborhoods in northern California seek to create networks of social connectedness and responsibility, particularly among alienated youth. In East San Jose Altman works with impoverished kids who have no sense of their future, many of whom belong to gangs. He encourages their involvement in "prosocial" gangs that foster the optimistic view that they can positively affect their own communities. The kids create murals in their neighborhoods with messages of hope and with calls for behavioral change in such areas as smoking and drugs. Altman's intervention research will eventually reveal whether these approaches are effective, but his preliminary findings suggests that they are.

Altman emphasized strategies that foster empowerment—a term he defined by redefining a lot of other familiar terms in the psychosocial lexicon. Empowerment, he said, comprises a sense of control, efficacy, mastery, connectedness, and the capacity to mobilize resources. According to Altman, all of these factors stem less from personality predilections than from people's sense that they can make a difference in their communities.

Nonetheless, Altman was not specific about how the community interventions he described could address the root causes he identified, namely, poverty, urban deterioration, racism, sexism, and structural unemployment. He painted a picture of interventions well integrated into communities, interventions that spoke to the real-life conditions people endure, but it is hard to imagine how the causes he pinpointed could be reversed even slightly by such interventions. Aren't massive political and economic

changes necessary to alter infrastructures of poverty that breed social isolation and despair—and ill health?

This question leads back, again, to the issue whether leading lights in
mind-body and behavioral medicine, as well as community health, should
get involved in campaigns to fight poverty, increase economic empowerment in blighted communities, and fund new educational and job-training
initiatives, all in the name of health. Such hard-core political issues may
seem far afield from the concerns of healthcare professionals and researchers, but Antonovsky would probably have said that it was high time
for them to tackle socioeconomic issues head-on.

The second talk on interventions, delivered by Kate Lorig, R.N.,
Dr.P.H., of the Senior Research Center at the Stanford University School
of Medicine, examined "Chronic Disease Self-Management: A Possible
Model for the Future." Lorig's focus is community-based self-management
programs for people with arthritis and other chronic diseases. She cited
1990 statistics on people in the United States with chronic diseases: 31
million with arthritis, 19.5 million with heart diseases, 10.5 million with
asthma, and 6.3 million with diabetes. The standard medical model, she
said, is better at rescuing people with acute illness than teaching people
how to manage long-term chronic illness.

Lorig described her own Chronic Disease Self-Management Program,
which provides group interventions in community settings to patients with
chronic health problems. The program teaches a range of skills: how to
develop disease-related, problem-solving communication skills; medication management; and nutritional information. Her treatment teams employ interactive teaching strategies, including skills mastery, modeling,
reframing, and persuasion.

Lorig's research shows that these interventions increase participants'
sense of self-efficacy, a concept elaborated by Albert Bandura, of the Stanford University School of Medicine (Bandura 1982). *Self-efficacy* refers to
the belief that one can perform a specific action or complete a task. When
older patients with chronic disease experience greater self-efficacy, Lorig
reports, they "get worse less rapidly." Lorig's previous research on arthritis patients showed that physical improvements were only weakly linked
to increases in any health-promoting behaviors, such as exercise and relaxation practices. However, a reduction of arthritis symptoms was
strongly related to increases in self-efficacy (Lorig et al. 1989).

The concept of self-efficacy is similar in many respects to Antonovsky's
sense of coherence, defined as "a global orientation that expresses the extent to which one has a pervasive, enduring though dynamic feeling of confidence that one's internal and external environments are predictable, and

54   that there is a high probability that things will work out as well as can reasonably be expected" (Antonovsky 1994). As Antonovsky points out, a
sense of coherence depends not only on one's ingrained personality or
worldview but also on structural (societal) sources. In other words, we can
develop a sense of coherence only when we receive coherent messages from
our environment and are granted the opportunity to cultivate the intellectual and emotional skills for interpreting them coherently. The latter
point does not disavow an individual's singular ability to develop such
skills; rather, it recognizes that over time one's native capacities for coherence and coping can be suppressed, deadened, or even destroyed by a
brutal environment.

Thus, it is possible to view Kate Lorig's program as a society in minia-
ture that offers elements that encourage health: a caring group of individuals who convey consistently coherent and even benevolent messages, create an environment of sensible feedback, and provide coping options. Such
a society does not exist for many people suffering with chronic illness.

HEALTH POLICY AND THE MULTIFACTORAL MODEL

The last section of the symposium examined health policy implications.
The first of two speakers, Dr. David Sobel, regional director of patient education and health promotion for the Kaiser Permanente Medical Care
Program in northern California, discussed how behavioral medicine
should influence health policy and the debate on healthcare reform.

Sobel focused on chronic diseases, which, he maintained, are addressed
by clinical behavioral interventions with far greater cost-effectiveness than
holds for many of the current high-tech treatments. (By implication, Sobel
was also calling for additional research funds for mind-body medicine,
whose search for treatments could help many patients as much as, or more
than, the ongoing biomedical searches for elusive "cures.") A majority of
medical patients—as many as 70–80 percent, he said—come to providers
with stress-related or self-limiting diseases that are better treated with educational and psychosocial support than with drugs and surgeries, the efficacy of which is questionable.

Cost-effectiveness was the crux of Sobel's argument. He cited studies
demonstrating that behavioral interventions significantly reduce office visits and treatment costs for chronic medical conditions. He stressed that
such interventions addressed more than the modification of health behaviors that either cause illness (such as smoking) or prevent it (such as a
low-fat diet). Such treatments also yielded health benefits by altering
people's social support, emotional states, attitudes, and coping behaviors.

Sobel specifically referred to personality styles such as *hardiness*—Suzanne Ouellette's term that encompasses a sense of commitment, control, and challenge (Maddi and Kobasa 1984). To enhance hardiness, Sobel indicated, is to enhance health. In his emphasis on preventive medicine, community-based interventions, and supportive group treatments Sobel did an excellent job of addressing the social dimension of the "biopsychosocial" model. But he did not touch on the suprastructural social factors that foster or undermine health-promoting mind states such as hardiness and a sense of coherence.

Given the focus of his talk—the potential of behavioral or mind-body medicine to increase medicine's cost-effectiveness—Sobel could not necessarily have been expected to address suprastructural factors. But his argument was weakened by his not doing so. For instance, it may be true that some citizens of our dangerous and depressing inner-city environs have high levels of hardiness, but their ability to remain "hardy" in mind and heart is determined less by the relative strength or weakness of their character than by the relative strengths and weaknesses evident in their family systems, neighborhoods, and economic infrastructures. While behavioral interventions may help people feel more confident and better supported, thus improving their health via mind-body interactions, a sociological critique posits a limit on their efficacy: economically impoverished individuals may become more empowered by these interventions, but their progress is likely to be undermined when they go back to homes and communities rife with stress.

To many, the idea of creating a socially conscious mind-body medicine might seem all too utopian. But a hard look at the data cited by Sobel and other participants at the symposium makes clear that socioeconomic status and psychological attitudes are inextricably intertwined in their influence on disease and health. Programs seeking solutions on both levels simultaneously therefore make simple sense.

One participant who suggested such a dual approach was the final speaker, George A. Kaplan, Ph.D., chief of the Human Population Laboratory at the California Department of Health Services. Kaplan, who also holds appointments in epidemiology at the University of California, Berkeley, and the University of Kuopio in Finland, has conducted population-based research on the behavioral, social, psychological, and socioeconomic factors in chronic diseases. In his talk, "Where Do the Shared Pathways Lead?: A New Research Agenda," he set forth a genuinely Antonovskian agenda for future health policy research: "I would argue that it is time for research on these shared determinants to follow a path that is guided more by social medicine than by clinical medicine, an approach

56   which is fundamentally based on public health, in which primary prevention holds the highest value." Kaplan began with a novel critique of much psychosocial research, including one sacred cow, its search for "a set of separate inputs that operate independently," stating that "most of our statistical models are based on such an approach, which is the health-sciences equivalent of Newtonian billiard ball physics." Indeed, when a variable is proven to lack an independent effect, it is often deemed unimportant.

To indicate the inadequacy of this standard approach, Kaplan discussed his recent reanalysis of data from the Alameda County study, which followed a group of almost seven thousand adults for more than twenty-nine years. People who were poor, isolated, and depressed were almost four times as likely to die early as people without these characteristics. "What's more, the pattern shows very clearly that these factors do not act independently of each other. Rather, there is one subgroup, defined by being at risk on all three factors, which is at dramatically increased risk of death" (Kaplan 1995).

Kaplan went on to cite similar findings from his large-scale Finnish study, which showed that people with low incomes, poor-quality relationships, or a sense of cynical mistrust all had an increased risk of mortality. But individuals who evidenced all three factors together were at a dramatically increased risk of death.

There are synergistic effects among these elements, Kaplan explained, that the language and methods of social science often obscure. If one thinks about it, it is easy to understand that people in poverty are likely to have impaired relationships and to mistrust others. Likewise, people who mistrust others are likely to have impaired relationships and will find it harder to make the considerable efforts needed to get out of poverty. But "as it stands now," said Kaplan, "the current strategy of attempting to identify independent risk factors, often leads to a 'risk factor of the month club,' widely covered by our friends in the press, confusing the public, and offering little guidance."

Kaplan embraced research on such health behaviors as smoking, diet, and exercise, as well as behavioral-medicine research on feelings, attitudes, and social support. But with regard to behavioral medicine, he criticized the current tendency to view emotions and attitudes (such as hostility or depression) as "properties of individuals, with little concern for their social and developmental roots." With Antonovskian zeal, Kaplan pointed to the macroeconomic, cultural, and social environments as root causes of illness, citing many of his previously published studies (Haan et al. 1987; Haan et al. 1989; Kaplan and Salonen 1990; Lynch et al. 1994). Our mental states and behaviors are mediators—pivotal ones, no doubt, but still just mediators.

Kaplan read his own data and the data of others to show that low income is the source of many behaviors and attitudes that are pathogenic. In his Alameda study virtually every disease risk factor—ranging from social isolation to smoking to feeling unappreciated to being a crime victim— was higher among people who were poorer. In his Finnish study the mind states thought to increase disease, such as cynical mistrust, helplessness, and depression, were far more prevalent among those with lower incomes. On the other hand, self-confidence and a sense of coherence increase with increasing income. Kaplan's data served to powerfully validate Antonovsky's sociological critique.

"The dramatic restructuring of the American economy which took place during the last ten to fifteen years, involving a substantial loss of secure jobs with benefits, presages important effects on the social, psychological, and physical health of the population and *these* should be studied by health researchers," said Kaplan. "We need to create a research agenda, I believe, that examines in greater detail the links between wealth and health."* Kaplan's agenda would have researchers identify "how socioeconomics get under the skin and into the body."

But what about interventions? Generally speaking, Kaplan spoke of the need for community health efforts to shift their attention from pharmaceutical and medical procedures to primary prevention efforts that involve community development and job creation. Here Kaplan was vague, perhaps partly because his talk was aimed at research priorities. But another possible reason for his vagueness may have been the sheer vastness of the problem as it was characterized, a vastness that would call for proposals to substantially reshape socioeconomic conditions.

In an interview conducted by me after his talk at the conference Kaplan was more specific. He spoke of the need for an ecological psychology that evaluates the health effects of environments and designs interventions that deal with the way people live in their residential settings. Urban environments that are rife with poverty and crime, inadequate housing, and high unemployment and that have only a few financial resources for develop-

---

*While dramatic improvements in the U.S. economy in the second half of the 1990s helped some on lower socioeconomic rungs, the persistence of poverty, the lack of access to healthcare, an ongoing disparity in wealth, and inner-city conditions that remain unacceptably poor must still be considered threats to the mind-body health of substantial numbers of Americans. For instance, 1999 poverty rates for African Americans and Hispanics stand at 23 percent (U.S. Census Bureau 2001), and child poverty rates have increased by 15 percent over the past nineteen years. One in three African American children, and one in six children of all backgrounds, currently lives in poverty (U.S. Census Bureau 2001).

ment would obviously be the first places in need of ecological psychologists. Kaplan wants experts to cross traditional academic boundaries to address the clustering risk factors of poverty, smoking, alcoholism, poor diet, social isolation, hostility, and despair. To do so, they must start by communicating with one another, which demands a common language. He encourages ecologists, psychologists, epidemiologists, urban sociologists, policy planners, politicians, and physicians to begin a dialogue on the creation of sustainable environments that foster health rather than disease.

Kaplan's approach is an immense corrective to trends apparent in mind–body medicine today. But he may be as guilty of reductionism as those scientists who tend to blame all disease on biomedical factors and those mind–body researchers who tend to blame all disease on psychological factors. Though he never discounted biology or psychology, the bottom line of his model was clearly socioeconomics—the "source," in his view, of everything above. But mind states, be they health-promoting or pathogenic, are not simply caused by one's environment, class, income, or educational opportunities. Nor are they simply caused by genes or upbringing. Just as health itself is a product of all these factors, the mind states that generate or undermine health are also multifactoral, and assignment of any one level as primary is a theoretical mistake that could carry over into proposals for practical solutions.

In my view, when helping people to develop a sense of coherence or confidence or hardiness clinicians must pay attention to environment *and* income *and* lifestyle habits *and* family dynamics *and* upbringing *and* cognitive coping strategies. (Such a multi-leveled intervention might be called *integral mind–body medicine*.) If they do this, a call for social medicine will never undermine a call to personal responsibility, and a call to personal responsibility will never blame the victim. A truly multifactoral model accepts the reality that one cancer patient, Treya Wilber, described in her memoir in response to friends' comments that she might have brought cancer on herself: "We are all too interconnected, both with each other and our environment—life is too wonderfully complex—for a simple statement like, 'you create your own reality' to be simply true" (Wilber 1992). I would add that life is also too wonderfully complex for a simple statement like "*they* create my own reality" to be simply true.

Not that Kaplan was ever that simplistic. But his model edged away from dialectical complexity when he spoke of macroeconomics as "the heart of the matter." Nonetheless, he trenchantly identified causal contributors to illness that academicians almost never speak about, thus properly pushing the pendulum toward social medicine—economic, political, and legislative changes designed to reshape structural conditions to favor health.

OPTIMISM AND HEALTH: HOW MUCH DOES EXPLANATORY
STYLE EXPLAIN?

In much of the rest of the joint conference the psychosomatic pendulum remained in its usual position—focusing on the individual, not on social factors. Many workshops on stress, coping, and health outcomes provided few social contexts, let alone social prescriptions. For the most part, the conference's treatment of variables typically considered in mind-body research—optimism, social support, depression, anxiety, and hostility—focused on the psychological. A good example was the discussion of optimism, which in a number of studies reported at the conference was shown to have a salutary effect on patients with heart disease, cancer, and even AIDS.

The research on heart disease was particularly compelling. At a session of the Society of Behavioral Medicine, Daniel B. Mark, M.D., MPH, a heart specialist at Duke University, reported that he followed the progress of 1,719 men and women who had undergone cardiac catheterization. After one year, 12 percent of people who were initially pessimistic about their health had died, while only 5 percent of the optimists had died. Nancy Frasure-Smith, Ph.D., of the Montreal Heart Institute presented data showing that heart patients who scored high on measures of pessimism and depression were eight times as likely as optimists to die over the course of a year and a half.

The presenters at another symposium, titled "Optimism, Coping, and Health," had studied whether optimistic attitudes influenced health outcomes of cancer patients, people undergoing surgery, and HIV-infected patients. Charles S. Carver, Ph.D., of the University of Miami, reported his findings that early-stage breast cancer patients who were optimistic experienced significantly lower levels of emotional distress over the course of a year than did those who were pessimistic (Carver et al. 1994). Richard Schulz, Ph.D., of the University of Pittsburgh, reported that of patients with recurrent cancer who were between the ages of thirty and fifty-nine those who were pessimistic were more likely to die than those who did not display pessimism within an eight-month timespan (Schultz 1996). Geoffrey Reed, Ph.D., of the University of California, Los Angeles, discussed three studies conducted with his colleagues on psychosocial factors in the progression of HIV disease. He reported that negative outcomes were predicted by negative mind states and experiences, specifically by an attitude of fatalism (the polar opposite of optimism) and by the loss of close friends or primary partners to AIDS. Patients who were bereaved and fatalistic in their attitude also had weaker measures of immunity and were more likely

60   to develop AIDS-related symptoms over the course of several years (Reed et al. 1999). Finally, and most tellingly, men with full-blown AIDS who had a fatalistic attitude had significantly shorter survival times.

These studies, which were later published, represented methodologically sound evidence of the extent to which attitudes such as optimism and pessimism may affect the physical course of diseases such as cancer and AIDS. Biomedical scientists still resist such findings, of course. (I am certain that most oncologists or AIDS specialists still remain largely unaware of this research.) While no reputable researcher would interpret such data to suggest that attitudes and coping styles are the *predominant* factor in the progression of cancer or AIDS, it is now impossible to refute that their influence is statistically and clinically meaningful.

But again, none of the researchers addressed the social dimensions of optimism and pessimism. They asked the following questions: Why do some people handle surgery better than others? Why do some patients with recurrent cancer live longer than others? Why do some HIV-infected patients resist AIDS longer than others? And to all three they gave the same answer: in part because they are optimistic. None of these researchers asked why some sick people are optimistic, while others are pessimistic, or more specifically, what social factors nourish attitudes of optimism or pessimism. Such a question would lead to a deeper understanding of interventions—both social and behavioral—that reinforce optimism, hope, and self-efficacy. When such questions are not asked and answered, says Antonovsky, the result is the development of treatments that exclusively call upon people to fix themselves.

For instance, cognitive-behavioral therapies designed to change people's minds about their experiences (from negative, unrealistic "appraisals" of stressful life events to positive, realistic ones) put the onus on individuals to lift themselves out of the muck of negativism by their cognitive bootstraps. These therapies are sometimes successful, I believe, because such intentional efforts, conducted with the aid of supportive caregivers, are an important aspect of healthy transformations. But the other part of the task, the creation of environments in neighborhoods and workplaces that generate optimism and self-efficacy, remains nearly absent from mind-body intervention research.

In *Learned Optimism* the psychologist Martin E. P. Seligman describes his impressive body of research and clinical work, all of which has led him to conclude that how people explain events to themselves—their "explanatory style"—determines whether they become depressed and/or physically sick under stress (Seligman 1990). But he writes not a word about social and economic conditions as shapers of optimism or pessimism. In Seligman's view, people's habitual thought patterns are independent, overriding factors in mind-body health. Helplessness can be learned, and it can be unlearned. Optimism can be developed with a set of skills. Physical health can thus be restored or maintained. The whole key is for people to change how they think about the bad things that happen to them.

No doubt that cognitive appraisal is an important factor in how people cope with stress. But Seligman's take on optimism ignores that when bad things keep happening to people, they become helpless, and it is not enough to exhort them to maintain a positive attitude in the face of traumas and tragedies. Ironically, Antonovskian principles may be found in the very experiments Seligman used to develop his theories of learned helplessness and optimism. He studied dogs who were yoked to each other in pairs. One dog in each pair was repeatedly administered shocks that the dog turns off by pushing a button. The other dog in each pair received the same shocks but had no access to a turn-off button. The dogs in the latter group eventually became helpless, lying down in their cages, because nothing they did mattered (Seligman 1990).

When he began conducting research on helplessness and optimism in humans, Seligman discovered the same phenomenon, but he also found that human cognition added a new level: how people interpreted their negative experiences played a part in whether they became helpless. But he lost sight of a lesson from his animal findings: take away control continuously and you still make people helpless—and pessimistic.

Many people in our society—the unemployed, the disaffected, and those who are discriminated against—get treated like the dogs in Seligman's experiments. They are shocked repeatedly, and they have no levers to push in order to remove the source of their pain. When they begin to think pessimistically, no one should be surprised. And while Seligman's cognitive therapy is undoubtedly helpful for many such individuals, as well as for more privileged people, more is needed to keep them in relative good health. The shocks must be turned off, or at least a lever of control must be provided. Yes, people can improve their lot by thinking, feeling, and behaving in more adaptive ways. But if people are asked to take greater responsibility for their attitudes and health, the social engineers, the politicians, the powerbrokers, and the medical establishment must also be asked to take greater responsibility for conditions that sometimes crush even the most resilient personalities.

CHRONIC FATIGUE SYNDROME AND THE SOCIAL
COURSE OF ILLNESS

Despite its basically psychological drift, the conference offered a few glimmers of social medicine. One concerned chronic fatigue syndrome (CFS), among the most perplexing problems facing medicine today. The condition is characterized by the sudden onset of debilitating fatigue that persists for months and includes a range of often severe psychological and physical symptoms, with no evidence of organic causes or severe psychiatric disorders other than depression.

The American Psychosomatic Society held a symposium titled "Update on the Chronic Fatigue Syndrome," which included talks by four experts on, respectively, the biomedical, immunological, social, and PNI aspects of the syndrome. It was clear, particularly from a talk on the "social course" of the illness, that a sociological perspective has begun to inform the study of this syndrome, perhaps because the disease is so unremittingly puzzling that scientists have had to look beyond the traditional "single disease agent" model, which has held sway since the days of Pasteur and Koch.

In instances where infectious illness is suspected as the source of a disease, as has been true for years with regard to CFS, the mainstream's modus operandi has been the biomedical equivalent of "rounding up the usual suspects" to see which pathogen can be pinpointed as the cause. In the case of chronic fatigue this approach has proved frustratingly inadequate. After years of study no single infectious agent has been found to cause this very real condition, which is neither a figment of patients' imaginations nor a veiled version of clinical depression. Other factors have been seriously sought and considered, and at least some doctors who are usually uncomfortable with psychiatry have acknowledged the role of psychosocial variables in the onset and course of chronic fatigue.

The first speaker, Antony Komaroff, M.D., director of the Division of General Medicine and Primary Care in the Department of Medicine at Brigham and Women's Hospital in Boston, and professor of Medicine at Harvard Medical School, provided a nuanced overview of research on the syndrome. The disease, he said, is not depression, but it is typically characterized by a depressive disorder that may sometimes trigger the syndrome and that often occurs on the heels of the syndrome's disabling physical symptoms (Komaroff and Buchwald 1991). People with severe chronic fatigue can barely function; their infirmity is certainly reason enough to become depressed.

Given uncertainties about the biochemistry of chronic fatigue, it is possible that neuroendocrine changes associated with depression help cause the physical syndrome and that neuroendocrine changes associated with chronic fatigue help cause the depression. It is probable that neuroendocrine alterations, whatever their origins, contribute to the disturbances of the immune system that characterize this disease. Contrary to popular opinion, the immune system of the chronic fatigue patient is hyperactive, not suppressed. Some event or combination of events, be they psychosocial or viral in origin, appear to trigger the disease process, which leads to what Komaroff described as a "chronically activated but tiring immune system."

Mary Ann Fletcher, Ph.D., head of clinical immunology at the University of Miami, expanded on Komaroff's talk with details about the immunology of CFS. Some individuals appear to be genetically predisposed to the condition. When these individuals contract CFS, their levels of cortisol (a stress hormone that can be immunosuppressive) drop, immune complexes circulate, their levels of cytokines (proteins such as interleukin-1 and tumor necrosis factor produced by the immune system) elevate, and their immune systems become so jazzed up that they eventually flag, allowing for reactivation of latent viruses such as Epstein-Barr and herpes simplex virus type 6.

Certain T-cell subpopulations and natural killer cells decline as the patients' cognitive and physical symptoms worsen. But Fletcher and Komaroff acknowledge that researchers still do not understand the initial triggering event(s). They do not think it is a virus, and they cannot say for certain whether it is psychological (a trauma, say), an ongoing stressor, or a long-lasting tendency toward depression. They admit that it could be a single factor, but the "trigger," they believe, is more likely a cluster of psychosocial and microbial factors in genetically susceptible individuals.

The next speaker examined the social dimension of chronic fatigue. Norma Ware, Ph.D., of the Department of Social Medicine at Harvard University, pointed out that CFS is not new and is not exclusively American. There have been similar combinations of somatic complaints and affective disorders under other names—*nervous*, common in Latin America; *neurasthenia*, widespread in East Asia; and *dhat* in India. The phenomenon may be on the rise, but it may also be a new name for a condition long observed in other cultures.

In her own preliminary study of fifty patients Dr. Ware found a clustering of stressful events leading up to the onset of illness, but as she notes, similar levels of stress have also been observed in healthy people. Other research of people with CFS has associated a large number of factors with poorer outcomes—psychiatric illnesses, certain personality traits, patients' belief in the strictly physical causes of their condition, attitudes by physicians that deny the patients' experiences, and the gloomy tone of media coverage on chronic fatigue. In her investigation, as yet incomplete, Ware is evaluating the possible effect of the attitudes of the patients' families, life events, social isolation, delegitimizing experiences (involving doctors, friends, or family members), coping strategies, and economic factors, including whether or not disability coverage is being provided. Her aim is to determine whether the "social course of the illness" is bound to its physical course.

Ware's study is striking in its fidelity to a multifactoral model of disease; she is trying to understand a bewildering illness by looking within and outside the individual. Thus, she appears to be heeding Antonovsky's call for social medicine, while retaining a regard for human intentionality. This was most apparent in her discussion of a key preliminary finding in her study. She said that 44 percent of the CFS patients (men and women) reported being incredibly busy, many of them involved in eighty hours a week of work, school, and caretaking responsibilities combined. These individuals led "overstimulated, exhausted lifestyles." According to Ware, one of her subjects described herself as "overdoing, overworking, over-trying-to-please people, and just over everything." It appears that the immune systems of these sufferers, who pushed themselves to the hilt under pressures we can presume are psychological, social, and economic, suffered along with their tired minds and bodies.

Ware's regard for intentionality was particularly apparent in her description of a significant "subset" of patients who used their illness as an opportunity to "take stock and reevaluate," leading to "abandonment of overwhelming jobs and reduced aspirations to high levels of achievement." These were "stories of liberation from exacting expectations," of changes that enabled the people to "reconstruct a more satisfying and comfortable social world."

Ware's acceptance of the social factors at play in CFS, as well as the individual changes possible among its sufferers, struck a delicate balance among biological, psychological, and social influences. Her discussion of the possibility of personal transformation, a reality she observed and recorded in her own research, put flesh onto Antonovsky's skeletal concept of *autopoiesis*, the capacity of human systems for self-reorganization.

But Ware also confirmed Antonovsky's principle that autopoiesis will be more likely and possible in a benevolent rather than a brutal environment. She implied that CFS patients confronting a hostile world that delegitimizes their experiences, either by shunning them for having psychiatric disorders or by discounting their physical symptoms ("It's all in your head"), suffer more in mind and body. Patients stricken with this illness will be more likely to change conditions that contribute to its progression—such as overwork or self-negating tendencies—when people around them validate the reality of their symptoms and their suffering.*

The final talk, by Michael Antoni, Ph.D., a PNI researcher at the University of Miami, demonstrated the subtle interplay among psychological factors, immunological abnormalities, and illness outcomes in patients with CFS. To test his hypothesis that various stresses, and the person's mental and behavioral responses to them, could influence the syndrome by causing neuroendocrine-mediated disturbances of the immune system, Antoni studied sixty-five white women, most of them highly educated, who had come to their doctors for treatment. He found that the people who experienced more stressful life events and who coped with their condition and their stressful lives with mental defenses of denial and disengagement had more severe symptoms.

As Antoni was conducting his study in 1991, the natural world presented him with a scientific *deus ex machina*: hurricane Andrew. Would this monstrous stressor affect the course of illness among CFS patients caught in its path? Antoni was able to compare CFS patients who lived in Dade County, where the damage was greatest, and those who lived in Broward County, where the damage was practically nonexistent. He found that patients in Dade were more likely to relapse and to experience the onset of worsening symptoms. But he also found that patients who were more emotionally distressed in the storm's aftermath—who were angrier, more disgusted, or more afraid of dying—suffered most from increasing fatigue. These emotional factors accounted for 29 percent of the variance in tests of people's "illness burden."

Antoni went further, discovering that people who maintained an attitude of optimism and who procured social support coped better with the hurricane and that these psychologically healthy responses translated into fewer immune abnormalities (poor natural killer cell function, higher levels of cytokines implicated in chronic fatigue, fewer flareups of the disease). However, the immune disturbances that did occur were associated with worsening symptoms. Thus, an objective stressor (hurricane Andrew) was linked through psychological attitudes to more or less immune dysfunction, which was linked to worsening symptoms in a population of individuals already beset by a bedeviling illness associated with the immune system.

---

*Overwork, to the extent that it contributes to CFS, is a truly psychosocial phenomenon. Psychologists who view overwork as strictly a result of personality predispositions, whether of the hard-driving Type A variety or the compliant Type C variety, and sociologists who view overwork as strictly the result of economic pressures are both overgeneralizing. Many people who overwork are subject to both internal psychodynamic and external economic pressures.

Antoni's elegant fabric of interacting psychological and immunological changes leading to clinically significant changes in people with CFS was a fine example of PNI research at its best—showing connections among levels of experience, doing justice to the complexity of mind-body interactions. But one social piece of the pattern was missing. Would income, job status, and insurance not have an impact on the extent of a patient's distress in the wake of a hurricane? If people lost the roofs of their houses, wouldn't their bank accounts or their insurance status powerfully influence the quality and degree of their emotional upset, and wouldn't that then influence their immune systems and physical symptoms?

Perhaps Antoni's research would benefit from Ware's perspective on the social course of illness, and perhaps Ware's research would benefit from Antoni's sophisticated PNI model. Maybe there is ultimately a limit to the number of variables any one study can gracefully entertain, but Antonovsky's critique challenges mind-body scientists to expand their vision.

One sign that the role of socioeconomic status in health may be touching the collective consciousness of academia was the first question from the audience at the end of these four talks: "What, exactly, is the socioeconomic makeup of people with chronic fatigue syndrome?"

Dr. Komaroff answered that a handful of studies have fed the cultural stereotype that most CFS patients are white and well educated, he said, because the studies have evaluated self-selected populations of people who sought medical treatment for their fatigue. Understandably, such patients are bound to be relatively well off and to have good health coverage. However, the federal Centers for Disease Control conducted a field study that revealed no skewing of CFS incidence toward wealthier patients. Moreover, in a community sample of four thousand randomly selected patients, not all of whom had sought medical care, Komaroff found that CFS patients had a lower socioeconomic status than healthy populations. Contrary to popular images, CFS patients may be *poorer* than average, not richer.

Which leads one to ask: If Michael Antoni's white, well-educated patients experienced such dramatic exacerbations in the wake of a hurricane, what must have occurred among the poor, who had fewer financial, social, and psychological resources for coping with destruction and disarray? Looked at through Antonovsky's lens, it is conceivable that state and federal funds targeted to help the poor during massive natural disasters not only enable people to put back the pieces of their lives but also stave off relapses of CFS and other immune-associated illnesses, not to mention the onset of new diseases. Socioeconomic policy *is* health policy, not in the direct sense of medical coverage and preventive health services, but in the indirect sense that socioeconomic supports keep people from free-falling into biologically damaging states of anxiety and hopelessness when they are subject to severe life stresses.

MINDFULNESS AND SOCIETY

Another glimmer of social medicine came from Jon Kabat-Zinn, Ph.D., who participated both in a workshop ("Boundaries of Behavioral Medicine: Do Alternative Therapies Belong?") and in a symposium ("Alternative Treatments: Fact or Fiction?"). Kabat-Zinn is well known for his Stress Reduction Clinic at the University of Massachusetts Medical Center in Worcester and for his two books on mindfulness meditation, *Full Catastrophe Living* (Kabat-Zinn 1991) and *Wherever You Go, There You Are* (Kabat-Zinn 1994). In both talks Kabat-Zinn described his implementation of stress reduction programs, with their emphasis on mindfulness meditation, in a community health center with a diverse, multicultural inner-city population with many non-English speaking Latinos. He also described his program within the state prison system, aimed at reducing hostility, substance abuse, violence, and recidivism. Kabat-Zinn said that his programs revealed signs that mindfulness, a mind-body treatment, had increased these individuals' sense of mastery and self-efficacy.

While mindfulness training obviously cannot redress poverty and unemployment, the notion of empowering individuals in harsh and even brutal social environments through mind-body treatments is radical in its implications. We tend to think of meditation, biofeedback, group therapy, and visualization—staples of clinical mind-body medicine—as necessarily the province of middle- or upper-middle-class individuals who turn within during a bout with chronic or life-threatening illness. Kabat-Zinn subverts these cultural stereotypes by showing that privileged people are not the only ones who need and deserve methods for self-renewal. People in harsh social conditions also need these techniques, perhaps even more so. And if we accept Antonovsky's concept of autopoiesis, or self-reorganization, then empowerment for individuals who wish to change their social conditions—on an individual or a political level—can start with methods for transforming their own consciousness and behavior.

Kabat-Zinn argues that self-reorganization begins with "living in the moment," and his clinical experience indicates that living in the moment increases people's sense of coherence and efficacy. Indeed, he's used Antonovsky's own concept of coherence and shown in careful research that mindfulness training increases it.

68

Social Change in the Service of Mind–Body Health

The introduction into mind-body research of new instruments for measuring the impact of social environment and economic well-being would enrich ideas such as social support, optimism, self-efficacy, and a sense of coherence. As George Kaplan has argued, such factors become more than single "variables" when studied as they really exist—embedded in a layered context of mind, body, and society. Just as great novelists give their readers a portrait of the social world in which their characters act and live, perhaps great psychosomatic researchers could strive for something similar—to provide a scientific portrait of the social world in which their subjects get sick or stay healthy.

And perhaps social changes that favor mind-body health will come when every imaginable resource is directed toward personal empowerment, as Jon Kabat-Zinn has been doing, and sociopolitical empowerment, as George Kaplan claims is essential. But the missing link, it seems to me, is an organized effort on the part of behavioral-medicine experts to educate the public—and the health policy planners—that poverty, social injustice, discrimination, racism, sexism, and social isolation are health issues, and not just because people at the bottom rungs do not receive the same healthcare. People at the bottom rungs do not get Antonovsky's "structural sources for salutogenic strengths," the social and economic supports that help to build a resilient character. Moreover, the influence of pathogenic social factors is as real and as deadly as smoking, alcoholism, drug abuse, a high-fat diet, and environmental pollutants. Society has waged wars on these addictions and chemical exposures with more or less commitment and success. Yet today a head-on war against poverty is deemed hopelessly passé. The surgeon general should be trumpeting the message that low socioeconomic status is a hazard to our health. But that day will not come unless leaders in mind-body and integrative medicine mount the barricades for social—not just individual—transformation.

REFERENCES

Adler NE, Boyce WT, Chesney MA, Folkman S, Syme SL. 1993. Socioeconomic inequities in health: no easy solution. *JAMA.* 269:3140–3145.

Adler NE, Boyce WT, Chesney MA, et al. 1994. Socioeconomic status and health: the challenge of the gradient. *Am Psychol.* 49:15–24.

Antonovsky A. 1994. A sociological critique of the "well-being" movement. *Advances.* 10:6–12.

Bandura A. 1982. Self-efficacy in human agency. *Am Psychol.* 37:122–147.   69
Berkman LF, Leo-Summers L, Horwitz RI. 1992. Emotional support and survival after myocardial infarction. *Ann Intern Med.* 117:1003–1009.
Carver CS, Pozo-Kaderman C, Harris SD, et al. 1994. Optimism versus pessimism predicts the quality of women's adjustment to early stage breast cancer. *Cancer.* 73:1213–1220.
Ekman P. 1984. Expression and the nature of emotion. In: Scherer K, Ekman P, eds. *Approaches to Emotion.* Hillsdale, NJ: Lawrence Erlbaum.
Fawzy FI, Fawzy NW, Hyun CS, et al. 1993. Malignant melanoma: effects of an early structured psychiatric intervention, coping, and affective state on recurrence and survival six years later. *Arch Gen Psychiatry.* 50:681–689.
Fox AJ, Goldblatt P, Jones D. 1985. Social class mortality differentials: artefact, selection, or life circumstance. *J Epidemiol Community Health.* 39:1–8.
Greer S, Morris T, Pettingale KW, et al. 1990. Psychological response to breast cancer and fifteen-year outcome. *Lancet.* 1:49–50.
Haan MN, Kaplan GA, Camacho T. 1987. Poverty and health: prospective evidence from the Alameda County study. *Am J Epidemiol.* 125:989–998.
Haan MN, Kaplan GA, Syme SL. 1989. Socioeconomic status and health: old observations and new thoughts. In: Bunker JP, Gomby DS, Kehrer BH, eds. *Pathways to Health: The Role of Social Factors.* Menlo Park, Calif: Henry J. Kaiser Family Foundation; 76–135.
Kabat-Zinn J. 1991. *Full Catastrophe Living: Using the Wisdom of Your Body and Mind to Face Stress, Pain, and Illness.* New York: Delacorte.
Kabat-Zinn J. 1994. *Wherever You Go, There You Are.* New York: Hyperion Books.
Kaplan GA. 1995. Where do shared pathways lead? Some reflections on a research agenda. *Psychosom Med.* 57:208–212.
Kaplan GA, Salonen JT. 1990. Socioeconomic conditions in childhood and ischaemic heart disease during middle age. *BMJ.* 301:1121–1123.
Kessler R, Neighbors H. 1985. A new perspective on the relationship among race, social class, and psychological distress. *J Health Soc Behav.* 27:107–115.
Kiecolt-Glaser J, Glaser R. 1995. Psychoneuroimmunology and health consequences: data and shared mechanisms. *Psychosom Med.* 57:269–274.
Komaroff AL, Buchwald D. 1991. Symptoms and signs of chronic fatigue syndrome. *Rev Infect Dis.* 13(suppl 1):S8–11.
Lorig K, Seleznick M, Lubeck D, et al. 1989. The beneficial outcomes of the arthritis management course are not adequately explained by behavior change. *Arthritis Rheum.* 32:91–95.
Lynch JW, Kaplan GA, Cohen RD, et al. 1994. Childhood and adult socioeconomic status as predictors of mortality in Finland. *Lancet.* 343:524–527.
Maddi SR, Kobasa SC. 1984. *The Hardy Executive: Health Under Stress.* Homewood, Ill: Dow Jones–Irwin.
Manuck SB, Kaplan JR, Adams MR, Clarkson TB. 1988a. Effects of stress and the sympathetic nervous system on coronary artery atherosclerosis. *Am Heart J.* 116:328–333.
Manuck SB, Kaplan JR, Adams MR, Clarkson TB. 1988b. Studies of psychosocial

70   influences on coronary artery atherogenesis in cynomolgus monkeys. *Health Psychol.* 7:113–124.

Pappas G, Queen S, Hadden W, Fisher G. 1993. The increasing disparity and mortality between socioeconomic groups in the United States, 1980 and 1986. *New Engl J Med.* 329:103–109.

Reed GM, Kemeny ME, Taylor SE, Visscher BR. 1999. Negative HIV-specific expectancies and AIDS-related bereavement as predictors of symptom onset in asymptomatic HIV-positive gay men. *Health Psychol.* 18:354–363.

Reed GM, Kemeny ME, Taylor SE, et al. 1994. "Realistic acceptance" as a predictor of decreased survival time in gay men with AIDS. *Health Psychol.* 13:299–307.

Scheier MF, Bridges MW. 1995. Person variables and health: personality predispositions and acute psychological states as shared determinants for disease. *Psychosom Med.* 57:255–268.

Schulz R, Bookwalla J, Knapp J, et al. 1996. Pessimism, age, and cancer mortality. *Psychol Aging.* 11:304–309.

Seligman MEP. 1990. *Learned Optimism.* New York: Alfred A. Knopf.

Slater P. 1974. *Earthwalk.* New York: Doubleday.

U.S. Census Bureau. 2001. *Statistical Abstract of the United States.* Washington, DC: U.S. Government Printing Office.

Wilber K. 1992. *Grace and Grit: Spirituality and Healing in Life and Death of Treya Killam Wilber.* Boston: Shambhala.

Williams RB, Williams V. 1993. *Anger Kills: Seventeen Strategies for Controlling the Hostility That Can Harm Your Health.* New York: HarperCollins.

Chapter 3

The Mindful Heart: Psychosocial Factors

in Heart Disease

The depth and scope of research on psychosocial factors in heart disease is breathtaking. But so is the lack of attention paid to it (and its clinical implications) by physicians, biomedical scientists, healthcare institutions, and even, in important ways, the mind–body investigators whose fine work has established the rich repository of findings about the role of the mind in heart disease. The public health ramifications of this research are monumental since heart disease remains the leading cause of mortality in the United States. According to the American Heart Association, in 1999 cardiovascular diseases claimed more than 958,000 lives, accounting for 40 percent of all deaths in the United States (American Heart Association 2002). Among these deaths, more than 529,000 were due to coronary heart disease (CHD), including deaths from heart attacks and sudden cardiac arrest (SCA).

In the case of CHD there is "clear and convincing evidence," to quote a recent review by three leading mind–heart investigators, that psychosocial factors "contribute significantly to its pathogenesis and expression" (Rozanski et al. 1999). Moreover, there is now overwhelming evidence that one specific psychological condition, depression, is a significant risk factor for recurrent disease and death after myocardial infarction (MI). These data would suggest a pressing need for psychosocial treatments for depression and distress among heart attack patients.

But the depression research is only one piece of the story of psychological factors in heart disease; the field is full of divergent findings that often seem hard to reconcile. Since the development and discovery of Type

72   A behavior in the early to mid-1970s the notion of "coronary-prone" behavior or personality has been superseded by relentless dribs and drabs of new data suggesting that every color and classification of negative emotion contributes to CHD. A broader theory is needed to explain these disparate findings, and it should begin with the question, Why are so many different states and traits linked to heart disease?

Is it really possible that a grab bag of purportedly negative attributes or psychological conditions—including stress, anxiety, Type A behavior, hostility, emotional nonexpression, vital exhaustion, depression, and hopelessness are all simply bad for our hearts?

It should be possible to *differentially* explain the contribution of each factor in heart disease—first, by defining which ones are clinically and statistically significant; second, by identifying the particular stage (or stages) of heart disease they tend to influence (i.e., etiology, progression, mortality); and third, by grasping the psychodynamic dimensions of each factor in a model that takes into account the meaningful arc of an individual life in transition. What is needed is an integrative *process model* (Lazarus and Folkman 1984), one that recognizes that people's characteristic emotional responses and perhaps even their personality traits change in response to life's vicissitudes, though not always for the better. Whether these changes are dramatic or barely noticeable, they can have important long-term effects on behavior and physiology.

My aim in this chapter is to set forth the findings that demonstrate the involvement of psychosocial factors in heart disease; to develop a theory that organizes and fits into one coherent picture the vast range of findings on psychosocial factors in heart disease; and to make the case that these findings provide ample evidence that psychosocial interventions for heart patients should be more intensively investigated and more broadly implemented.

In the first section I examine the psychosocial data, using as my organizing principle the natural history of heart disease. That is, broadly speaking, I first look at the psychosocial factors that contribute to the emergence of heart disease and then examine factors that contribute to its progression, to heart attacks, and to recurrence and mortality. In the second section I examine the findings that link psychosocial factors to physiological mechanisms implicated in CHD. Again, the presentation is organized following the natural history of heart disease. In the third section I offer the integrative process model as a theoretical framework for interpreting disparate data in this field. And in the fourth section I present the data on psychosocial interventions for heart disease, highlighting the consistently beneficial effects of these interventions. The fourth ends with a consideration of interventions that are most likely to be effective, drawing insights from the theoretical model presented in the prior section.

Psychosocial Factors in CHD: The Findings

FROM TYPE A BEHAVIOR TO HOSTILITY

In the 1970s the cardiologists Meyer Friedman and Ray Rosenman proposed the notion of coronary-prone Type A behavior, a constellation including time urgency, competitiveness, hard striving for achievement, and free-floating hostility (Friedman 1974). They used a structured interview (SI) to ferret out Type A behavior, and in a prospective study of three thousand middle-aged men lasting eight and a half years, the Western Collaborative Group Study, they found that Type As were roughly twice as likely as Type Bs (nonhostile, noncompetitive, relatively calm subjects) to suffer from a CHD-related event (Friedman et al. 1974). (The effect remained significant after investigators controlled for all known risk factors for coronary artery disease [CAD], the most common type of heart disease, the one that leads to most heart attacks.) Other studies that used coronary angiography to evaluate the degree of CAD among patients found more severe CAD among Type As (Blumenthal et al. 1978; Frank et al. 1978; Zyzanski et al. 1976); and autopsy studies revealed more severe CAD among Type As than among Type Bs (Friedman et al. 1968).

But in a development that has been widely documented, subsequent studies failed to support the Type A hypotheses (Williams 1987). In the Multiple Risk Factor Intervention Trial (MR-FIT) Type A patients were no more likely than Type Bs to develop CAD, whether their behavior was assessed by an SI process (as it had been in Friedman and Rosenman's research) or by a standardized questionnaire developed by C. D. Jenkins (Jenkins 1978; Shekelle et al. 1985). Furthermore, in a study involving 2,289 patients who underwent coronary angiography, Redford Williams and his colleagues at the Duke University Medical Center found a relationship between Type A behavior, as measured by the SI, and the presence of more severe CAD, but only among patients aged forty-five or younger (Williams et al. 1988). And this relationship was statistically much weaker than the link between smoking or hyperlipidemia and more severe CAD.

Williams, along with his colleagues John Barefoot, James Blumenthal, and Theodore Dembroski, among others, proceeded to study—and affirm—the hypotheses that the Type A constellation was a statistically unreliable measure of coronary-prone behavior because it was unwieldy and imprecise. Specifically, they theorized that only one element of Type A behavior—hostility—was a reliable predictor of CAD or CAD severity, and they deemed hostility the "toxic core" of the Type A behavior pattern. In an important summary paper Williams reviewed research leading to "the emergence of the hostility complex" as the toxic core of Type A and the true psychological contributor to CHD (Williams 1987). Relying upon aspects of the SI and the Cook-Medley Hostility Scale of the Minnesota Multiphasic Personality Scale (MMPI) to measure hostility, Williams and colleagues pursuing similar lines of research at other institutions proceeded to study hostility as a singular dimension and found more reliably robust relationships with CHD. For example, in a reanalysis of SI data from 131 patients who had undergone coronary angiography, Dembroski and colleagues (1985) found that only hostility and anger-in (the tendency to feel anger but not to express it openly) were significantly associated with CAD severity.

Larger prospective and matched-control studies followed:

- The epidemiologist Richard Shekelle and colleagues reviewed the original Cook-Medley hostility scores of patients enrolled in the Western Electric Study of 1,877 middle-aged employees at the company. They found that hostility was a clear factor in heart disease risk: the ten-year incidence of major CHD events (MI and CHD death) was lowest in the first quintile of the hostility scale's distribution, highest in the middle quintile, and intermediate in the other three quintiles (Shekelle et al. 1983).
- John Barefoot conducted prospective studies of doctors and lawyers and found significant associations between hostility measured when individuals attended medical or law school and their CAD incidence more than twenty years later. Doctors who scored high on the Cook-Medley Hostility Scale were four to five times more likely to develop CAD. Among the most dramatic findings in these studies were that among doctors 14 percent of those with high hostility scores had died by age fifty, compared with only 2 percent of those with low scores; and among lawyers 20 percent of the highly hostile had died by age fifty, compared with only 4 percent of the minimally hostile. Most of the early deaths were due to heart disease (Barefoot et al. 1983; Barefoot et al. 1989).
- Behavioral-medicine investigators at the SRI International laboratory in Menlo Park, California, matched 250 CHD cases with 500 matched controls from the Western Collaborative Group study to assess the 8.5-year prospective relationship between psychosocial factors and clinical CHD. They reevaluated the data from the original Type A structured interviews, and they were able to develop twelve categories of behavior under the Type A rubric. When all twelve categories were included in a multivariate model,

only one—hostility—remained a significant risk factor for clinical CHD (relative risk [RR] = 1.93; degree of significance, p = .045).* In other words, those who evidenced hostility at the study's outset had approximately a twofold increased risk of developing heart disease over eight and a half years (Hecker et al. 1988).

• Theodore Dembroski and colleagues at the University of Maryland reanalyzed data from the MR-FIT study, matching 192 cases of coronary death and nonfatal MI to 384 matched controls. Only two of eight characteristics in the Type A behavior pattern were significant predictors of these coronary events, and both were hostility parameters: potential for hostility and the antagonistic interpersonal component of hostility. After adjustment for traditional CHD risk factors, only potential for hostility showed a significant RR (1.5; p = .032) (Dembroski et al. 1989).

Other studies conducted in the 1980s and early 1990s revealed no link between hostility and heart disease, though several of these studies had notable flaws, and others were relatively smaller than the positive studies (Williams 1993). More recently, however, the hostility hypothesis has received renewed support. John Barefoot and colleagues evaluated a sample of 730 Danish men and women over 50 years old at study initiation, and after a twenty-seven-year follow-up they found that subjects with higher hostility scores (2 standard deviations higher) than others had an RR of 1.53 (Barefoot et al. 1995), a statistically significant though modest risk factor when compared with similar kinds of data for heavy smoking (RR = 2.8) or high blood pressure (RR = 3.1 [untreated] or 2.0 [treated]) (Whiteman et al. 1997). In an analysis of the Veterans Administration Normative Aging Study, Ichiro Kawachi and his colleagues in the Harvard School of Public Health and the Harvard Medical School evaluated the responses of 1,305 men aged sixty-one and older to the MMPI-2 Anger Content Scale, which taps an inability to control expressions of anger. The men were followed for an average of seven years, and those who evidenced the highest levels of anger were more than three times (RR = 3.15) as likely to suffer a nonfatal heart attack or a fatal coronary event than men with low levels of anger (Kawachi et al. 1996). This study was notable in its use of the MMPI-2 questionnaire, with its emphasis on angry emotions and expressions, which according to the authors is distinguishable from the cynical mistrust and hostile attitudes measured by the Cook-Medley Hostility Scale.

*Relative risk (RR) is a measure of the increased risk relative to others who do not evidence a given variable; for example, an RR of 2.0 indicates a twofold elevated risk. The p value is the measure of statistical significance; any value below .05 is considered a statistically significant finding.

76   The former measures emotional states and expressive tendencies, while the latter measures a characteristic cognitive and attitudinal mind-set.

All the above-cited studies controlled for known CHD risk factors, including age, smoking, hypertension, and high cholesterol levels, and found that hostility remained a significant predictor of CHD. In only one major prospective study were positive findings essentially nullified by confounding variables. Investigators from the Human Population Laboratory of the Public Health Institute in Berkeley analyzed data from 2,125 men aged forty-two to sixty in the Kuopio Ischemic Heart Disease Risk Factor Study. While high hostility scores result in a greater than twofold risk of cardiovascular mortality (RR = 2.30), the relationship was substantially weakened when the researchers controlled for smoking, alcohol, exercise, and body mass index (Everson et al. 1997).

How robust and consistent is the overall relationship between hostility and CHD risk? Perhaps the best answer comes from a rigorous meta-analysis of forty-five studies published in 1996 by T. Q. Miller and colleagues at the University of Texas Medical Branch, along with Timothy W. Smith and Charles Turner of the University of Utah (Miller et al. 1996). Using state-of-the-art statistical methods, the researchers concluded that hostility is a meaningful, independent risk factor for CHD. (Specifically, for structured interview indicators of "potential for hostility," the weighted mean *r* [WMR, a measure of effect size] was .18. The Cook-Medley Hostility Scale and other cognitive-experiential measures of hostility were modestly predictive of CHD [WMR = .08], though this scale was more powerfully predictive of all-cause mortality [WMR = .16]). But Miller found a stronger link between hostility as measured by the structured interview technique than as measured by the Cook-Medley Hostility Scale or by self-report measures of hostile emotions or behaviors. According to Miller and colleagues (1996), the SI is more likely to tap expressive or outward manifestations of hostile affect than is the Cook-Medley Hostility Scale, which, as noted above, measures hostile or cynical attitudes toward others and the world, a more cognitive, internal ("experiential") classification than an expressive-behavioral one.

Overall, the meta-analysis showed that hostility influenced the development of CHD independent of other known risk factors. This held true across most studies, but here again the statistical independence of hostility was more consistently apparent in studies that used the SI measures. Finally, the increased risk of CHD associated with hostility, particularly as measured by the SI, was considerable, as Miller and colleagues (1996) noted: "The effect sizes for SI measures of hostility are equal to or greater in magnitude to those reported for the traditional risk factors for CHD—

elevated serum cholesterol, elevated blood pressure, and cigarette smoking." The conclusions of this meta-analysis have not been contradicted by a group of more recent negative studies. Arguably, this meta-analysis represents the definitive statement to date about the role of hostility in CHD risk.

One recent study adds to our understanding of how chronic hostility may physiologically set the stage for long-term development of CHD. In a prospective evaluation of 374 men and women aged eighteen to thirty, participants in the Coronary Artery Risk Development in Young Adults (CARDIA) study in Chicago and Oakland in the mid-1980s, subjects were tested at baseline for hostility and followed for ten years with electron-beam computed tomography scans (EBCT) to determine the presence of any coronary artery calcification and to quantify the extent of coronary artery calcium. (Arterial calcification represents any early stage of plaque development and is a risk factor for CHD and CHD-related events.) In a logistic regression analysis, the investigators found that subjects with hostility scores above the median were more than 2.5 times as likely to have any coronary artery calcification after ten years; they were also 9.5 times as likely to have calcium scores greater than 20, a predetermined cutoff for high calcium (Iribarren et al. 2000). The results held strong after adjustment for demographic, lifestyle, and physiological factors. The study, published in the *Journal of the American Medical Association*, suggested that high hostility predisposed young adults to coronary artery calcification, which, as measured by EBCT, may be a stronger predictor of CAD than standard risk factors (Kennedy et al. 1998; Secci et al. 1997).

Type A Behavior, Hostility, and CHD Progression and Mortality

The preponderance of evidence suggests an uncertain link between Type A behavior and the incidence of CHD and a strong, fairly reliable association between hostility—the putative toxic core of Type A—and the development of CHD. The relative risks for hostility range roughly between 1.5 and 3.0, which suggests that it is a clinically significant risk factor for CHD. But what about the link between Type A behavior or hostility and the clinical course of CHD, including mortality among those diagnosed with CHD? Here the data are sketchy at best.

"Although there is good evidence that type A behavior, and especially the hostility and anger components of such behavior, predispose to an increased risk of suffering an initial CHD event, there is considerably less epidemiological evidence that these factors adversely affect prognosis once clinical CHD is present," wrote Redford Williams and Andrew Littman in 1996. Indeed, they cited two studies in which Type A heart patients were at less risk of dying than type B patients (Barefoot et al. 1989; Ragland

78   and Brand 1988), though they also cited studies linking hostility to a decrease in a key index of the heart's pumping ability, left ventricular ejection fraction (Ironson et al. 1992), and to the degree of myocardial ischemia among patients with existing CHD (Helmers et al. 1993), which suggested possible mechanisms for a relationship that had not yet been established.

On the positive side, a few studies suggest that people who exhibit hostile traits after an MI have a worse prognosis. One prospective study involving 104 Finnish men previously treated for ischemic heart disease found that high hostility ratings predicted subsequent coronary attacks (RR = 14.6 after standardization for CHD risk factors) (Koskenvuo et al. 1988). Three other studies including cohorts between 150 and 250 CAD patients found relative risks of coronary death, MI, or progressive CAD ranging from 1.7 to 2.1 (De Leon et al. 1996; Dembroski et al. 1989; Hecker et al. 1988).

Among heart patients, however, negative studies on Type A behavior or hostility and poor outcomes (i.e. recurrent and/or fatal events) are slightly more prevalent:

- In a prospective evaluation of 516 MI patients evaluated for Type A behavior within two weeks of suffering heart attacks and then followed for one to three years there was no relationship between Type A scores and total mortality, cardiac mortality, time to death for nonsurvivors, or duration of stay in the cardiac unit (Case et al. 1985).
- Among 1,467 patients with documented CAD, Type A behavior did not predict the subsequent incidence of nonfatal MI (Barefoot et al. 1989). Moreover, among patients with poor left ventricular function (an established negative prognostic indicator) those who evidenced Type A behavior had better survival odds than those categorized as Type Bs.
- In a study carried out at the Pennsylvania State College of Medicine 331 MI patients were prospectively evaluated for depression as well as hostility (measured by the Cook-Medley Hostility Scale). Patients were evaluated at six and twelve months after discharge; those who initially evidenced depression were significantly more likely to have died at twelve months (p = .04) (Kaufmann et al. 1999). However, hostility was not found to be a predictor at either six or twelve months.

Why is it that Type A behavior and, more reliably, hostility are involved in the etiology of CHD, while neither Type A nor hostility has consistently been shown to influence disease outcome in patients with existing CHD? The answer undoubtedly has to do, at least partially, with the differential pathophysiological mechanisms involved in CHD initiation and development and in progression to recurrent coronary events (i.e., repeat heart attacks, restenosis, fatal coronary events) or mortality. While the mechanisms involved in the development of ischemic heart disease, the primary causes of coronary events, may overlap those involved in recurrent disease or death, the natural history of CHD involves phases with distinct, albeit overlapping pathophysiological pathways. I will return to the question of mechanisms, but different psychosocial factors are involved more or less prominently in different stages of CHD. And certain maladaptive coping styles and damaging emotional states are more likely to occur at different times in the course of CHD progression. For instance, characteristically defensive or hostile types are more likely to maintain their defensive or hostile behavior when coronary disease is silently developing without their knowledge and less likely to exhibit this behavior, at least with the same intensity, after being diagnosed with CHD or after a heart attack. I return to this argument ahead.

Anger, Anxiety, and Incipient CHD

Contrary to some popular confusion, Type A behavior and hostility are not synonymous with anger per se. Anger is an emotion; Type A behavior is a coping style or personality trait involving a constellation of characteristics; and hostility is a complex of attitudes, cognitive predilections, and expressive tendencies. Type A or hostile individuals may either suppress anger or express it openly. Put differently, they may either seethe or explode, but on some level anger is apparent. (Even those who seethe exhibit noticeable behavioral signs that they are seething, signs that can be detected in SIs [Haney et al. 1996].) These distinctions may be important for understanding the dynamic role of hostility and anger in CHD, as I will show.

Is anger the underlying problem in the development of CHD? The question remains unresolved because the most impressive data link hostility, not anger per se, with CHD. It seems clear to most researchers of Type A behavior and hostility in CHD that in such individuals anger is just below the surface and either explodes episodically in angry outbursts or continues to simmer below the surface. The exploders (anger-out) are people whose anger never appears to resolve, and therefore never abates, by virtue of their outbursts. (The vulnerability of these individuals calls into question the superficiality of the once-popular idea that simply venting anger relieves the emotion. Undiluted rage cannot be considered a healthy expression of anger.) Among those who seethe (anger-in) attitudes of hostility and cynical mistrust belie a sense of bitterness, resentment, and, one can only surmise, an unprocessed well of angry feelings and im-

80   pulses. Such observations have led some researchers to suggest that anger is the toxic emotion in CHD.

This idea is buttressed by studies showing that the emotion of anger, while not a measure that has been as widely investigated in most epidemiological studies of CHD risk, is a conspicuous factor in short-term risk, preceding coronary events by hours. In the Determinants of Myocardial Infarction Study, a case-crossover study of 1,623 patients, episodes of anger were found to be powerful triggers of MI (Mittleman et al. 1995). The relative risk of MI in the two hours after an anger episode was 2.3, a result consistent with those of other studies showing that extreme emotional stress can trigger acute coronary events (Kop 1997).

But anger is not the only episodic emotion associated with incipient MI; anxiety has also been implicated. Evidence from the Determinants of Myocardial Infarction Study reveals that the relative risk for MI associated with an anxiety attack occurring within two hours of onset is 1.6 (Mittleman et al. 1995). While this association is not as very strong, anxiety may be a long-term risk factor for CHD (Kubzansky and Kawachi 2000).

That anger or anxiety may be involved in the onset of a heart attack suggests that these emotions may influence the pathophysiology of MI as a discrete "biopsychosocial" event and, further, that longstanding coping styles in which anger or anxiety is present below the psychic surface, as with Type A and hostile persons, may contribute to the long-term pathogenesis of underlying atherosclerosis. But the sudden breakthrough of "toxic emotions" under stressful circumstances may represent the proverbial straw that breaks the camel's back, in this case an emotional "event" that rapidly precipitates neuroendocrine, inflammatory, and arterial events leading directly to a heart attack in people whose coronary arteries are already occluded or to sudden cardiac death (SCD) in people vulnerable to arrhythmias.

ANXIETY AND LONG-TERM CHD DEVELOPMENT

Studies on the relationship between anxiety and the long-term risk of CHD have been mixed, although recent reviews (Kubzansky and Kawachi 2000; Kubzansky et al. 1998) suggest that methodologically stronger studies support anxiety as a risk factor. Kubzansky and Kawachi (2000) cite three studies with null results (Algulander and Lavori 1991; Martin et al. 1985; Wheeler et al. 1950) that dashed interest in the anxiety-CHD relationship, but they suggest that other findings, including several from recent investigations, have stirred renewed interest in the matter. The primary positive studies are:

- In the Health Professionals Follow-Up Study (of the Harvard School of Public Health), a cohort of 33,999 male health professionals without CHD were followed for two years. At baseline, they were administered the Crown-Crisp Index, a short self-rating measure of phobic anxiety. Compared with men who reported little anxiety, men who scored high on this index were three times as likely to die of coronary disease (Kawachi, Colditz, et al. 1994). (When investigators adjusted for a range of CHD risks, the relative risk was still 2.45.) Most of the CHD deaths associated with high anxiety were sudden. To quote the researchers: "The specificity, strength, and dose-response gradient of the association, together with the consistency and biological plausibility of the experimental and epidemiologic evidence, support a strong causal association between phobic anxiety and fatal CHD."
- In the Northwick Park Heart Study, 1,456 healthy men were tested for phobic anxiety using the Crown-Crisp Index and then followed for a decade. Compared with low-anxiety subjects, those with the highest levels of phobic anxiety had a relative risk of fatal CHD of 3.77 (Haines et al. 1987).
- In the Normative Aging Study (involving 1,305 community-dwelling men followed for seven years) five domains of worry were evaluated: about social conditions, health, finances, self-definition, and aging. The researchers found associations between three of these domains (worry about social conditions, finances, and health) and CHD (Kubzansky et al. 1997). For example, compared with men who worried least about social conditions, men who worried most were 2.41 times as likely to suffer a nonfatal MI, and there was a dose-response relationship between level of worry and overall CHD risk. In the same study men reporting symptoms of anxiety (i.e., an affirmative answer to the question "Are you considered a nervous person?") were four and a half times more likely than nonanxious subjects to die suddenly of heart disease.
- In twenty-year follow-up data from the Framingham Heart Study, analysis of female subjects ($N = 749$) revealed a significant association between anxiety symptoms and the risk of CHD, but only among homemakers, not among women employed outside the home (Eaker et al. 1992). Among the homemakers, women who reported any symptoms of anxiety, as compared with those who reported none, had a relative risk of 7.8.

In their review of this evidence Kubzansky and Kawachi (2000) note that "the relative risk estimates in studies of anxiety and CHD have been imprecise, due in part to the small numbers of events occurring." They also assert that studies with null findings were methodologically "weaker in design" than the above-cited studies showing positive associations. One conclusion from their careful reviews is that evidence for an anxiety-CHD link is relatively strong and growing; more prospective studies in this area should provide more clarification, including which types of anxiety disorder (generalized, phobic, panic, social phobia, etc.) may be most strongly correlated with CHD. It will also be incumbent on future researchers to determine whether state or trait anxiety is a root factor in CHD, though measures used in the positive prospective studies are suggestive of trait anxiety. If this bears out, trait anxiety may join hostility—a psychosocial variable that is also more trait than state—as a verifiable CHD risk factor.

TYPE D BEHAVIOR: A NEW PSYCHOSOCIAL CONSTRUCT FOR CHD RISK

Since it appears that anger, hostility, anxiety, and, as I will shortly discuss, stress and depression, all play some role in CHD risks, a clear picture of causal factors in different stages of CHD seems ever harder to paint. The "hodgepodge of negative emotions" theory would seem to prevail, and this is not a particularly coherent construct. A thoughtful and methodologically fine-tuned effort to cut through the confusion has been made by the health psychologist Johan Denollet of the University Hospital in Antwerp, Belgium.

In studies with heart patients Denollet and colleagues (1995, 1996, 1998, 2000) have developed the concept of a distressed personality type—also dubbed Type D—as an independent risk for poor outcome. The Type D individual scores high on *negative affectivity*, the tendency to experience a range of negative emotional states, including anxiety, anger, worry, and depression, but also high on social inhibition, the tendency to inhibit expression of emotions (Denollet 1998). Denollet's theory fits with other research on the health-damaging influence of emotional inhibition (Pennebaker and Susman 1988), based on the notion that nonexpression of strong negative feelings requires intense physiological work that strains a variety of biological systems, especially the cardiovascular system. (This inhibition research does not lead to the simplistic, now spurned recommendation that mere outbursts of anger are healing; most experts in emotional expression and health view healthy expression as a matter of constructive communication and internal resolution of anger, not "discharge" per se.) In Denollet's theory the hostile, anxious, and depressed individual is at greatest risk if he or she also keeps a perpetually tight lid on these emotional states.

In one of Denollet's studies eighty-seven post-MI patients with a decreased left ventricular ejection fraction (LVEF), a strong predictor of poor prognosis, were studied psychologically and tracked for a mean of eight years. At follow-up, twenty-one patients had experienced a cardiac event (including thirteen fatal events), and Denollet and Dirk Brutsaert found that patients who conformed, on standardized tests, with the Type D profile were significantly more likely to experience an event over time than non–Type D patients (52% versus 12%; $p = .00005$) (Denollet and Brutsaert 1998). After controlling for risk factors, they found that the risk of a cardiac event in patients with an LVEF of less than 30 percent had increased threefold, while the risk in Type D personalities had increased nearly fivefold.

While the study was small, the degree to which Denollet's findings fit his hypothesis was stunning. Specifically, CHD patients who scored high in negative affectivity—they experienced anxiety, depression, anger, etc.—but low in social inhibition—they tended to express emotions—did *not* have an increased rate of cardiac events; only one of thirteen such patients, or 8 percent, experienced a coronary event. But patients equally beset by negative emotion who also *inhibited* them—the Type Ds—had a strikingly higher rate: fourteen of twenty-seven, or 52 percent ($p = .01$). According to this finding, the toxic psychosocial factor is not negative emotions per se but intense negative emotions combined with strenuous efforts (conscious or unconscious) to suppress them.

To briefly summarize Denollet's other study findings:

- After a six- to ten-year prospective follow-up of 268 men and 35 women with documented CHD, 38 patients died; among them 24 died of cardiac events (Denollet et al. 1996). The mortality rate was higher for Type D patients than for other patients (27% versus 7%; $p < .00001$). When biomedical predictors were controlled for (in a multiple regression analysis), the impact of Type D remained significant (odds ratio [OR] = 4.1; $p = .0004$).* In this group of CHD patients a Type D personality was an independent predictor of both cardiac and noncardiac mortality. Social alienation and depression were also related to mortality but did not add to the predictive power of a Type D personality.
- In a study of 105 post-MI males followed for a mean of 3.8 years the mortality rate for Type D patients was 39 percent, compared with 5 percent for patients with other personality types ($p < .0001$) (Denollet et al. 1995). Type D patients also exhibited high levels of depression, stress, and somatization, though these factors did not add to the predictive value of a Type D personality. Among the most striking findings was that of twenty-four

*The odds ratio (OR) is a statistic reflecting the increased odds of an outcome depending upon a variable.

patients who scored high in anxiety but *low in inhibition* not one died during follow-up. By contrast, eleven of twenty-eight Type Ds (high anxiety, *high inhibition*), or 39 percent, died during follow-up.

• In a five-year prospective study of 319 CHD patients a multivariate analysis revealed the following factors as independent predictors of cardiac events: LVEF < 50 percent (OR = 3.9; p = .009); age < fifty-five (OR = 2.6; p = .05); and Type D personality (OR = 8.9; p = .001) (Denollet et al. 2000). A convergence of these risks predicted the lack of an expected positive response to medical treatment, which occurred in 10 percent of the patients.

While none of Denollet's studies involved large populations with high numbers of cardiac events after follow-up, their statistical power was arguably sufficient, and the degree to which his findings matched his theories is notable, to say the least. Based on their body of work, Denollet and colleagues developed a concise clinical and diagnostic portrait of the Type D individual (see table 3.1).

For now, it appears that a Type D personality is a risk factor for worsening, recurrent, or fatal CHD among patients already diagnosed. The same can be said for depression, as I will shortly detail, so the question arises, Is there a relationship between a Type D personality and depression? Denollet believes that they are related: "The characteristics that define this personality type (i.e., high levels of social inhibition and negative affectivity) have been linked to the onset of depression. In fact, research indicates that patients with coronary disease with a distressed personality are prone to depression and life stress, as well as other characteristics associated with increased risk for mortality after MI" (Denollet et al. 1995). While an association was found between depression and Type D personality in several of his studies, a Type D personality was more predictive, suggesting that nonexpression of emotions in concert with negative affectivity puts patients at risk for both depression and CHD progression. In the absence of larger studies on the Type D personality, it remains uncertain whether, as Denollet might argue, a Type D personality is a more significant psychological cause of worsening CHD than depression per se.

Also, Denollet has not conducted long-term studies of healthy patients to determine whether a Type D personality is a risk factor for *developing* CHD. If this were shown, the findings would have to be reconciled with the convincing data on hostility as a CHD risk factor. Do hostility and Type D personality traits overlap? What, if any, is the relationship between these constructs? Denollet's portrait of the Type D person suggests some-

TABLE 3.1
Type D Personality

	PERSONALITY TRAIT	
	NEGATIVE AFFECTIVITY	SOCIAL INHIBITION
Definition	Tendency to experience negative emotions across time/situations	Tendency to inhibit emotions and behaviors in social interactions
Clinical Picture	Often feels unhappy; tends to worry; is pessimistic; easily irritated; lacks self-esteem/assertiveness; has symptoms of depression and anxiety	Feels insecure in social interaction; tends to keep others at a distance; tends to be closed and reserved; reports low levels of social support
Diagnosis	High on Negative Affectivity Scale (Type D Scale 16)	High on Social Inhibition Scale (Type D Scale 16)
Prognosis	Type D, defined by high scores on negative affectivity and social inhibition: independent predictor of long-term mortality in patients with CHD; associated with cardiac events in post-MI patients with LVEF ≤ 50%.	

one who is irritable, anxious, isolated, and insecure though not necessarily overtly hostile. The Type D personality is more consistent with the anger-in variety of hostility than with the anger-out variety (Dembroski et al. 1985). Several analyses of extant data, most notably those of Dembroski, suggest that the tendency to feel anger but not express it (a Type D–like trait) is indeed strongly associated with CHD risk. On the other hand, Miller's meta-analysis suggests that expressive indices of hostility—anger-out—are better predictors.

In toto, however, hostile individuals, whether they seethe or explode, are at increased risk for developing CHD. It is not yet clear whether being classified as Type D—a "negative emotions-in" classification—means that one is at risk for *developing* CHD, but it does appear to be a powerful risk factor for *worsening* CHD among patients already diagnosed. Thus, if we rely on Miller's analysis of hostility studies and Denollet's Type D work, we can make a fairly clear set of distinctions: anger-out is a strong CHD risk factor; anger-in is also a risk factor, though not quite as reliable; and holding in negative emotions—the distressed Type D pattern—is a risk for worsening disease or death among individuals already diagnosed with CHD.

VITAL EXHAUSTION: PRELUDE TO A HEART ATTACK

It has been frequently observed by doctors, patients, and family members alike that individuals who suffer a heart attack or other dire cardiac event are physically exhausted and emotionally deflated prior to the event. In a series of studies Ad Appels of the Department of Medical, Clinical, and Experimental Psychology at the University of Maastricht, Netherlands, identified a confluence of psychophysical symptoms preceding the onset of MI, SCA, or recurrent cardiac events among patients with existing CAD (Appels and Mulder 1988). The symptoms include extreme fatigue, irritability, and feelings of demoralization, a complex he terms *vital exhaustion.*

Appels's research on vital exhaustion (VE) reveals that it frequently precedes cardiac events by days, months, or perhaps a few years but not by longer than that. (By contrast, men who are highly hostile may be at greater risk than nonhostile males for many years or even decades.) In 1988 Appels and Mulder published the results of a four-year prospective study of 3,877 men; VE was predictive of a future MI after controlling for blood pressure, smoking, cholesterol, age, and the use of antihypertensive drugs. In a later reanalysis Appels used factor analysis to validate the three key dimensions of VE—fatigue, irritability, and demoralization—which involve some depressive symptoms.

In later studies Appels confirmed and expanded upon his original findings. Regarding where along the continuum of heart disease VE is most apparent as a risk, he was able to be precise. In 1992 he published results from a prospective study of 3,365 men who were measured at baseline for VE and were then followed for an average of 9.5 years (Appels and Otten 1992). The results showed "a highly significant interaction between duration of follow-up and exhaustion upon the risk of cardiac death." The *hazards ratios* (HR) for exhaustion were 8.96, 6.33, 4.47, and 3.16 for the first ten, twenty, thirty, and forty months of follow-up, respectively.* Thereafter there was no significant association. Put differently, compared with other subjects, those who said they were vitally exhausted were nine times as likely to die from heart disease within ten months; six times as likely to die within twenty months; and so on. It seemed that Appels and his colleagues had taken a snapshot of men at a particular moment in time, and those who were exceedingly exhausted were at a much greater risk for a period of months or a few years. They did not do serial follow-ups to see which men continued to be vitally exhausted, but if they had, the VE hy-

*The hazards ratio (HR) reflects the increased hazard of an outcome depending upon a variable.

pothesis would suggest that men who overcame their vital exhaustion would have a lesser risk of cardiac events, while men who remained exhausted would be in greater cardiovascular peril.

Based on his view of VE as a prelude to cardiac events, Appels began studying CHD patients undergoing balloon angioplasty (percutaneous transluminal coronary angioplasty, or PTCA), who often have relapses or cardiac events within a limited time frame, to determine whether VE influenced their near-term outcome. In several studies he and his colleagues showed that VE was a significant factor in recurrent events (Appels et al. 1995; Kop et al. 1994; Mendes de Leon et al. 1996). For instance, among 127 subjects (105 men, 22 women) 35 percent of patients who were vitally exhausted experienced a cardiac event (repeat angioplasty, bypass surgery, MI, cardiac death, documented ischemia, etc.) within eighteen months, while only 17 percent of the nonexhausted patients experienced such events (OR = 2.7; p = .02) (Kop et al. 1994). In an attempt to reconcile research on anger or hostility and VE, Mendes de Leon, Appels, and colleagues studied 149 postangioplasty patients, and they found that a composite index of psychosocial risk based on anger and VE was significantly related (p = .02) to cardiac events after controlling for standard CHD risk factors (Mendes de Leon et al. 1996).

But is VE just a symptomatic stand-in for worse or worsening CHD rather than an independent contributor to the disease? To address this issue, Appels, along with W. J. Kop and others in the Uniformed Services University of the Health Sciences in Bethesda, studied 307 patents undergoing coronary angiography. The conclusion: "Neither the extent of CAD nor impaired cardiac pump function is related to feelings of exhaustion in patients referred for coronary angiography. Therefore, the previously reported association between exhaustion and future MI is not likely to be caused by underlying coronary disease" (Kop et al. 1996).

Bearing in mind Denollet's research on the Type D personality, Appels speculated that vitally exhausted individuals who also inhibited emotion might be at greater risk for CHD or, more specifically, SCA. He embarked on a case-control study of 99 people who had died from SCA, comparing them with a control group of 119 patients with CHD, matching them by age and gender (Appels, Golombeck, et al. 2000). In order to analyze the mind-body states and emotional styles of deceased individuals they questioned their closest surviving family members (mainly spouses) using structured interviews, including Appels's standard inventory for VE rephrased for loved ones, focusing on the subjects' degree of exhaustion during the eighteen months prior to their cardiac arrest. They also asked these family members about their loved ones' "openness" versus "closedness,"

88   a measure of emotional expression or disclosure. For those members of the control group who were still alive, questions were again posed to loved ones rather than to subjects, a research method that at least one other investigator (Nellison–de Vos 1994) had found to be valid, meaning that spouses' views dovetailed with those of subjects. The results confirmed Appels's hypothesis: according to spouses and close family the victims of SCD were more often exhausted and closed than were the control subjects. Apparently, the interaction of these two factors was like that of a lit match and a time bomb: the vitally exhausted subjects who also inhibited emotions had seven times the risk of SCA.

This study confirmed an aspect of the Type D hypothesis: closedness (or nonexpression of emotion) is toxic to the heart when it coexists with VE. There are certainly differences between VE and Type D personality: the former emphasizes fatigue, while the latter emphasizes a greater range of negative affects. But there are also similarities: the emotional coloration of both types suggests irritability, inner conflict, resignation, low energy, and emotional withdrawal. But at present we only have evidence that VE presages heart attacks, and we only have evidence that a Type D personality is a negative prognostic indicator after a heart attack or diagnosis of heart disease.

Thus, it is not clear whether VE plays a role in outcome *after* a heart attack. However, we know that depression does play a role, and Appels maintains that VE is not synonymous with depression. Subjects in his studies who were vitally exhausted were demoralized, and they may have evidenced some symptoms of depression, but they do not appear to have been beset by the guilt and sadness often apparent among clinically depressed people (Kop 1997). It appears, therefore, that VE and depression are not the same, that the former heralds a heart attack, while the latter predicts a worse outcome after a heart attack. I try to shed light on these distinctions below.

DEPRESSION: MAJOR RISK FOR THE HEART PATIENT, MODEST RISK FOR THE HEALTHY

The accumulating evidence that depression is a risk factor for recurrent disease or death among heart patients can now be reasonably described as overwhelming. There is also solid though less robust and voluminous evidence that depression is a risk factor for the development of CHD among otherwise healthy people.

Among the most important studies have been those conducted by Nancy Frasure-Smith and her colleagues at McGill University in Montreal. In their first investigation, published in the *Journal of the American Medical Association* in 1993, the team studied 222 patients who had suffered a heart attack (78% of whom were male), interviewing them and testing major depression from five to fifteen days after their MI (Frasure-Smith et al. 1993). The patients were tracked for six months, at the end of which depression was found to be a significant predictor of cardiac mortality: those who had been seriously depressed were more than five times as likely to have died (HR = 5.74; p = .0006). This robust influence of depression on cardiac death remained after the researchers controlled for such prognostic indicators as left ventricular dysfunction and previous MI, and the statistical impact of depression was deemed to be "at least equivalent" to both of these biological predictors.

After this study was published, to much fanfare in the biomedical and behavioral-science communities, Frasure-Smith continued her investigations, first by following the original 222 patients for an additional year. While major depression was the significant predictor at six months, less severe depressive symptoms were significant predictors of coronary death at eighteen months—an almost eightfold increase among these patients (OR = 7.82; p = .0002) (Frasure-Smith et al. 1995). After controlling for a range of established biological predictors, the findings held up: depression was associated with a more than sixfold increased risk of death (OR = 6.64; p = .0026.) In 1999 Frasure-Smith and colleagues published a study of 896 patients (283 of them women) who were tested for depressive symptoms before leaving the hospital and then tracked for one year. Even after controlling for biological prognostic indicators, high depression scores were significantly related to cardiac mortality for both genders: the odds ratios were 3.29 for women and 3.05 for men (Frasure-Smith et al. 1999). In a later study of 887 patients the team found that elevated depression scores were again related to cardiac mortality at one year (p = .0006) but that measures of social support were not (Frasure-Smith et al. 2000). However, the link between depression and cardiac mortality dwindled among those with higher levels of social support. Not only did depressed patients with more social support sidestep the otherwise substantial increased risk of death but they were more likely to overcome their depression during the year after their heart attack. Social support was found to be a buffer, protecting patients from deteriorating emotional and physical health.

How did Frasure-Smith's surviving subjects do many years later? In her most recent study she and François Lesperance followed all patients from their two large studies and found that after four years elevated depression scores at baseline were still associated with a roughly twofold in-

90   crease in cardiac mortality (HR = 1.91; p < .0001), and so was depression after one year (HR = 2.09; p = .0007) (Lesperance et al. 2002). But a critical finding was that patients at the highest long-term risk were those who were depressed at baseline *and* at one year. Patients who were depressed after their heart attack and who survived for one year had no increased long-term risk—as long as they were not depressed a year later. Frasure-Smith concluded that "prevention of depression recurrence and chronicity may be particularly important clinical goals for post-MI patients" (Lesperance et al. 2002).

Investigations with even longer follow-ups reveal depression as a long-term risk factor for recurrence or death after a MI. A research team from the Heart and Lung Institute of Göteborg University in Sweden tracked 275 MI patients (including 45 women) for a decade; depression was associated with a threefold increased risk of coronary mortality (RR = 3.16; p = 0.0007), and lack of social support was almost as risky (RR = 2.75) (Welin et al. 2000). After controlling for medical risks (left ventricular failure, dysrhythmias, etc.), depression and lack of social support were still found to be independently associated with higher mortality. Importantly, the Swedish investigators looked at a range of other psychological variables, including mental strain at work or in marriage, anxiety, dissatisfaction with family life or finances, Type A behavior, anger-in, irritability, and locus of control, and none of them were linked to a lesser or greater likelihood of mortality.

The clear majority of studies have shown positive associations between depression, measured in a variety of ways, and poor prognosis or death, with relative risks (or odds ratios) ranging from modest (RR = about 1.5 [Barefoot et al. 2000]) to robust (OR > 6.0 [Frasure-Smith et al. 1995]). However, a few negative studies have also been published (e.g., Mayou et al. 2000), including a recent study by Diane Lane and colleagues at the University of Birmingham, Edgbaston, United Kingdom (Lane et al. 2001). They measured depression and anxiety among 288 patients hospitalized for MI, and after twelve months follow-up analyses demonstrated that symptoms of depression and anxiety predicted quality of life but did not predict cardiac or all-cause mortality (Lane et al. 2001). The researchers acknowledged their failure to use measures of major depression (as opposed to depressive symptomatology) as one possible weakness, though they pointed out that a number of other studies using the same symptomatic measures elicited positive results.

As for the relationship between depression and the risk of CHD among otherwise healthy individuals tracked prospectively for extended periods of time, the data are compelling though not conclusive both because the

relative risks are generally more modest than those found in the prognosis studies and because there are more negative or null findings (Kubzansky and Kawachi 2000). Among the positive findings are the following:

- Investigators from the Ohio State University College of Medicine and Public Health analyzed data from the National Health and Nutrition Examination Survey (NHANES I), involving 5,007 women and 2,886 men who
  were followed for ten years (or until the occurrence of a CHD event) after
  baseline testing (Ferketich et al. 2000). After adjustment for standard CHD
  risk factors, the relative risk for a CHD event among depressed women,
  as compared with the nondepressed, was 1.73; the same figure for men was
  1.71. Depression did not predict eventual CHD mortality among women,
  but it did among men (adjusted RR = 2.34).
- In a community-based longitudinal study a team of researchers from the
  University of Maastricht and its Academic Hospital in the Netherlands
  evaluated a cohort of 2,847 men and women aged fifty-five to eighty-five
  (Penninx et al. 2001). After four years of follow-up they found that subjects who did not have CHD at baseline but did evidence minor depression
  had a relative risk of cardiac mortality of 1.5, while those with major depression had a four times greater risk of cardiac death.
- In a six-year prospective study of 4,493 individuals over sixty-five and free
  of CHD at baseline, researchers at the Johns Hopkins University and Wake
  Forest University found that every five-unit increase in depression scores
  resulted in a 15 percent increased risk of CHD (adjusted R = 1.15) (Ariyo
  et al. 2000). Comparing those having the highest cumulative mean depression scores with those having the lowest, investigators found a 40 percent
  greater incidence of heart disease among the former.

Several other positive studies have revealed similar, modestly increased
risks of coronary events or deaths among subjects with no evident CHD
at baseline. In a study by John Barefoot of 730 men and women followed
for several decades a specific increase in depression scores (of two standard
deviations) was associated with a relative risk of 1.71 for MI and of 1.59
for deaths from all causes. Barefoot concluded that "the graded relationships between depression scores and risk, long-lasting nature of the effect,
and stability of the depression measured across time suggest that this risk
factor is best viewed as a continuous variable that represents a chronic psychological characteristic rather than a discrete and episodic psychiatric
condition" (Barefoot and Schroll 1996). The idea of coronary-prone depression as a "chronic psychological condition" offers both insight into
the nature of emotional factors in CHD and a beacon for clinicians (med-

ical or psychological) who might identify this condition in patients who may, for other reasons as well, be vulnerable to coronary disease.

But there have also been negative studies of depression and coronary risk. Vogt and colleagues followed 2,573 men and women for fifteen years; in their study the highest level of depressive symptoms was not associated with a greater increase in the risk of ischemic heart disease than was the lowest level (Vogt et al. 1994). Two studies of hypertensive subjects also failed to find an increased risk of MI or coronary deaths among depressed individuals (Simonsick et al. 1995; Wasshertheil-Smoller et al. 1996), although one did find a link between increasing depression scores over time and a raised risk of stroke or MI (Simonsick et al. 1995). However, another prospective study of hypertensives, with a less reliable measure of depression but with a much larger population (5,564 patients in a worksite hypertension control program), turned up positive results. The subjects were asked at baseline if they had ever been treated for depression, and those who reported prior treatment were more than two times as likely to suffer a heart attack (HR = 2.10) during the approximately 4.9 years of follow-up (Cohen et al. 2001).

In studies of both CHD incidence and prognosis a relatively consistent finding has been that the risks associated with depression exist along a continuum, according to the magnitude of depressive symptoms (Rozanski et al. 1999). Also, a particular shading of depression—hopelessness—has received increasing attention. Two prospective epidemiological studies published in the 1990s reported a link between symptoms of hopelessness and the development of CAD (Anda et al. 1993; Everson et al. 1996). In one of these studies subjects were asked, "During the last month, have you felt so sad, discouraged, hopeless, or had so many problems that you wondered if anything was worthwhile?" A positive answer to this one question was associated with a greater than twofold increased risk of CAD (Anda et al. 1993).

The ramifications of the data on depression and heart disease have largely been overlooked by institutional biomedicine. The studies are published in peer-reviewed journals of psychology and medicine, and editorials are written, but few concerted efforts are made to evaluate and treat depression either in healthy populations at risk or in CHD patients. That the hazard is so apparent among CHD patients makes this oversight particularly appalling. Because the population at risk is already being treated in clinics or hospitals where risk factors for poor outcome (smoking, high-fat diets, no exercise, etc.) are often addressed by physicians or practitioners in cardiac rehabilitation programs, screening and treatment for depression could rather easily be included.

Why is the relationship between depression and poor prognosis among CHD patients more robust than the link between depression and the development of CHD? Only a process model can address this issue. Suffice it to say for now that *overt* depression will not be as apparent in otherwise healthy individuals at risk (both for depression and heart disease) as in patients who have been diagnosed with heart disease. As I will argue, the healthy "at-risk" person may suffer from latent depression, which is difficult to detect with most standard instruments. Depression may "break through" into more clinically overt and detectable forms once a life-threatening disease has been diagnosed, often after a cardiac "event," typically a heart attack, which can be traumatic.

STRESS, SOCIOECONOMIC FACTORS, AND SOCIAL SUPPORT

Stress, socioeconomic status (SES), and social support all play significant roles in the development and progression of cardiovascular disease. While all of these factors contribute to psychosocial CHD risks, they are almost certainly not the nub of the matter. With regard to stress, coping capacities are usually more influential than stress levels or stressful life events since adaptive copers can often withstand high levels of stress without succumbing to chronic or life-threatening diseases (Dreher 1995). Which is not to say that hardy copers are indomitable, since everyone has a stress threshold, but coping and personality variables are more important in mind-heart interactions than stress measures, which helps explain why variables such as hostility and depression have taken precedence over life events or stress in the literature of psychosocial factors in heart disease.

That said, acute stress may be associated with cardiac events, including SCD (Jiang et al. 1996), and a compelling body of research has focused on the impact of work-related stress. In literature on the latter, significant associations with heart disease have been identified when measures of work stress were combined with other measures of job role characteristics, such as "decision latitude" (Karasek et al. 1981), "low reward" (Siegrist et al. 1990), or "low job control" (Johnson et al. 1996). Studies that have evaluated this dual dimension of job stress—i.e., high demands and little control or few rewards—have shown elevated risks of CHD (Bosma et al. 1998; Johnson et al. 1996; Karasek et al. 1981; Siegrist et al. 1990). While these data are convincing, studies that do not show a significant correlation between work-related stress and CHD have also been reported (Bosma et al. 1998; Hlatky et al. 1995).

Another primary contributor to CHD incidence and mortality is SES, as a number of epidemiological studies have demonstrated (Adler et al.

1994; Kaplan and Keil 1993; Lynch 1997; Williams et al. 1992). For example, Redford Williams and his colleagues at Duke Medical Center evaluated social factors in 1,368 patients after cardiac catheterization had documented CAD (Williams et al. 1992). After five years 90 percent of patients with an annual household income over $40,000 were alive, compared with 76 percent of those with an annual household income under $10,000, a finding that was independent of all known medical prognostic factors. While studies have linked low SES and income with high-risk behaviors (Winkleby et al. 1990), others have related SES to psychological risk factors such as hostility (Barefoot et al. 1991), and still others suggest that SES may be an independent factor in its own right (Adler et al. 1994; Marmot et al. 1978).

From the perspective of sociological critiques of mind-body studies (Antonovsky 1994; Dreher 1995b; Kaplan 1995), SES is indeed a fundamental factor in many diseases, including CHD, since varieties of stress (work, finances, family) and even psychological states and traits, or *person variables,* to borrow a term from the researcher Michael Scheier (Scheier and Bridges 1995)—e.g., hostility, Type A behavior, Type D coping styles—can be shaped by social class. Low SES, racism, and sexism are often the unseen and unacknowledged roots of job strain, family dysfunction, distressing social environments, social isolation, health-damaging behavior patterns (addictions, smoking, alcoholism, etc.), impoverished self-esteem, feelings of helplessness, an external locus of control, chronic anger, and despair. Thus, a genuinely comprehensive integrative medicine must target the socioeconomic factors that produce the pathogenic psychosocial conditions leading to CHD. Certainly, my purpose here is to explore person variables; to set forth a process model that explains how psychodynamic and psychobiological mechanisms intertwine in CHD; and to evaluate psychological interventions that reduce CHD risks. But intervention on a much broader social scale is surely needed to address the superstructural contribution of SES to CHD, and that suggests a massive political effort to reduce poverty, transform inner-city environments, and mitigate the impact of racism and sexism on the work and family lives of minorities and women—all under the rubric of public health.

A lack of social support—due to socioeconomic factors, person variables, or a confluence of both—is also a powerful risk factor for CHD incidence and progression. Conversely, strong social networks may help prevent CHD and also protect CHD patients against recurrent disease and mortality. In their exhaustive overview of psychosocial factors in CHD, Rozanski, Blumenthal, and Kaplan identified fifteen epidemiological studies of social support, all of which showed an association between low levels of social support and coronary disease, all-cause mortality, or coronary mortality. (In a number of studies the outcome was all-cause mortality, which included a high percentage of coronary deaths.) Across these studies, a comparatively small social network was found to be associated with a two- to threefold increase, on average, in the incidence of CAD over time (Rozanski et al. 1999).

Rozanski and colleagues also identified eleven studies evaluating the link between social support and prognosis among patients with existing CAD, all but one of which revealed a prognostic relationship between low social support and poor medical outcomes. For instance, in a study of 194 male and female MI patients led by Lisa Berkman, of the Yale University School of Medicine, those who reported a lack of emotional support were three times as likely to have died after six months of follow-up (Berkman et al. 1992). In the above-cited study by Williams et al. (1992) of economic and social resources among patients with CAD, unmarried patients without a confidant had a five-year survival rate of 50%, as compared with an 82 percent survival rate among those who were married, had a confidant, or both. In the one-year prospective study of 887 MI patients conducted by Frasure-Smith and her colleagues social support was not directly related to survival (Frasure-Smith et al. 2000). However, subjects with very high levels of social support experienced reductions in their depressive symptoms, and according to Frasure-Smith, this support "appeared to buffer the impact of depression on mortality."

An analogy might help put the social and environmental variables of SES, stress, and social support in proper context. One could personify the coronary threat posed by low SES (and other social factors) as a gunman with a pistol aimed at the individual at risk for CHD. This vulnerable person is confronted by the gunman, a symbolic representative of particular threats, namely poverty, demoralizing residential conditions, low-wage or low-level jobs, unemployment, the dehumanization of racism and sexism, etc. The pistol is pointed, the trigger pulled, and the bullet fired represents "stress." In other words, all the SES-related threats cause stress, which can enter the body and "wound" the heart through various biological pathways. But the person can dodge the bullet of stress by taking assertive action or deflect it by wearing the armor of his or her coping defenses. It is often impossible to avoid being nicked, grazed, or even wounded, but actions may be taken to avoid chronic or mortal injuries. Social support is an essential part of the protective armor—or *buffer*, to use the social science term—since turning to family, friends, and coworkers can ease the stress of traumatic life events or demoralizing social conditions. But person variables are still pivotal since individuals may compensate for deficits in their social environments, at least partially, by using personal strengths to draw upon existing social resources, for instance, by actively seeking practical and emotional support from friends and family. In other words, people can use volition to don the protective armor of coping defenses and social support.

Such a model posits person variables not necessarily as *primary* but rather as *pivotal,* which means that people can be helped, often through psychosocial intervention, to cultivate their internal coping resources, to seek and utilize support, and to transform behavior patterns in ways that reduce CHD risks. While challenging social conditions (e.g., poverty, disrupted family life, poor educational opportunities, etc.) make such changes vastly more challenging, the view that psychosocial interventions cannot help individuals to even partially overcome the inimical impact of low SES is a form of social determinism. A dynamic biopsychosocial model would have it that both societal and individual transformation are needed to promote health optimally and that such changes can act synergistically. But health-promoting changes on the microlevel of the individual and the macrolevel of SES do not depend upon each other in some mechanistic fashion; they can unfold independently. Put differently, a person can exercise some degree of empowerment with regard to his or her emotional life and behavior patterns even when his or her socioeconomic environment seems fixed.

Psychobiological Mechanisms of Mind–Heart Unity

No single biological pathway explains the relationships between coronary-prone psychosocial factors, including person variables (Type A behavior, Type D personality, hostility, etc.), emotional states (depression, anger, anxiety), and social factors (stressful events, low SES, low social support), on the one hand, and heart disease risks, on the other. These relationships are exceedingly complex on both psychological and biological levels, and reflecting this complexity, many labyrinthine biological pathways are involved. Rather than reviewing this entire field of inquiry, I highlight the most important pathways, emphasizing how they link particular psychosocial factors with particular CHD outcomes; I focus especially on the recently recognized psychoimmunological pathways that appear to play a surprisingly significant part in heart disease. (Research on the role of immunity, inflammation, and even infection in the etiology and progression of heart disease has virtually exploded over the past decade.)

TYPE A AND HOSTILITY: MULTIFARIOUS PATHWAYS TO THE HEART

As is true of the relationship between every psychosocial factor and CHD, the relationship between Type A behavior or hostility and disease involves two broad pathways: Type A or hostile individuals engage more prevalently in lifestyle habits (i.e., smoking, poor diet, lack of exercise, alcoholism) that contribute to CHD, and hostile traits may also influence internal pathophysiological mechanisms in CHD. I focus here on the latter, since the signal studies of Type A behavior or hostility (and the other psychosocial factors to be discussed here) controlled for the lifestyle factors, suggesting that internal pathways can operate alongside but independently of the lifestyle factors associated with these personality traits and emotional states. (This may explain why some hostile, anxious, or depressed individuals who sustain healthy lifestyle habits may still be at risk for CHD.)

Compared with nonhostile persons, hostile individuals have higher ambulatory blood pressure levels in daily life (Suarez and Blumenthal 1991), and they exhibit what is known as high *cardiovascular reactivity* (heart rate, blood pressure, stress hormone production) in response to experimental stress (Suls and Wan 1993). Specifically, they are more likely than nonhostile people to have high blood levels of the stress hormones cortisol and the catecholamines (adrenaline, noradrenaline) (Pope and Smith 1991; Suarez and Blumenthal 1991), as well as reduced beta-adrenergic receptor function (Suarez et al. 1997). The high level of catecholamines in hostile reactors may intensify blood coagulation (through platelet aggregation, a risk for thrombosis in narrowing coronary arteries); increase circulating lipids and assist their deposit in arteries, leading to the formation of plaque; and cause injuries to arterial endothelial linings (Kop 1999; Suarez 1991b; Suarez et al. 1991). Also, hostile individuals exhibit reduced heart rate variability (HRV) in response to stress, which suggests that their heartbeats are not being properly regulated by the autonomic nervous system; reduced HRV is another indicator of CHD risk (Gorman and Sloan 2000). In sum, hostile individuals have volatile sympathetic nervous systems. And according to Willem Kop and Nicholas Cohen, "Direct effects of elevated sympathetic tone include damage of vasculature due to arterial lipid deposition and elevated intraarterial pressure that promote *early stages of CAD*" (Kop and Cohen 2001, italics mine).

But hostile personality traits may also influence immune factors in the pathogenesis of heart disease. According to a paper by Fricchione and colleagues from Brigham and Women's Hospital in Boston, hostility may be associated not only with higher catecholamines but also with higher levels of serum lipids, which are processed by macrophages (immune scavenger cells) and endothelial cells into oxidized low-density lipoproteins (LDLs) (Fricchione et al. 1996). Oxidized LDLs are a prime culprit in the formation of atherosclerotic plaques, the hallmark of CAD. Once plaques have begun to form, macrophages and endothelial cells appear to regulate nitric oxide production in a manner that causes vasoconstriction, a further development in the pathogenesis of CAD (Fricchione et al. 1996).

Recently, teams of researchers have validated that homocysteine, a sulphur amino acid, is strongly positively associated with cardiovascular disease, and cardiologists are now beginning the routine practice of testing homocysteine levels and recommending vitamins (i.e., vitamin B_6, folic acid) to reduce blood levels. Some argue that homocysteine will prove to be a prognostic factor as critical as cholesterol. Catherine Stoney of Ohio State University has initiated studies of the relationship between psychosocial variables and homocysteine levels; in one recent study she and T. O. Engebretson focused on measures of hostility and anger expression in a sample of healthy middle-aged men and women. They found significant correlations between hostility (measured by using the Cook-Medley questionnaire) and homocysteine levels for all participants and significant positive correlations between a measure of anger-in tendencies and homocysteine among male participants (Stoney and Engebretson 2000). In a separate study, in which subjects were exposed to experimental stress, Stoney found that homocysteine levels jumped during stressful procedures, as did blood pressure and heart rate (Stoney 1999). She concluded that "the rise in homocysteine levels may have been sympathetically mediated." While these studies are not conclusive, homocysteine may soon be added to the list of biological mechanisms in CHD that are sensitive to stress, hostility, and other person variables.

When the immunology of heart disease is debated, a central question arises: Is CHD an infectious disease? Data have accumulated on the presence of certain pathogens in atherosclerotic plaques, especially *Chlamydia pneumoniae* and cytomegalovirus (CMV) (Kop and Cohen 2001). But there is currently more convincing evidence for systemic, or low-grade, inflammation in the pathogenesis of CHD than for direct involvement of microbial pathogens (Kop and Cohen 2001). That said, the infectious theory of CHD remains a distinct possibility, whether such organisms are primary causal agents or secondary invaders of arterial endothelium "weakened" by plaque formation, injury, and inflammation. To the extent that bacterial or viral organisms play an important role, the possibility exists that immunosuppression allows for bacterial invasion or viral reactivation, which in turn sets off—or exacerbates—the inflammatory responses (activation of macrophages and lymphocytes, acute-phase proteins, and proinflammatory cytokines) that definitely contribute to atherogenesis, plaque disruption, and excessive coagulation involved in coronary syndromes and incipient heart attacks.

How might hostility influence these processes? In a study by Margaret Kemeny and her colleagues at the University of California, Los Angeles, of thirty-six patients with recurrent herpes simplex virus (HSV) (Kemeny et al. 1989) the subjects who were most depressed, anxious, and hostile had a lower proportion than others in the study of CD8+ cells, which possess the dual abilities of vanquishing bacterial or viral invaders and suppressing excessive immune responses. (Both functions could be helpful in warding off CHD.) Moreover, subjects with depressive symptoms had a particularly high rate of HSV recurrence. While HSV is indeed one of many pathogens suspected in CHD pathogenesis, Kemeny's work is more important for the general principle it underscored: immune mechanisms that keep viruses from reactivating are compromised in depressed or hostile individuals. If reactivated viruses are ultimately proven to cause heart disease, this psychoimmune finding must be revisited.

While the infectious-invader theory of CHD remains somewhat controversial, the inflammation theory is no longer controversial, and there is little doubt that psychosocial variables can influence inflammatory cells and cytokines through the actions of neuroendocrine mediators. (While data on hostility as an instigator in this cascade are modest, the evidence for depression is more substantial.) We now know that inflammation contributes to virtually every stepwise stage in the pathogenesis of CAD and MI, but more multileveled studies that specifically measure hostility, neuroendocrine mediators, inflammatory markers, and disease processes and then track them all prospectively in the same group of patients are needed. The incomplete data on the psychoimmune model of heart disease should not overshadow the substantial evidence that nonimmune mechanisms— cardiovascular reactivity, high catecholamine levels, sympathetic tone, lipid deposition, homocysteine, and subsequent plaque disruption—are critically involved in CHD and are powerfully influenced by chronic anger and hostile personality traits.

ACUTE ANXIETY AND ANGER: LINKS TO SUDDEN CARDIAC ARREST

Anxiety has been associated with sudden cardiac death. In two key studies the link to SCD was clear, but no relationship was shown to MI or "non-sudden" cardiac death (Kawachi, Colditz, et al. 1994; Kawachi, Sparrow, et al. 1994, 1995). Such findings suggest that ventricular ar-

100   rhythmias are the most important cause of cardiac death among people subject to acute anxiety. The recent publication of prospective studies suggesting that anxiety is implicated in long-term CHD pathogenesis means that mind-body scientists must also investigate atherosclerotic mechanisms related to anxiety—as they have investigated atherosclerotic mechanisms related to hostility. But these findings are not yet as strong as the findings linking acute anxiety and SCA.

In support of the theory that anxiety increases the risk of arrhythmias that cause sudden death, studies have shown that individuals with anxiety disorders have reduced HRV (Kawachi et al. 1995). Indeed, people with reduced HRV during stress tests have reactive sympathetic nervous systems (Lown et al. 1973) and impaired *vagal* control of the heart (referring to the innervation and regulation of the heart by the vagus nerve) (Rich et al. 1988), both of which are associated with increased cardiac mortality. One recent study concentrated on a key index of impaired vagal control, namely, reduced baroreflex cardiac control, and found it significantly more prevalent in people with anxiety (Watkins et al. 1998).

We can infer links between anxiety and specific mechanisms from biological studies of stress and CHD. These studies reveal that stress causes both sympathetic arousal and *parasympathetic withdrawal,* the reduced capacity of the parasympathetic nervous system to becalm the cardiovascular system. This dynamic taxes the heart by increasing cardiac demand while decreasing the coronary blood supply (Jiang et al. 1996), a dangerous state that can incite cardiac arrhythmias (Verrier 1987).

Is there an immune connection between acute anxiety or stress and acute coronary syndromes? In theory, yes. Acute psychological challenges activate the immune system, which includes brisk enhancements of CD8+ T cells, inflammatory cytokines, acute-phase proteins (e.g., C-reactive protein and fibrinogen), and circulating adhesion molecules (Kop and Cohen 2001). (Note that C-reactive protein, a measure of systemic inflammation, is now being used by mainstream cardiologists as a significant prognostic risk factor.) As Kop and Cohen noted in their superb overview of psychoimmunology and CHD (2001), "These immune system changes may be relevant with respect to triggering acute coronary syndromes because increased immune activation may lead to activation and subsequent rupture of vulnerable atherosclerotic plaques."

Indirectly, immune activation may also promote thrombus (blood clot) formation in coronary arteries by up-regulating blood-clotting factors, and it can choke off perfusion (the passage of blood) through of coronary arteries near occluded sites in these arteries (Entman and Ballantyne 1993). One of the final stages leading to MI is plaque disruption. In his paper on the role of inflammation in this process P. K. Shah of the UCLA Medical School noted that "inflammatory cells may play a critical role in plaque disruption" and that "surges in sympathetic activity provoked by sudden vigorous exercise, emotional stress—including anger—may also trigger plaque disruption" (Shah 1998). In the event that immune factors are proven to be important in the link between acute emotional arousal (i.e., anxiety attacks or anger outbursts) and cardiac events, an activated immune system, rather than a weakened one, may be the source of the problem.

TYPE D: TAXING THE CARDIOVASCULAR SYSTEM

According to Johan Denollet, developer of the Type D personality concept, Type Ds are highly susceptible to stress. Though he does not make it explicit, one can presume that Type Ds, who experience chronic irritability, unhappiness, and distress ("high negative affectivity") but are also inhibited (they do not share these emotions) are psychobiological pressure cookers: they cannot sustain mind-body homeostasis because they have few, if any, constructive outlets for negative thoughts and feelings. In Type Ds, stressful life events cause internal distress that cannot readily be relieved by emotional expression or resolved through social engagement and assertive action. Thus, while Denollet has not studied specific psychophysiological mechanisms in the link between Type D and heart disease, he theorizes that Type Ds, who evidence high levels of internal distress in response to stressful events, are subject to the same cardiovascular perturbations observed when people experience chronic or acute stress. Specifically, people exposed to stress in life or under laboratory conditions may be subject to increased platelet aggregation (Grignani et al. 1991), coronary spasm (Yeung et al. 1991), or ventricular arrhythmias (Myerberg et al. 1992). Several important laboratory studies in which patients with CAD were exposed to stressful mental procedures revealed measurable degrees of myocardial ischemia during the testing (Blumenthal et al. 1995; Rozanski et al. 1988), and in one study the same reduced blood flow to the heart was demonstrated in daily life through ambulatory monitoring (Blumenthal et al. 1995). In sum, Type D traits and the internal stress they engender may tax the cardiovascular system via several pathways.

In their psychoimmunological review Kop and Cohen (2001) divide psychosocial variables in CHD into three categories: chronic (more than ten years in duration; they include hostility and low SES here), episodic (less than two years, including depression and exhaustion), and acute (less than one hour, including anger and mental activity, as in mental stress tests). Kop and Cohen relate each of these temporal categories to fairly

102   distinct sets of immune changes that they associate with different phases of CHD. As a personality type, Type D ought to be categorized as a chronic condition, although one might argue that this longstanding trait can also yield episodic states of stress. Thus, it is difficult to identify specific immune perturbations in CHD that may be caused by Type D behavior. But it is conceivable that Type D coping may contribute in several ways: as a chronic factor it may weaken immune defenses (e.g., macrophages) against pathogens implicated in atherosclerosis; as an episodic factor it may boost platelet aggregation and proinflammatory cytokines; and as a trait that makes people susceptible to acute distress it may raise catecholamines, increase cardiac demand, and jump-start inflammation, which in differing but overlapping ways can contribute to plaque rupture, ischemia, and arrhythmias. This unfolding cascade of mechanisms is certainly speculative, but it is consistent with Denollet's construct and the psychoimmune model elaborated by Kop and Cohen.

VITAL EXHAUSTION: STRESS HORMONES AND INFLAMMATORY CYTOKINES

Vital exhaustion, which precedes MI and other cardiac events by a few months to a year and a half, is associated with a host of biological perturbations involved in heart disease. In the psychoimmune model of CHD proposed by Kop and Cohen (2001), VE and depression are considered together as "episodic factors," meaning that they predate the onset of clinical CHD by less than two years. While Kop and Cohen acknowledge that depression and VE are not entirely congruent and have different biological substrates, they do not specify the differences in terms of immune factors or other CHD mechanisms. (I would also question whether depression should be categorized solely as an episodic factor in CHD, since chronic depression or dysthymia that lasts years or decades may contribute to the gradual development of atherosclerosis and coronary syndromes.)

In a fascinating paper, Ad Appels, the pioneer in VE research, collaborated with Karl Goodkin of the University of Miami to theorize about the biological correlates of VE and to plot a psychobiological time line with regard to initiation of CHD and onset of cardiac events (Goodkin and Appels 1997). In their view, the irritability associated with VE overlaps hostility, both psychologically and in terms of their biological correlates: both are associated with jumps in catecholamine secretion, which stimulates vasoconstriction, platelet clumping, and smooth muscle proliferation, all factors in CAD. But they also posit an indirect affect: such individuals have a hyperactive hypothalamic-pituitary-adrenal (HPA) axis, a key feature of a hair-trigger sympathetic nervous system, which generates chronic increments in catecholamines, particularly noradrenaline. These stress hormones dampen certain immune functions, such as lymphocyte proliferation and natural killer (NK) cell activity, defenses that otherwise prevent microbial infections, including reactivation of viruses such as CMV and HSV, that may contribute to CAD. Goodkin and Appels are persuaded by both the infectious and inflammatory theories of CHD; they believe that a compromised immune system allows for viral reactivation and bacterial invasion, the "first stage" in their two-stage model of CHD pathogenesis.

The second stage occurs when the individual becomes increasingly irritable and demoralized when beset by stressors, such as painful life events or prolonged overwork, and finally lapses into VE. Just as the person has been on overdrive, so has the HPA axis, and as the person becomes worn out, so too does the HPA axis. This is accompanied by a significant drop in the HPA signaling molecules corticotropin-releasing hormone (CRH, produced by the hypothalamus) and adrenocorticotropic hormone (ACTH, released by the pituitary), the stress hormone cortisol, and the glucocorticoids (Goodkin and Appels 1997). These biological characteristics are shared by other conditions of fatigue, including chronic fatigue syndrome and post-traumatic stress disorder (PTSD). Thus, under cumulative or severe stress the chronically hostile or irritable person becomes vitally exhausted, and his usually hyperactive sympathetic nervous system undergoes a concomitant collapse in the months prior to a cardiac event.

But what is the relevance of this collapse to CHD? Since chronically high levels of catecholamines, cortisol, and other stress hormones have been shown to contribute to CAD, would not a sudden reversal help the heart? According to Goodkin and Appels, the answer is no: the long-term damage caused by an overactive HPA axis and its by-products (excess stress hormones) has already been done; atherosclerotic plaques have flourished in the coronary arteries. But now the collapse leads to a new set of immune and cardiovascular conditions that are tantamount to pulling the trigger on a loaded gun.

Once a pathogen (bacteria such as *C. pneumoniae* and *Helicobacter pylori*, reactivated CMV or HSV, etc.) has been introduced into the body (and the coronary arteries), activated macrophages secrete proinflammatory cytokines, especially interleukin-1 (IL-1), interleukin-6 (IL-6), and tumor necrosis factor–alpha. These cytokines can enter the brain, where they interact with neurons, and at sufficiently high levels each of them can invoke fatigue. IL-1 effectively stimulates the HPA axis, but chronic stimulation eventually causes the HPA axis to wear down, leading to reductions in CRH, ACTH, and cortisol that are characteristic in people with VE

104   (Goodkin and Appels 1997). IL-6 is involved in the inflammatory response to tissue damage, including ulcerated arterial plaques; this inflammation may worsen the hazardous narrowing of coronary arteries. IL-6 is also a powerful inducer of acute-phase proteins, such as C-reactive protein, which is found in patients with acute coronary syndromes and predicts future risk in healthy people (Yudkin et al. 2000). This cytokine also activates monocytes (immune sentries) in the vessel wall, causing deposits of fibrinogen, a strong risk factor for CHD. Tumor necrosis factor–alpha (TNF-alpha) is not only associated with inflammation and fatigue; it is also linked to a rise in triglycerides (Dezube et al. 1993). In one recent study Ad Appels compared fifteen exhausted and fifteen nonexhausted patients about to undergo angioplasty and found that only the exhausted patients had elevated levels of IL-1 beta and TNF-alpha (Appels 1999). It is important to note that not only may VE "cause" excess proinflammatory cytokines but the release of these cytokines in response to pathogens may also "cause" VE. This insight exemplifies mind-body unity, since bidirectional relationships between psychological and physiological states are dialectical, not causal in the traditional, one-way model of cause and effect.

Another cytokine, interferon–alpha, is also elevated in people with chronic fatigue, and it too may have a role in CHD. It lowers corticotropin-releasing hormone in the body, which in turn depresses glucocorticoids, our natural anti-inflammatories (Saphier et al. 1993). By lowering glucocorticoids, elevated interferon-alpha may ultimately contribute to the low-grade inflammation that many investigators suspect in atherosclerosis and plaque disruption.

How important are proinflammatory cytokines in the development and course of CHD? Here is a sampling of the evidence:

- In a controlled study at Tel Aviv University patients with CAD had significantly higher serum levels of IL-1 beta than healthy matched control subjects (Hasdai et al. 1996).
- Investigators at the University of Colorado Health Sciences center excised fresh samples of heart muscle tissue from patients undergoing open-heart surgery, then suspended them in organ baths. They stimulated the live tissue with an electrical charge and measured the force with which it contracted. Next they added TNF-alpha and IL-1 beta to the bath, separately and then together, and remeasured the heart muscle responses. Both cytokines, separately and synergistically, were found to markedly depress human myocardial function (Cain et al. 1999).
- Italian researchers studied angina patients and conducted biological studies during the first two days after they were hospitalized. The patients with

unstable angina and/or a complicated in-hospital course had higher levels of IL-1 and IL-6 than those who had stable angina and/or an uncomplicated course (Biasucci et al. 1999).

Goodkin and Appels (1997) also believe that VE, like depression, is a condition in which the functions of the neurotransmitter serotonin are compromised. According to Redford Williams, reduced serotonin is behind a range of behavioral risk factors for CAD and MI, including addictive behaviors (smoking, excessive eating, and alcohol consumption) as well as chronic hostility, a hyperactive sympathetic nervous system, and a sluggish parasympathetic system (Williams 1994). Serotonin also stimulates the HPA axis, and people with a dearth of serotonin may be vulnerable to the HPA-depletion syndrome that Goodkin and Appels observe in vitally exhausted patients at risk for CHD. Goodkin and Appels also suspect a chain linkage between psychological distress, fatigue, low serum cholesterol, and biological events triggering MI, though their argument that low cholesterol is involved in the late stages of CHD does not appear to be well substantiated (Goodkin and Appels 1997).

Although Goodkin and Appels have written a speculative paper, the puzzle pieces fit together neatly, and a vast variety of studies—many of which they do not even cite—support their view that the biological concomitants of VE detonate the final processes leading to a heart attack, including neuroendocrine perturbations, excessive cytokine release, systemic inflammation, and possibly myocardial dysfunction. If chronic hostility and irritability set the stage by generating atherosclerosis, VE is the denouement, contributing to inflammation in the coronary arteries, thrombus formation, and plaque disruption, the immediate biological precursors of a heart attack.

DEPRESSION: THE ROLE OF NEUROHORMONE AND IMMUNE MECHANISMS

Just as the data on depression and CHD are the most substantive among all the psychosocial data, research on depression's role in the pathogenesis and progression of CHD is also, arguably, the most substantive among the biological studies.

To identify depression's role in CHD mechanisms, we can start by temporarily borrowing Goodkin and Appels's two-stage model, in which hostility and irritability (the latter being one feature of VE) contribute to atherosclerotic processes (stage 1), and a lapse into extreme fatigue and demoralization (full-fledged VE) accompanies the late phase in the pro-

106   gression of CHD, leading right up to a heart attack (stage 2). Depression has an impact on biological processes in both stage 1 and stage 2, but it also has a powerful influence in stage 3, the crucial period after a heart attack, which is not addressed by Goodkin and Appels.

Regarding stage 1 (the long-term development of atherosclerosis), there are ample data that depression is accompanied by high levels of cortisol (Gold et al. 1986; Yeith et al. 1994). (Researchers have shown that depressed individuals have elevated levels of CRH, which in turn raises their cortisol [Kop and Cohen 2001; Nemeroff et al. 1984]). As with hostility, irritability, and Type D distress, depression may be associated with sympathetic hyperactivity and decreased parasympathetic activity (Carney, Freedland, et al. 1995). Also, depressed people evidence greater platelet aggregation, and the combination of high cortisol (hypercortisolemia) and stickier platelets can promote development of atherosclerosis (Rozanski et al. 1999).

Conceivably, depression can also influence immune processes relevant to stage 1, the early to middle phases in the development of atherosclerotic plaques. (And there are some epidemiological data, cited above, linking depression and CHD risk in healthy populations.) Many studies have correlated depression with immune dysfunction, including a rise in peripheral leukocytes, decreased lymphocyte responsiveness, and weakened NK cells (Maes 1995). Clinically depressed patients also have raised antibodies to herpes viruses, including CMV, the viral infections that have been implicated (by some investigators) in the etiology of CAD. (This high level of antibodies is not a sign of adequate defenses; on the contrary, it indicates that T-cell immunity has faltered, viruses have reactivated, and antibodies are being produced in an effort to fight them.)

To a large extent, stage 1 depression is associated with immuno*suppression;* this may allow bacterial or viral infections involved in atherosclerosis to take root in the coronary arteries and perhaps in other tissues of the cardiovascular system. And those immune components that are *activated* during depression do not help; rather, they tend to make matters worse: greater numbers of leukocytes bind to the coronary artery endothelium via the action of adhesion molecules, a process that contributes to atherosclerosis (Kop et al. 1998). Platelets become stickier, and the complex process of fibrinolysis, the body's natural check against clot formation in the arteries, is impaired. For example, Parisian investigators found that clinically depressed CHD patients had significantly higher levels of plasminogen activator inhibitor ($p = .02$), a proven sign of impaired fibrinolysis (Lahlou-Laforet et al. 2001).

The role of depression shifts, at least partly, in stages 2 and 3. In a rough parallel to the model presented by Goodkin and Appels for VE, the depressed person may at first have an overactive sympathetic nervous system tied to a sluggish immune system, but this state of affairs gradually gives way to an "exhausted" sympathetic nervous system and an immune system that is hyperactive in some domains. As infectious processes take hold in the coronary arteries and elsewhere in the body, certain elements of the immune system try to compensate for the failures of antimicrobial defenses: macrophages become extremely active, and the proinflammatory cytokines are released by macrophages and other immune cells. Macrophages, which may also contribute at earlier stages of plaque development, produce enzymes (proteases) that lead to unstable coronary lesions (Kop and Cohen 2001), and these immune cells also secrete factors that promote thrombus formation (Libby and Hansson 1991).

In the section on VE I described the biological role of proinflammatory cytokines in the later stages of CAD. The data showing an inextricable link between depression and high levels of these cytokines are impressive. In a recent review paper Licinio and Wong, of the Clinical Neuroendocrinology Branch of the National Institutes of Health, noted that "over the years a body of evidence has been accumulated suggesting that major depression is associated with dysfunction of inflammatory mediators," and they cited "several lines of evidence that brain cytokines, principally IL-1 beta and IL-1 receptor antagonist may have a role in the biology of depression, and that they might additionally be involved in [its] pathophysiology and somatic consequences" (Licinio and Wong 1999). Licinio and Wong went so far as to say that inflammatory processes "could explain the biology of this disorder" and its "waxing and waning course."

What about a link between depression and elevated proinflammatory cytokines *specifically* in patients with CAD? One study addressed this very issue. In their comparison of fifteen exhausted and fifteen nonexhausted patients undergoing angioplasty (see above) Appels and colleagues also gauged depression, both as a general measure of distress and as a psychiatric disorder. Both indices of depression were associated with high levels of IL-1 beta, IL-6, and antibody titers to CMV, indicative of viral reactivation. A subset of patients with major depression had mean values of IL-1 beta, IL-6, antibodies to CMV, and antibodies to *C. pneumoniae* that were significantly higher than those of all other patients, including those who were exhausted but not overtly depressed (Appels, Bar, et al. 2000). The researchers concluded that "major depression in coronary patients is associated with markers of inflammation" and signs of infection with the very pathogens commonly implicated in CHD.

Such patients are at stage 2: they already have CAD, and they are at risk

108   for MI and CHD-related mortality. Exhaustion and depression are the best-studied risk factors at this stage. And depression is clearly the best-documented risk for poor outcome at stage 3, after a person has suffered a heart attack. (Note that Appels has not followed heart attack patients to see whether VE is a further risk for recurrence or fatality, as has been shown for depression. It remains to be seen whether VE is a true post-MI risk factor.) Biologically speaking, stages 2 and 3 overlap, because factors that cause vascular endothelial inflammation, thrombus formation, plaque rupture, and destabilizing arrhythmias can contribute to an initial MI, a recurrent or fatal MI, and SCA. The salient point here, as stated succinctly by Kop and Cohen (2001), is that "low-grade inflammation may alter the stability of atherosclerotic plaques . . . and increase the risk of plaque rupture leading to acute coronary syndromes."

But there is yet another mechanism that links depression with poor outcomes among MI patients: reduced heart rate variability. Compromised HRV has been shown to be a strong predictor of fatal outcome after MI (Bigger et al. 1992; Kleiger et al. 1987; Vaishnav et al. 1994). What is reduced HRV? According to the Swedish researchers Myriam Horsten, Kristina Orth-Gomer, and colleagues, "Decreased HRV could be conceptualized as a lack of ability to respond by physiological variability and complexity, making the individual physiologically rigid and, therefore, more vulnerable" (Horsten et al. 1999). Such patients have an underactive parasympathetic nervous system, which is supposed to govern the body's relaxation response—the counterbalance to sympathetic "fight or flight" stress responses. Poor *parasympathetic tone* is a signal finding among people with reduced HRV, whose autonomic nervous system is strikingly unbalanced in favor of sympathetic responses, and this is reflected in rigid (inflexible or invariable) cardiac function. This rigidity is a clear-cut contributor to ventricular arrhythmias. Put differently, we need parasympathetic tone and proper HRV to maintain the electrical stability of the heart (Hughes and Stoney 2000) and thus to prevent life-threatening arrhythmias.

Decreased HRV has been demonstrated in depressed psychiatric patients as well as in depressed cardiac patients (Carney, Saunders, et al. 1995; Dalack and Roose 1990; Krittayaphong et al. 1997; Rechlin et al. 1994). (Recall that other psychosocial predictors of CHD incidence or outcome have also been linked to decreased HRV, including Type A behavior or hostility and stress.) Even physically healthy individuals with depressed mood have reduced parasympathetic cardiac control (Hughes and Stoney 2000).

When HRV is dysfunctional in patients who have suffered an MI, electrical instability can lead to arrhythmias that are especially dangerous in these patients, who have significant coronary artery occlusion and compromised myocardial function. (This is why reduced HRV is a risk for poor outcomes after MI.) While not every facet of the depression–reduced HRV–arrhythmia risk–post-MI mortality equation has been proven, Frasure-Smith of McGill University came close in her eighteen-month follow-up of MI patients. She found that mildly to moderately depressed patients who also exhibited premature ventricular contractions (arrhythmias more common in people with reduced HRV) had an especially high risk of post-MI mortality (Frasure-Smith et al. 1995).

The intersecting pathways between depression, CHD incidence, MI risk, and poor MI outcome are inordinately complex, but the roads are being mapped, the street signs clarified, and the time course for each separate route estimated. No one pathway represents the clearest connection, since the most crowded (multifarious) routes are the ones that cause the most trouble, for example, when hemodynamic, hemostatic, neuroendocrine, immunological, and arrhythmogenic mechanisms coalesce, sequentially or coincidentally, in ways that cause the most "traffic" in the coronary arteries and the most breakdowns in myocardial function. While the maps are still being drawn, understanding that depression fuels much of this dangerous traffic is enough to help prevent catastrophic mishaps on the roads between the mind and the heart.

STRESS, SOCIAL SUPPORT, AND SES: TRIGGERS, BUFFERS, AND BACKDROPS

As noted above, stress, social support, and SES play different sorts of roles in CHD than those played by personality traits, emotional states, and emotional proclivities. Stress is a direct trigger; social support a potential buffer (and its lack a potential indirect risk); and SES a significant background variable causing chronic stress and emotional distress.

Mental stress can directly influence myocardial ischemia in the laboratory, although according to Rozanski and colleagues such ischemia is "usually electrocardiographically and clinically 'silent,' and generally occurs at relatively low heart rate elevations compared with exercise testing" (Rozanski et al. 1999). Moreover, mental stress tests do not yield nearly as much evidence of abnormalities in left ventricular wall motion (a key index of myocardial function) as do emotionally laden stress procedures, such as a speaking assignment concerning personal faults (Rozanski et al. 1988). Overall, only about half of CAD patients with exercise-induced myocardial ischemia also exhibit ischemia during mental stress testing. Relative to these findings, blood pressure elevations among CHD patients are

110   more consistently observed and often more dramatic during mental stress tests in the laboratory (Gottdiener et al. 1994; Rozanski et al. 1988). But do such laboratory fluctuations have much clinical relevance? One particularly impressive study showed that CAD patients who evidenced ischemia induced by mental stress were significantly more likely to suffer subsequent fatal and nonfatal cardiac events, above and beyond all medical predictors (Jiang et al. 1996).

Also, a range of animal and human studies demonstrate that acute stress can trigger cardiac arrhythmias. While electrical instability may be involved in many phases of CHD, it often plays a decisive part in post-MI recovery, and it is almost always the cause of SCA. In a review of his own research and of the vast literature in this area the renowned cardiologist Bernard Lown identified three primary conditions that contribute to arrhythmias: (1) an electrical instability of the myocardium, usually due to CAD; (2) an acute triggering event, often related to mental stress; and (3) a chronic, pervasive, intense psychological state, often including depression and hopelessness (Lown et al. 1977). While Lown's third condition, chronic stress, is difficult to study in the laboratory, it has been associated with elevated blood pressure (Schnall et al. 1990; Schnall et al. 1998) and higher levels of catecholamine and other stress hormones generated by the sympathetic nervous system (Cobb 1974; Theorell et al. 1988), factors especially implicated in the early to middle phases (stage 1) of atherosclerosis and CHD initiation.

The cardiovascular perturbations seen in socially isolated people or in people whose networks provide little emotional support are similar to those observed in both chronic and acute stress: high catecholamine levels (Seeman et al. 1994); elevated resting heart rates, a sign of sympathetic nervous system overactivation (Unden et al. 1991); and high blood pressure and an elevated heart rate in response to stressful stimuli (Gerin et al. 1992; Kamarck et al. 1990). These findings underscore that social support acts as a buffer against the cardiovascular ravages of severe short-term stress or persistent, emotionally debilitating stress. Perhaps the most convincing evidence comes from a study of post-MI patients in which those with high levels of life stress and social isolation had a twofold increased risk of recurrent cardiac events, while people with *both* high stress and low support had a fourfold increased risk (Freeman et al. 1987). The same negative synergy was observed among healthy people, who were significantly more likely to die from heart disease if they were both stressed and isolated (Rosengren et al. 1993).

While little research has directly evaluated the specific pathophysiological mechanisms linking low SES and heart disease, it is certain that low

SES contributes to social isolation, acute and chronic stress, hostility, anxiety, and depression. Therefore it is not difficult to theorize that the ways in which low SES gets "under the skin" and into the heart are directly related to mechanisms associated with isolation, stress, and profound emotional distress.

A Process Model of Psychosocial Factors and Heart Disease

The purpose of the process model presented here is to clarify and reconcile the disparate findings, data, and theories regarding psychosocial factors in heart disease. As I have argued, without such a model one is left with a grab bag of negative emotional states, psychiatric disorders, and maladaptive personality traits, as if any or all could influence heart disease at virtually any stage in its pathological unfolding. In the first two sections of this chapter I painstakingly laid out the scientific evidence regarding psychosocial influences on CHD because the model I present is founded on this evidence, and without a map based on data this model would be pure theoretical speculation. Though I will rely on speculative theory to fill in gaps and to flesh out psychodynamics that have not (and perhaps cannot) be studied in experimental, cross-sectional, or prospective studies, I believe the model is justified by scientific evidence as well as by the theories of seminal figures in psychoanalysis and psychosomatics.

I call this model an *integrative* process model because it attempts to explain disparate findings in mind-body-cardiology research by integrating multiple factors, primarily social or situational factors, psychological factors, and the psychobiological (or mind-body) mechanisms that connect mind and heart (see fig. 3.1). The notion of a *process* model, which emphasizes the unfolding of coping processes over time, is based largely upon the work of Susan Folkman and Richard Lazarus (1988). But the particular process model presented here is also greatly influenced by Lydia Temoshok's visionary 1987 paper, in which she attempted to elucidate (and integrate) disparate findings in psychosocial research on cancer by showing how characteristic coping processes are multileveled; subject to changes with the vicissitudes of stress, life events, and illness itself; and inextricably bound to biological processes.

The process model seeks to reconcile discrepancies and resolve uncertainties in the annals of mind-body-heart research. Surveying this literature, one is struck by the current state of the evidence: hostility is well documented as a fairly strong risk factor for developing CHD, while depression is moderately well documented as a modest risk factor. There are now substantial data that depression is a powerful risk for recurrence

Psychobiological [Mind-Body] Mechanisms

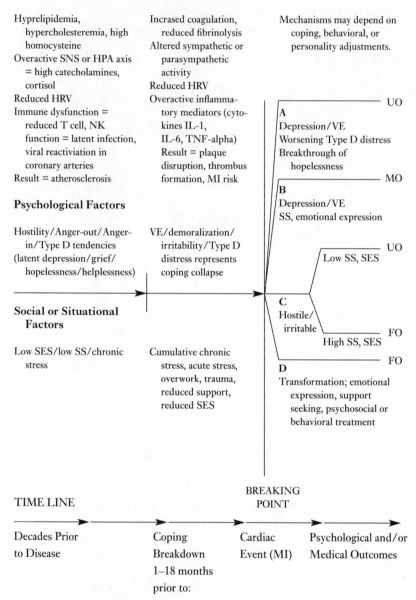

Hyprelipidemia, hypercholesteremia, high homocysteine
Overactive SNS or HPA axis = high catecholamines, cortisol
Reduced HRV
Immune dysfunction = reduced T cell, NK function = latent infection, viral reactiviation in coronary arteries
Result = atherosclerosis

Incrased coagulation, reduced fibrinolysis
Altered sympathetic or parasympathetic activity
Reduced HRV
Overactive inflammatory mediators (cytokines IL-1, IL-6, TNF-alpha)
Result = plaque disruption, thrombus formation, MI risk

Mechanisms may depend on coping, behavioral, or personality adjustments.

—————————— UO

A
Depression/VE
Worsening Type D distress
Breakthrough of hopelessness

—————————— MO

B
Depression/VE
SS, emotional expression

Psychological Factors

Hostility/Anger-out/Anger-in/Type D tendencies (latent depression/grief/hopelessness/helplessness)

VE/demoralization/irritability/Type D distress represents coping collapse

—————————— UO

Low SS, SES

Social or Situational Factors

Low SES/low SS/chronic stress

Cumulative chronic stress, acute stress, overwork, trauma, reduced support, reduced SES

C
Hostile/irritable

High SS, SES

—————————— FO

—————————— FO

D
Transformation; emotional expression, support seeking, psychosocial or behavioral treatment

BREAKING
POINT

TIME LINE

Decades Prior to Disease

Coping Breakdown 1–18 months prior to:

Cardiac Event (MI)

Psychological and/or Medical Outcomes

Key: FO = favorable outcome; HRV = heart rate variability; MO = mixed outcome; SES = socioeconomic status; SNS = sympathetic nervous sytem; SS = social support; UO = unfavorable outcome; VE = vital exhaustion

FIGURE 3.1 Process Model of Psychosocial Factors in Coronary Heart Disease

or death after a heart attack; there is some evidence, but not much, that hostility is a risk for poor outcomes after an MI. The evidence that VE precedes a heart attack by a few months to a year and a half is highly persuasive, and there are solid data that Type D traits—the copresence of negative emotion and inhibition—pose another risk for poor outcome after a diagnosis of CHD.

How does all this piece together? Why is hostility a risk for developing CHD, and why is depression a risk for poor post-MI outcomes? And why is hostility only a questionable risk for poor post-MI outcomes, and depression only a modest risk for developing CHD? Finally, given the increased CHD risk associated with hostility, clearly some (if not many) hostile individuals become depressed after an MI and consequently have a poorer outcome. What, if any, is the connection between pre-MI hostility and post-MI depression?

An integrative process model that is avowedly interpretive yet consistent with the extant data can explain these seeming discrepancies by demonstrating the following:

1. Cardiovascular health depends upon maintenance of mind-heart homeostasis.
2. Hostility, anxiety, Type D coping, VE, and depression disturb mind-heart homeostasis through differing (and sometimes overlapping) psychobiological mechanisms, some of which are more relevant to particular stages in the development of CHD.
3. Hostility, a proven CHD risk factor, is a defensive way of being in the world that often masks latent depressive tendencies, including unconscious hopelessness, helplessness, fear, or grief. Also, hostility is not synonymous with anger; indeed, it represents unexpressed or unresolved anger and can show itself as a tendency to either seethe or explode.
4. Anxiety, a less proven but still compelling risk factor for CHD, may cover the same latent depressive tendencies underlying hostility. (It may also overlap hostile "seething" tendencies.)
5. Type D personality—negative emotions coupled with social inhibition—is a construct consistent with dispositional hostility, anxiety, and latent depressive tendencies and may be present in some form during every phase of CHD development and progression.
6. Depression or hopelessness plays a role in the etiology of the disease, but long-term studies of physically healthy people have shown mixed results because in this population depression is frequently *masked* by anxiety, irritability, or hostility and therefore often is not detected by standard depression scales.

114   7. Over time, painful life events, social stressors, and cumulative stress in work
or relationships can strain hostile, anxious, or defensive coping to the
breaking point, until the individual lapses into VE. Low SES exacerbates
all of these environmental factors. VE may occur when a traumatic event
or sudden confluence of stressful events tear at the fabric of the person's
basic coping structure.

8. VE—fatigue, irritability, demoralization—represents a nearly total (and in
some cases total) collapse of hostile, anxious, or defensive coping mechanisms that helped the person maintain a superficial psychosocial and biological homeostasis. (Hostile or defensive coping is associated with relational instability, as well as with the silent pathogenesis of coronary artery
disease. One can get by with these simmering troubles for a long time, but
probably not forever.)

9. There are two common, related scenarios for heart attacks during a period of vital exhaustion, a fragile mind-body state in which MI risk factors (sympathetic hyperreactivity followed by underactivity, subclinical infection, low-grade inflammation, and reduced HRV) are dangerously
intensified. The exhausted person can suffer an MI when a confluence of
these mechanisms leads to thrombus formation, plaque disruption, or malignant arrhythmias. The second scenario is roughly the same, except here
an acute attack of anxiety or unbridled anger suddenly provokes sympathetic nervous system–mediated mechanisms, leading to plaque disruption
or cardiac arrhythmias. The result is incipient MI or SCA.

10. While VE represents a serious disruption of the person's characteristic coping capacities, the collapse is often complete with the onset of a heart attack and sometimes even with a diagnosis of severe CHD. This is the breaking point, a pivotal time when already strained coping capacities are
severely challenged by a life-threatening circumstance. The individual may
follow several paths toward recovery (e.g., restructured or transformed coping and restoration of homeostasis) or ill health (e.g., further coping collapse, psychophysiological imbalance, and a perilous disease course).

11. After a heart attack or diagnosis of severe CHD there are roughly four different psychological paths the person may take, with differing biological substrates and likely psychological as well as medical outcomes. They include:

A. After the trauma of a heart attack, which may occur after months of fatigue and demoralization, latent depressive tendencies emerge in the
form of depressive symptoms or major depressive disorder. VE continues or worsens. The individual, once an anxious or hostile coper, may
not have sought social support as a habitual means of handling stress.
A continuing inability to procure support exacerbates the depression by

fostering further isolation and reducing his or her ability to get practical and emotional help. The individual is therefore troubled by negative feelings that he or she is unable to share or express (Type D). Under conditions of low SES, stress and isolation are intensified. Such depression is associated with specific coronary perturbations that increase the risk of poor medical outcomes.

B. After the trauma of a heart attack, the latent depressive tendencies emerge in the form of depressive symptoms, and VE continues. The person, once an anxious or hostile coper, has not habitually sought social support but, because of the dire nature of his or her condition, reaches out to others for emotional support, which represents a change from his or her Type D tendency of social inhibition. (Alternatively, the person may not have been as socially isolated to begin with and therefore seeks support in this time of intense emotional distress and physical infirmity.) Denial can also be an effective stopgap measure in the postcrisis period. Moderate to high SES may also buffer the stress of illness. It may not eliminate depressive symptoms, but it can prevent severe, unremitting clinical depression. Thus, despite the breakthrough of latent depression, social support and favorable social or situational variables provide the person with somewhat more favorable psychological and medical outcomes.

C. After the trauma of a heart attack, the person continues to engage in hostile or defensive coping and remains in a state of VE (which includes irritability and demoralization), though he or she may not lapse into clinical depression. There are two tributaries within this coping pathway. In the first, the person is also beset by conditions of low SES and social isolation. If he or she does not (or cannot) change sufficiently to express emotions and seek social support, the distress will be neither relieved nor resolved (characteristic Type D behavior). Such an individual, while not clinically depressed, may still have an unfavorable psychological and medical outcome. In the second tributary, the person also remains hostile or defensive and continues with Type D behavior but is not beset by conditions of low SES and is more socially integrated. He or she receives more support to buffer his or her distress and may also use denial as an effective stopgap in the aftermath of medical crisis. Such an individual has a relatively more favorable outcome.

D. After the trauma of the heart attack, latent depressive tendencies and underlying emotional states (fear, grief, sadness, anger, regret) may come to the fore, but the health crisis motivates a transformation. Recognizing the brush with mortality, the person acknowledges his or her primary emotions, seeks social support, and pursues active efforts to

116   change behavior, relationships, work life, and so on. Put differently, the individual recognizes aspects of his or her prior defensiveness and Type D tendency and now seeks to loosen the grip of social or emotional inhibition on his or her own psyche and behavior. The person may pursue behavioral or psychological treatments that further facilitate his or her efforts to express emotions, manage stress, seek meaning in work and relationships, or engage in spiritual growth. This transformative path is associated with the most favorable psychological and medical outcomes.

These eleven points represent the essence of the process model. In the following section I paint a fuller portrait of the coronary-prone individual and differentiate those people with favorable outcomes from those people with mixed or unfavorable outcomes. A process model must account for the fact that people at risk for CHD, like any population, are complex individuals with multileveled personalities and layers of emotionality whose behavior and emotional states change in response to life events, social environment, and stress, including the stress of illness itself. In the case of the coronary-prone individual, he or she brings fairly stable traits (person variables) to any encounter or stressful occurrence, such as hostility or a Type D tendency toward negative affectivity and inhibition. In the wake of a coronary event the person may persist with these characteristic coping styles; make minor shifts; or make significant alterations (Folkman and Lazarus [1988] call this "coping as a process").

How the person handles novel challenges is based not on a rigid equation (coping trait + stressor = coping reaction) but rather on an understanding of the subtle interplay of traits, states, and social circumstances, with due deference to the possibility of surprising outcomes, as when people dramatically alter their usual coping style after a life-threatening diagnosis. Indeed, how a person copes with uniquely challenging circumstances may, in turn, mediate how he or she responds emotionally. (Folkman and Lazarus [1988] call this "coping as a mediator of emotional states.") These ongoing changes in coping, be they perceptible or imperceptible, adaptive or maladaptive, conscious or unconscious, regressive or transformative, will simultaneously influence emotional states and cardiovascular health via psychobiological pathways that are increasingly well understood.

THE DRAMA OF THE CORONARY-PRONE PERSONALITY

An integrative process model such as the one shown in figure 3.1 is essentially a chronological narrative rendered in a biomedical context. It is an unfolding story with a setup, a climax, a denouement, and an ending that can be tragic, triumphant, or ambiguous. The model presented here must account for different sorts of "protagonists," characters with unique traits who may ultimately take different paths. However, like dramatists, I am primarily concerned with certain universal truths. In this instance I focus on how the psyche is involved in heart disease, and the data support a narrative consistent with the stories of heart patients who are subject to strikingly similar psychological conflicts and coping conundrums. In this model, which deals with people who do develop CHD, the greatest variance occurs after the breaking point of a heart attack or cardiac event, when patients can proceed in a variety of directions that help determine how the story will end.

The process model is summarized by the eleven points listed above; the following sections flesh out the "story" of the mind's complex role in heart disease.

HOSTILITY, TYPE D DEFENSIVENESS, AND ANXIETY COVER LATENT DEPRESSION

Based on the extant data, it is my contention that hostility, defensive (Type D) coping, and anxiety, separately and in various admixtures, are the primary psychosocial risk factors for developing CHD, enduring traits and chronic states associated with the development of CAD over years and decades. While the data on anxiety as a long-term risk are not as substantial as those on hostility, the research focus on anxiety is more recent, so fewer studies have been conducted. (I will return to anxiety's role with an argument that anxiety and hostility share psychodynamic and psychobiological features that help explain why both are CHD risk factors.)

What is hostility, and why is it a risk factor for CHD? These elementary questions are too often neglected. As I argued in a previous section, hostility is frequently confused with anger, a primary emotion. But hostility is not a primary emotion; it is a complex of attitudes, a cognitive style that both contains and distorts emotion. When anger is consciously recognized as a signal of something amiss in one's internal or external environment, and constructively expressed, it can be a positive psychic force, enabling the person to maintain mind-body homeostasis (Temoshok and Dreher 1992). In *Freedom and Destiny* Rollo May (1981) distinguishes between anger and forms of hostility:

> In our society, we confuse anger with resentment, a form of repressed anger that eats steadily at our innards. In resentment we store up "am-

munition" to get even with our fellows, but we never communicate directly in a way that might solve the problem. This transformation of anger into resentment is, as Nietszche so emphatically proclaimed, the sickness of the middle class. It corrodes our stature as human beings.

Or we confuse anger with temper, which is generally an explosion of repressed anger; with rage, which may be a pathological anger; with petulance, which is childish resentment; or with hostility, which is anger absorbed into our character structure until it infects every act of ours.

When anger is repressed below the level of awareness; misconstrued; turned against the self; or turned against others—which is a fair description of hostile or defensive traits—in time it becomes a deleterious psychic force, one that ultimately disrupts mind-body (and cardiovascular) homeostasis. Whether the hostile person holds anger in (resentment) or acts it out (rage), he or she does not constructively manage, express, or resolve anger. For the hostile individual, anger is a dangerous powder keg rather than a useful set of psychophysical signs guiding him or her towards adaptive means of expression (emotion-focused coping) and problem-solving. The person either sits on the powder keg or allows it to intermittently explode, but he or she never subdues the threat, which is often intrapsychic rather than external. In his book about heart health the psychiatrist Alexander Lowen (1988) describes the various distortions of anger in the hostile personality: "When anger is suppressed, resentments build up. When they, too, are denied, the underlying anger smolders like a slumbering volcano, manifesting its existence by little puffs of steam—in the form of irritability or critical remarks—that escape through the cracks in the crust. But in many of these people, continued frustrations can raise the energy of the inner fire to an explosive level, resulting in the breakthrough of an irrational and exaggerated response. Expressing their rage doesn't free them, because their reaction is so arbitrary it makes them feel guilty, which fans the flames of their hostility all over again."

That said, hostility may enable a person to maintain superficial psychic stability for a long time. As noted earlier, hostile types either seethe (anger-in) or explode (anger-out), but these behavior patterns are rarely so unfettered that they prevent the person from functioning. On the contrary, the hostile individual who is flooded by angry impulses (among other emotions) may gain stability by keeping these impulses at bay (anger-in) or letting off steam (anger-out). Moreover, since he or she may be threatened by feelings of helplessness or hopelessness, all stemming from disappointments in past or present relationships, the person gains a measure of stability by keeping people at bay. With his or her simmering resentments and sense of victimization, the hostile person surely has trouble sustaining relationships rooted in trust. (Hostility researchers often use the term *cynical mistrust* to characterize the relational dimension of hostility.) Thus, for the hostile individual, intimacy can be a threat, so maintaining social distance is actually a coping strategy, albeit a short-sighted and ultimately detrimental one.

The process model reveals that a coping style that maintains psychic, biological, and social homeostasis at one stage of life can outlive its utility. Under changed circumstances this same coping style becomes explicitly maladaptive. Most often this occurs when the original adaptation is a response to extreme stress or trauma. The coping mechanism helps sustain psychic equilibrium for a prolonged period, but when the person is far removed from the trauma by time, the original strategy becomes more of a hindrance than a help (Dreher 1995a; Temoshok 1987). A perfect example is dissociation: a person whose life has been threatened by physical or sexual abuse often splits off overwhelming emotions (i.e., rage, grief, and terror) that threaten to cause psychic disintegration. Here, dissociation is a psychic survival strategy, but if it continues for years, it becomes the very source of severe emotional and relational disturbance, as well as psychiatric disorder. So it is with hostile or defensive coping. Strained to the breaking point by cumulative stress, trauma, profound disappointment, or extreme overwork, hostile or defensive coping outlives its (fragile) functionality. It may even become wholly ineffective at helping the person maintain a semblance of psychic stability.

Although Johan Denollet does not explicitly try to reconcile hostility and the Type D personality, it seems apparent that Type D negative affectivity includes irritability and that Type D social inhibition includes keeping others at a distance, being closed and reserved, and so on. These traits are often observed among hostile or defensive personalities, particularly the anger-in types described in heart disease studies. Denollet also captures the tension within the coronary-prone personality, who experiences negative emotions but is socially inhibited, defensively disinclined to express or communicate his anger, unhappiness, or sense of isolation.

While everyone's psyche is layered (if one accepts the tenets of ego psychology as opposed to animal psychology), mind-body-heart research suggests that certain prototypical layers—hostility, anxiety, covert depression—are shared by these individuals. (I use the word *suggests* because biobehavioral studies are not designed to tease out these psychodynamic layers; for the most part, they must be inferred.) What do I mean by layers? For instance, I have asserted that the hostile individual is likely to have latent depressive tendencies as a result of unconscious hopelessness, help-

120 lessness, fear, or grief. I base this assertion on psychoanalytic thinking, particularly from the schools of object relations and self-psychology, but this requires some elaboration.

While debates abound among members of differing schools, many thinkers (such as Fairburn, Kohut, Guntrip, and Suttie) regard hostile aggressiveness not as a biological drive or instinct (as did Freud and many of his acolytes) but rather as a frustrated assertiveness in early relations with love objects (mother and father, usually in that order). In his overview of psychoanalytic theories of aggression Salman Akhtar (1999) cites the theories of Ian Suttie: "Suttie proposed that after an early phase of 'infantile solipsism,' the child undergoes a process of 'psychic parturition' through which it becomes capable of independent existence. During this process, the need for the mother's love is intense, hence the vulnerability of separation anxiety. Anger or hate is 'a development or intensification of separation-anxiety which in turn is roused by a threat against love. It is the maximal ultimate appeal in the child's power. . . . Its purpose is not death-seeking or death-dealing, but the preservation of the self from the isolation which is death, and the restoration of a love relationship.'"

Hence the original hate-filled impulse is a response to "a threat against love" and an effort on the part of the child to exercise his or her power to "restore" the "love relationship." Unless that exercise of power is met with gratification, and the separation anxiety is ultimately resolved through an affirmed attachment, the anger or hate reaction can become "absorbed into [the] character structure." When childhood experiences of attempted attachment to love objects are ultimately frustrating, if not traumatic, hostility may indeed become anchored in the person's character structure (Lowen 1988). The relational psychoanalyst Stephen Mitchell says that aggressive traits develop early in defense of an "endangered self" (Mitchell 1993).

From a different perspective, cognitive-oriented researchers have come to fairly similar conclusions about the origins of hostility. Houston and Vavak (1991) acknowledge that hostility begins in childhood as feelings of insecurity coupled with negative attitudes toward others. They further contend that such attitudes are a consequence of parental behavior that (1) lacks genuine acceptance; (2) is overly strict, critical, and demanding of conformity; and (3) is inconsistent with regard to discipline. Meyer Friedman, developer of the Type A construct, increasingly came to view childhood losses as the psychic source of hostility and time urgency: "We now believe that one of the most important influences . . . is the failure of the Type A person to receive unconditional love, affection, and encouragement from one or both parents" (Friedman and Ulmer 1984).

In psychoanalytic parlance, a person may develop trait hostility due to a range of disturbances in early bonding with parents. A number of clinicians and researchers working with heart patients have identified "heartbreak," usually stemming from childhood experiences but also stemming from recent losses, at the core of the hostile patient's character structure (Lowen 1988; Lynch 1977; Sinatra 1996). In their view, hostility is both an expression of and a defense against a deeper disappointment, and its growth is fueled by a learned conviction that one cannot trust love objects to sustain attachment. In time the hostile or defensive person shields from his own consciousness a profound hopelessness that relationships can bestow emotional gratification. (Such hopelessness may be even more profound when the person is subject to early physical or sexual abuse.) Now, the notion of hostility as a psychological defense goes well beyond the constructs measured and tested in biobehavioral studies of heart disease. But I believe this leap is necessary to understand the temporal arc of the drama of the coronary-prone individual. Turning to the psychoanalytic literature, it is entirely plausible that coping styles and emotions can be defenses against other emotions. As Leo Rangell (1995) writes:

> Affects, in addition to being motives for defense, can also themselves be defended against as derivatives of instinctual drives. They can serve as defenses as well as be defended against. Lewin . . . has described the utilization of screen affects as a defense against other repressed elements, and Greenson . . . has written about the defensive aspects of moods clinically and in life. Affects can also become ego-dystonic symptoms in their own right, coming about, like other symptoms, by compromise formations between the id and the ego. *As symptom complexes they can be further repressed, so that a person may, for example, become aware only during analysis, following the undoing of defenses, of the existence of chronic depression or an anxiety state.* (italics mine)

This leads me to the avowedly theoretical but nevertheless psychologically grounded contention that most temperamentally hostile and/or defensive individuals (and, as I will argue shortly, those beset by anxiety) suffer from latent depression. Before defining this term, I reiterate that clinical depression has in some epidemiological studies been shown to increase the risk of developing CHD. But these studies are fewer and less robust than studies linking depression and poor post-MI prognosis, supporting the theory that since high-risk individuals are more likely to have *latent* (rather than overt) depression, it would not likely be detected by standard depression scales. Depression may indeed contribute to the onset of CHD, through mechanisms I have cited, but for most people the effect

122   would be subterranean: the depression is underground, and so are the pathways linking it to CAD. Therefore, one would find some (weak, modest, or inconsistent) associations between depression and incident CHD, reflecting the presence of subjects with severe clinical depression and not those (in the majority) with subclinical or latent depression.

Support for this thesis comes from a study of 114 patients with diagnosed CAD (but not MI) in which researchers at the Washington University School of Medicine in St. Louis concluded that the patients' depressive symptoms, measured by a standard questionnaire, were "relatively mild and nonspecific"; they even found this to be true among a subgroup with major depression diagnosed by a psychiatrist (Freedland et al. 1992). The finding suggests that many pre-MI heart patients have "mild" depression and that pencil-and-paper depression tests will not adequately detect subclinical or latent depression.

What is meant by *latent depression?* The comparable idea of "masked depression" has been propounded for decades, mostly in the context of somatization, the condition of patients with chronic illness or unexplained physical symptoms found to suffer from a subclinical depression of which they are unaware (Bschor 2000; Posse and Hallstrom 1998; Verster and Gagiano 1995). More recently, the *Diagnostic and Statistical Manual of Mental Disorders, Third Edition (DSM-III)* has subsumed what once was called "masked depression" under other categories, including "non-melancholic depression" (Parker et al. 1998). But one investigator argues that masked depression is still relevant, as a "condition in which the classic affective and cognitive symptoms of depression are hidden behind a variety of somatic complaints or behavioral problems" (Verster and Gagiano 1995). After examining these studies, I concluded that hostility represents just such a complex of cognitive-behavioral problems that mask underlying depression.

The hostile or defensive person, whose relational stance is one of cynical mistrust, is likely to have suffered in childhood from disturbed or nonexistent attachment to love objects that left him with unresolved grief, the psychic wellspring of depression. The notion that early unresolved grief is a contributor to adult depression is well founded (Luecken 2000; Zisook and DeVaul 1985), and most psychoanalytic theorists believe that grief in response to disturbed or missing attachments can be as powerful a shaper of adult personality and behavior as the actual loss (death) of a parent or caregiver. In Luecken's study of thirty university students who had experienced the death of a parent before age sixteen, along with thirty-one control subjects, there was a significantly higher level of depression, poor social support, and hostility among subjects who not only had lost a parent but also reported poor-quality family relationships in childhood (Luecken 2000). Those students who had lost a parent but reported good family relationships did not display these maladaptive traits—strong evidence that attachment quality is critical: it can enable a child to psychically overcome the actual death of a parent.

The hostile character does not readily become aware of his or her depression (and the underlying, unresolved grief); it threatens to disintegrate the internal psychic barriers he or she has unconsciously erected in order to remain in that strenuous state of homeostasis, what Lydia Temoshok, referring to the putative cancer-prone pattern, calls "a fragile accommodation to the world" (Temoshok and Dreher 1992). When the person's hostile or defensive coping is severely strained by external circumstances, the latent depression begins to emerge. (This depression is not the same as the primary emotions—grief, sadness, or anger—associated with childhood losses; depression is the affective and vegetative result of unprocessed, deflected, or repressed primary emotions [Lowen 1993]). This emergence frequently occurs in two stages: first, when life events overwhelm the person's coping capacities, and second, when the person suffers a heart attack.

In sum, hostility develops as both a coping strategy and a defense against early losses, or, put in psychoanalytic terms, disordered or nonexistent attachments to primary objects (i.e., parents). The initial aggressive impulse is a howl of protest, an effort to meet relational needs. This changes across developmental stages: among anger-out types the childhood aggression gives way to chronic anger, in which the typical response to stressful (and eventually even nonstressful) encounters is reactive rage. Among anger-in types aggression goes underground, but the person seethes with hostile thoughts and fantasies. In both cases the person's relational stance—shutting people out—leaves him more isolated, reinforcing cynical mistrust and loneliness. And in both cases the person repetitively overreacts to stressful stimuli, and so does his sympathetic nervous system, which eventually goes into perpetual overdrive, with all the attendant neuroendocrine and immune dysregulation (described above) involved in long-term CAD development.

Whether the resentment simmers or explodes, it covers a grief or sadness that had been banished to the unconscious and was therefore never "worked through." The ongoing hostile or defensive or Type D behavior becomes locked in; attitudes of cynicism, wariness, victimization, and wounded narcissism take deeper root in the personality. (By all accounts, conditions of low SES cause or exacerbate early losses, reduce social support, and foster traits of hostility and anxiety [Williams 1998].) The un-

124   conscious hopeless-helpless complex never comes fully into awareness, where it might be explored and perhaps resolved. In time, it transmogrifies into a chronic, latent (or masked) depression. This depression and the range of emotions it deflects (primarily grief but also authentic anger and sorrow) may only emerge when the hostile or defensive or Type D coping structure becomes ineffective under the weight of cumulative or traumatic stress.

Finally, anxiety may turn out to be as powerful a risk factor for CHD incidence as hostility. If it holds up as a CHD risk in further longitudinal studies, it may be that anxiety (including the major disorders—phobia, panic, social anxiety, obsessive-compulsive disorder, PTSD, and generalized anxiety) is similar to hostility in the following respects: (1) it is both an affective symptom of and a defense against deeper emotions of fear, anger, and grief that have been banished to the unconscious; (2) these underlying affects stem largely from early loss, abuse, or frustrated attachments; (3) it is consistent with Type D irritability, defensiveness, and difficulty procuring social support; and (4) its chronic forms are associated with easy arousal of the sympathetic nervous system, impaired immune functions, reduced serotonergic function, increased stress hormones, impaired autonomic control of the heart, and heightened cardiovascular reactivity to stress—all physiological factors in CHD.

It remains to be seen what types of anxiety contribute significantly to the onset of CHD. The largest studies showing a positive relationship have linked phobic anxiety (Kawachi, Colditz, et al. 1994; Kawachi, Sparrow, et al. 1994) and generalized worry (Kubzansky et al. 1997) to incident CHD. Several early studies correlated the coronary-prone Type A complex with high trait anxiety, an ingrained tendency toward anxious responses to stress (Langeluddecke and Tennant 1986; Smith et al. 1983). Conceptually, coronary-prone anxiety may be consistent with the personality construct identified by Weinberger et al. (1979) as "defensive high-anxious," which combines high manifest anxiety with high scores on a social desirability scale. Based on descriptions in the literature, these are anxious, often irritable individuals who closely resemble Denollet's Type Ds: they combine strong negative emotional states with social inhibition. By definition, this form of anxiety, a state of psychobiological tension, is clearly associated with the biological risks cited in the mechanisms section, above. And depending on a host of genetic, familial, and social factors, defensive high-anxious individuals may also evidence hostility. But whether or not they are also hostile, defensive high-anxious individuals have a mind-body profile that is consistent with unresolved underlying affects and with biological mechanisms implicated in CHD.

Further long-term studies ought to evaluate CHD risk among people who evidence high anxiety (particularly Type D or defensive high-anxiety), among people who score high on hostility measures, and those who score high in both. In my view, studies that give weight to measures of both anxiety and hostility may find an even more robust set of predictors for CHD. Put differently, if people who exhibit anxiety, people who exhibit hostility, and people who exhibit both are placed into one pool, the relative risks may be considerably higher than those found in previous efforts to uncover psychosocial traits in the onset of CHD.

VITAL EXHAUSTION, A BREAKDOWN IN COPING, SETS THE STAGE

The strong evidence that a heart attack or other cardiac event is preceded by vital exhaustion—extreme fatigue, irritability, and demoralization—suggests that the person's characteristic coping style is no longer working. This hypothesis was set forth explicitly by Goodkin and Appels (1997): "An enduring state of exhaustion as opposed to chronic hostility—a long term risk factor—has been found to be a more proximal precursor of myocardial infarction. The strength of the association with exhaustion suggests that this behavioral factor reflects not only a breakdown in adaptation but also the disease process itself." Goodkin and Appels present evidence for a reverberating circuit between coping breakdown and its psychological correlates, on the one hand, and CHD development and its biological correlates, on the other. (This raises chicken-or-egg questions about whether psychological factors drive physiology, or vice versa. But Goodkin and Appels, appropriately, opt for a "mind-body unity" answer: the relationships are dynamic, bidirectional, and simultaneous; in other words, mind and body respond in a unified, organismic fashion to the internal and external flow of events.)

Psychologically, the hostile or defensive individual may be able to function adequately for prolonged periods of time. But the person is vulnerable to coping breakdowns because his or her character defenses are often too rigid to allow him or her to acknowledge and work through denied affects; seek adequate social support; or develop problem-solving strategies that depend on social integration, such as cultivating teamwork with colleagues in a stressful work environment. These vulnerabilities set the individual up for vital exhaustion. This thesis is largely similar to one posited by a leading investigator in psychosocial CHD research, Timothy W. Smith of the University of Utah. Smith posits a number of models to help explain how hostility influences CHD, including the "psychosocial vulnerability model," the "psychophysiological reactivity model," and lastly,

126 a synthesis of the two, the "transactional model" (Miller et al. 1996; Smith 1994). The psychosocial vulnerability model "suggests that adults with hostility have lower levels of social support, higher levels of intrapersonal stress, and more stressful life events." What is important here is that hostile or defensive coping causes a range of difficulties in relationships that exacerbate intrapsychic distress. A longitudinal study by Todd Q. Miller and colleagues found that high scores on an irritability scale, which taps dimensions of hostile or defensive behavior, predicted heavy levels of drinking, somatic symptoms associated with depression (more evidence of the "latent depression" thesis), negative feelings associated with intrapersonal stressors, divorce, marital separation, not being married at follow-up, and the dissolution of serious nonmarital relationships (Miller et al. 1995). Smith's psychophysiological model identifies heightened sympathetic reactivity as the link between hostility and heart disease, while his transactional model integrates and extends these two models into a coherent picture of mind-body factors in CHD. As a summary statement (Miller et al. 1996) reveals,

> For [the transactional] model, hostile cognitive-emotional states (e.g., mistrust and expectations of hostility from others) are expected to lead to antagonistic and aggressive behaviors that produce intrapersonal conflict and hostility from others, which, in turn, leads to a reduction in social support and more negative affect. Thus, hostile attitudes serve to create a self-fulfilling prophecy for the mistrusting, hostile individual by producing a hostile environment that is a result of their own initiation of intrapersonal conflict and aggressive reactions from others.
>
> The transactional model also extends the cardiovascular reactivity model by suggesting that hostile individuals not only have increased reactivity under stress but display increased reactivity to self-imposed stressors (Smith 1994). For example, they may display reactivity when individuals are present whom they mistrust. Thus, the transactional model suggests that a hostile individual's negative thoughts and actions toward others produce CHD by increasing the number of heightened cardiovascular reactivity responses and episodes of intrapersonal conflict.

As Smith's model shows, the hostile person sows the seeds of his own homeostatic undoing by engaging in behaviors that reinforce his alienation, isolation, and distress. The above is an elegant description of how hostile or defensive copers function for decades until their social fabric is badly shredded, if not wholly destroyed, leaving them with cumulative internal distress. While Smith describes the cardiovascular consequences of this pattern, he does not extend his model to explain other psychosocial variables on the CHD time line, including VE and depression. But one can draw clear inferences from his work to make these connections. Specifically, hostile individuals frequently lack the personal and social resources that would enable them to make fundamental changes in coping style, leaving them vulnerable to the coping breakdown described so graphically by Appels in his work on vital exhaustion: a wholesale lapse into exhaustion, irritability, and demoralization. The same vulnerability applies to anxious and defensive high-anxious individuals, who may not experience the same levels of intrapersonal stress delineated in Smith's models of hostility but who create a different set of self-fulfilling prophecies: persistent fears, phobias, and worries may extend to the social realm, disabling the person from pursuing social support (e.g., due to fear of rejection or alienation) and assertive problem solving. And the defensive high-anxious person, in particular, lives with high-wire tension. As Larry Jamner, Hoyle Leigh, and Gary Schwartz (1988) have noted, "The defensive high-anxious group may represent repressors whose coping mechanisms are failing and have become ineffective."

Smith's transactional model implies that personality or coping variables interact with social factors to yield the psychophysical reactivity (and other biological mechanisms) involved in CHD progression. For the hostile or anxious person, life stressors; losses; age-related change or upheaval (i.e., retirement); low SES conditions, including poverty; social factors, including racism and sexism; low social support; job strain; and chronic overwork can stretch his or her often maladaptive coping mechanisms to the limit. An accumulation of such stresses or a disruptive event of high-stress magnitude (divorce, job loss, death of a loved one) can cause the collapse of these mechanisms, leaving the individual exhausted, irritable, and demoralized (VE).

I have already described the immunological and cardiovascular correlates of VE, which set the stage for myocardial infarction. But Goodkin and Appels (1997) capture dimensions of an integrative process model when they summarize their two-stage thesis on the role of the psyche in the pathogenesis of CHD:

> We propose a long-term first stage consisting of chronic hostility, prolonged occupational over-exertion, and exposure to other life stressors, terminating eventually in a much shorter second stage of "vital exhaustion." Stressor-associated neuroendocrine changes result in immunosuppression leading to reactivation of latent system infections (such as cytomegalovirus) and potentially to autoimmune reactions as well. This consequent release of pro-inflammatory cytokines exacer-

bates fatigue and induces a stimulus for cytokine production in the brain. This cytokine production stimulates a chronically activated, over-compensated limbic-hypothalamic-pituitary-adrenal axis, resulting in a dampened response, continued exhaustion, and a potential "reverberating circuit" between behavior, neuroendocrine change, cytokine release and coronary artery occlusion, culminating in myocardial infarction.

One piece missing from Goodkin and Appels's model is the role of acute anger and anxiety attacks in the onset of MI. This represents a subcategory of hostile, defensive, or vitally exhausted individuals who already evidence both psychosocial vulnerability and (diagnosed or undiagnosed) atherosclerosis or cardiac arrhythmias. Among these individuals an acute anxiety attack or an outburst of severe anger may trigger plaque disruption, thrombus formation, or malignant ventricular arrhythmias leading to sudden cardiac arrest and death.

Overall, however, Goodkin and Appels have rendered a complex and compelling theoretical picture of mind-body unity as it relates to MI. But their telling of the story includes the beginning and middle but not the end, which entails the mind-body interactions involved in post-heart-attack recovery—or relapse. The "third act" in the drama of the coronary-prone person hinges on this question: Will the agitated, exhausted, and now fearful heart patient lapse further into full-scale depression, or will he or she develop new coping capacities in the face of life-threatening illness?

HEART ATTACK AS BREAKING POINT: THE FOUR PATHS

The coping breakdown apparent in pre-MI exhaustion contributes to the coronary event, usually a heart attack. The MI itself can be traumatic, depending on the severity of the attack. Whether or not the MI is classified as severe, the person is still confronted by mortality, and how he or she perceives and manages this frightful (if not cataclysmic) event contributes to his or her psychological and medical outcome. Thus, the heart attack is indeed a breaking point: if the already exhausted and demoralized person cannot seek support, reframe hostile cognitions, and find ways to constructively express emotion (i.e., anger, fear, sadness), he or she will be vulnerable to depression. Support for this contention comes from an important study by B. H. Brummett and his colleagues at Duke University: 506 patients hospitalized for coronary angiography were tested for trait hostility and social support while hospitalized. Patients with less social support and higher hostility were significantly more likely to suffer depressive symptoms one month after hospitalization (Brummett et al. 1998).

Put differently, unless the vitally exhausted and now frightened heart patient can modify his or her coping style in the aftermath of MI, he or she will be vulnerable to depression. As noted above, post-MI depression may be associated with high cortisol and other stress hormones; suppression of antimicrobial and antiviral immune defenses, increasing susceptibility to infectious causes of atherosclerosis; increased platelet aggregation and impaired fibrinolysis; release of proinflammatory cytokines that contribute to thrombus and plaque formation and plaque disruption; and reduced heart rate variability. Thus, any psychosocial path that attenuates or prevents depression may also reduce activation of these detrimental mind-body pathways. Certainly, when the heart patient uses the event to conduct a reappraisal of her coping and life circumstances, seeking more support and constructively expressing emotion, she can (more likely) prevent severe depression and find her way toward mind-body homeostasis and recovery.

Thus, I have posited four common mind-body paths taken by people after a heart attack. As noted above, they include (1) a coping collapse that results in major depression and heightened risk of recurrent or fatal MI; (2) a lapse into depression followed by a change: the person seeks more social support and begins to process emotions (e.g., fear, anger, sorrow), including those associated with his or her medical condition, which may herald a more favorable outcome; (3) a continuation of hostile behavior and irritable mood, with two different tributaries: lower SES or support leading to unfavorable outcomes, or higher SES or support leading to more favorable outcomes; and (4) a transformation, including cognitive reappraisal and emotional awakening, in which the person recognizes deficits in his or her coping style and initiates change, that is, expressing emotion, seeking support, engaging in psychosocial treatment, modifying lifestyle factors associated with CHD.

As I have shown, there are ample data to support my contention that the first path—coping collapse and depression—presages a poorer psychological and medical outcome. But what is the nature of the depression arising after a heart attack, and why does it portend a worse outcome? First, a number of investigations have shown that post-MI risks correlate closely with the *severity* of the depression (Anda et al. 1993; Everson et al. 1996; Pratt et al. 1996): mild post-MI depression, which may be situational, is associated with far less risk than is major depression, which I view as the pathological result of coping collapse. In other words, some degree of depression may be normal after a heart attack, but major depressive disorder suggests a nontherapeutic dissolution of psychic defenses. Therefore, the process model detailed here is required to determine why some

130   patients respond with mild and transient depression, an understandable response to a life threat, while others become severely clinically depressed. The person's latent depression and hopelessness, previously masked by hostile or anxious traits, emerges after cumulative or acute stress; a premonitory stage of vital exhaustion; and the final breaking point, a heart attack. How the person handles this post-MI depression may determine his or her psychological and medical outcome.

With regard to the second path, strong supporting evidence comes from Frasure-Smith's recent analysis of data from her two large studies revealing depression as a risk for poor post-MI outcomes. She and François Lesperance retested 91 percent of the persons studied ($N = 1,367$) for depression at one year, and only those who were depressed at baseline (post-MI) *and* at one year were at significantly increased risk for coronary mortality (Frasure-Smith and Lesperance 2001). Put differently, patients experiencing only transient post-MI depression, including those who may have developed adaptive coping strategies to mitigate depression were not at increased risk beyond one year. This is a critical point: depression does not have to herald recurrent disease or death when it is transient or when patients find ways to ameliorate depressive symptoms. Regarding social support, Frasure-Smith evaluated the long-term impact of both depression and perceived social support in 887 of the patients from her initial studies. Those with high depression in the hospital had a threefold increased risk of cardiac mortality, but among these depressed subjects those in the highest quartile of perceived social support had no significant increase in mortality.

Regarding the third path, there is some evidence, but not much, that hostility after a heart attack is a risk for poor outcome. Based on these mixed data, I surmise that post-MI hostility is a less common path since the predominant risk-elevating states preceding and following MI are exhaustion and depression, respectively. This can be explained largely by the mind-body dynamics highlighted above: the shift from hostile or defensive coping (which correlates with atherosclerotic mechanisms) to VE and depression (which correlate with final-stage mechanisms in MI) as coping defenses falter and break down. Thus, hostility may be less overtly apparent after a heart attack even among previously hostile personalities. The cumulative weight of stress and, finally, a heart attack may simply leave the individual too tired and scared to be mean, not unlike a fighter felled by a vicious punch.

That said, some individuals still exhibit characteristic hostility after an MI, and this can be a negative prognostic indicator. But the relative weakness and inconsistency of this evidence may be interpreted thusly:

people who persist in their hostile coping may retain some degree of homeostasis, more at least than those who lapse into major depression. I hypothesize that among the persistently hostile, those with relatively higher SES or high social support will do better, while those with low SES or low support have a less favorable outcome. A recent German study and an earlier Type A study indirectly support this theory. Angerer and colleagues (2000) studied 223 patients with documented CAD who had follow-up angiograms two years later. The only significant correlation was found among patients with high anger-out and low social support, who had a threefold risk of disease progression. Blumenthal and colleagues (1987) found that Type As with low social support had significantly more severe CAD than those with high social support.

While neither study involves post-MI outcomes, the finding that hostile types with more support had less progressive or severe CAD suggests that social factors can moderate CHD outcomes. Also, the weakness of hostility in post-MI outcomes may relate to mechanisms: the immune and cardiac substrates of depression (inflammatory cytokines, reduced HRV, etc.) appear more likely to push the heart attack patient toward fatal recurrence than do those associated with hostility. More research is needed on hostility, social factors, biological mediators, and post-MI outcome to validate my hypotheses about this third pathway and its two tributaries.

Finally, the fourth path of transformation involves cognitive reappraisal of one's coping style and life circumstances; greater emotional awareness; more appropriate expression of emotion; support-seeking behaviors; and lifestyle changes. All of these shifts can be expected to prevent or reduce the severity of post-MI depression, the prominent factor in poor medical outcomes. The strongest evidence for the salutary effect of this pathway comes from psychosocial intervention trials. In the next section I briefly review the clinical trial findings, but here I highlight the most compelling single study of the transformative path: Friedman and colleagues' Recurrent Coronary Prevention Project (RCPP). The RCPP investigators randomized 1,013 post-MI patients into two groups for (1) Type A behavioral counseling and group cardiac counseling (an educational intervention) and (2) group cardiac counseling alone (Friedman et al. 1986); a nonrandomized control group was followed as well. After four and a half years of follow-up the cumulative cardiac recurrence rate was 12.9 percent in the Type A counseling group, 21.2 percent in the educational intervention, and 28.2 percent in the control group ($p < .005$). After the first year, the researchers found a significant difference in the number of cardiac deaths between the Type A counseling patients (3.4%), on the one hand, and the education group (6.4%) and the nonrandomized controls (9.2%), on the other.

132   Thus, a program designed to change the behavior of Type As—Friedman and his colleagues demonstrated significant reductions in hostile, time-urgent, anxious, and isolating tendencies among participants—dramatically improved their odds of recovery after MI. The program was also designed to generate tranquility, empathy, forgiveness, and a willingness to seek emotional support (Friedman and Ulmer 1984). While those studying Type As did not specifically measure improvements in depression, a host of other intervention studies have shown reductions in depression in tandem with improved medical outcomes (Linden et al. 1996).

As several meta-analyses demonstrate, there are substantial data showing that various psychosocial treatment programs for heart patients can demonstrably reduce the risks of recurrent heart attacks and death (Dusseldorp et al. 1999; Linden et al. 1996). These studies offer powerful proof that merely addressing the psychological issues faced by the heart patient is enough to make a significant difference in clinical outcomes. We now need more analysis concerning the kinds of interventions that produce the most salutary (and potentially life-saving) transformations in these patients, who are so often debilitated, depressed, and frightened. Based on this process model, it is my hypothesis that treatments addressing not only current anxieties about the heart attack but also the person's characteristic coping style and the origins of his or her emergent depression will be most effective in alleviating depression and promoting full medical recovery.

Psychosocial Interventions for Heart Disease: Neglected Evidence

A thoroughgoing review of research on psychosocial interventions for heart disease patients is beyond the scope of this chapter. But even a glancing overview, based on two recent meta-analyses of intervention trials, makes a strong case for the value, even the vital necessity, of psychosocial treatments for heart patients.

The first meta-analysis, led by psychologist Wolfgang Linden, of the University of British Columbia in Vancouver, was published in 1996 in the *Archives of Internal Medicine* (Linden et al. 1996). Numerous reviews and meta-analyses had already established the value of cardiac rehabilitation programs in reducing post-MI mortality and recurrence. These programs generally had involved education about heart health, including instructions on diet, exercise, and medication. Linden wondered whether rehabilitation programs that included psychosocial intervention—to manage stress, reduce anxiety and depression, enhance coping, and so on—would improve patient outcomes above and beyond the standard cardiac reha-

bilitation programs. He therefore performed a meta-analysis of twenty-
three randomized controlled clinical trials, each of which evaluated the additional impact of psychosocial treatment on cardiac rehabilitation for CAD and MI patients. All told, the twenty-three studies included 2,024 patients who received psychosocial treatment and 1,156 who did not.

The results were striking: during the two years of follow-up, the psychosocially treated patients showed greater reductions in psychological distress, systolic blood pressure, heart rate, and cholesterol, with effect sizes of −0.34, −0.24, −0.38, and −1.54, respectively. With regard to psychological outcomes, Linden and colleagues concluded that the interventions were associated with "significant improvements on psychological measures suggesting, on the whole, improvements in quality of life and reductions in distress, i.e., anxiety and depression." What about medical outcomes? Patients who received psychosocial treatments experienced a 46 percent reduction in recurrent cardiac events (including heart attacks) and a 41 percent reduction in coronary-related deaths, both statistically significant findings. Importantly, Linden's statistical findings remained essentially the same whether or not the large number of patients from one seminal (and positive) study, the above-mentioned RCPP, were excluded or included in the analysis. Linden's conclusion is worth quoting:

> The findings suggest that psychosocial interventions deserve routine inclusion in cardiac rehabilitation programs in addition to drug therapy and exercise regimens. The benefit is not only apparent for targeted psychosocial end points like depression and anxiety but could also be demonstrated for biological risk factor reductions, and even more importantly, for improving the odds ratios for mortality and nonfatal and other cardiac recurrence. The consistency of the positive outcome associated with psychosocial treatment across different classes of end points is encouraging.
>
> What is striking about the current results is that the nature of the psychosocial interventions was diverse in terms of length, target behavior, and the type of person delivering them; yet the effects were almost universally positive. Practitioners and health care policymakers who want to act on our recommendation to include routinely psychosocial treatments in cardiac rehabilitation may also want to know which kind of treatment and how much is needed for maximum benefit.

There should be little doubt, then, that psychosocial treatments for heart disease and heart attack patients make a meaningful difference by measures of psychological, biological, and medical outcomes. But as Linden states, which treatments work best remains an open question. A more recent meta-analysis also yielded strong results, but differences in the study's purview and findings may provide clues to the answer to this question.

Elise Dusseldorp and her colleagues at Leiden University in the Netherlands conducted an analysis of thirty-seven studies of psychoeducational (health education and/or stress management) programs for heart patients (Dusseldorp et al. 1999). In her breakdown of the studies included, Dusseldorp distinguished programs that included health education (HE), stress management (SM), and exercise (E); HE and SM together; HE and E together; and HE or SM alone. (Follow-up ranged from six months to ten years; the final post-test results from each study were used for the meta-analysis.) The results of all these studies, taken together and computed from effect sizes, demonstrated a 34 percent reduction in cardiac mortality and a 29 percent reduction in recurrent MI (Dusseldorp 1999). These effects were significant for long-term follow-up (more than two years) but not for shorter-term results. Overall the studies showed significant positive effects on blood pressure, cholesterol, weight, smoking, exercise, and eating habits ($p < .025$) but, somewhat surprisingly, no significant reductions in anxiety or depression.

While Dusseldorp's results are encouraging, two aspects are noteworthy: the reductions in cardiac mortality and recurrence were not as striking as those found in Linden's analysis; and there was no across-the-board reduction in anxiety and depression—also distinct from Linden's findings. One possible reason for these discrepancies is that only seven studies (out of Dusseldorp's thirty-seven and Linden's twenty-three) were shared by both meta-analyses, so that for the most part they evaluated different sets of studies. And the interventions included in the two analyses differed in character. In Dusseldorp's own words, Linden's analysis "included all interventions that appeared psychological or of a counseling nature while excluding studies of educational interventions" (Dusseldorp et al. 1999). By contrast, Dusseldorp included six studies with no "stress management" component, the term she used to characterize purely psychosocial interventions. Moreover, nine of her studies packaged "stress management" with "health education" and exercise programs, and it is not clear whether these particular programs put relatively less emphasis on the psychosocial component.

In a later review of CHD intervention research Wolfgang Linden paid special attention to a key statistic buried in Dusseldorp's meta-analysis: "Most striking was a comparison of those studies in which psychological treatment failed to produce psychological changes with those in which it succeeded. When psychological distress was not reduced by treatment, patient mortality was higher than that of controls (odds ratio: 0.88:1) and MI recurrence was not affected (odds ratio 1.03:1); however, when psychological distress was reduced, the odds ratio for mortality was 1.52:1 and for MI recurrence was 1.69:1" (Linden 2000). In other words, the medical outcome benefits found in Dusseldorp's analysis were due entirely to studies of interventions that had successfully treated anxiety and depression.

These findings are consistent with the process model presented here. Interventions without an explicit psychosocial component or with an inadequate one would not help patients work through depression or hopelessness in a therapeutic fashion nor teach coping skills to help them procure social support. Such programs would be less likely to ameliorate anxiety and depression and therefore less likely to yield optimal results in terms of medical recovery. Health education, with or without exercise, will unquestionably reduce recurrence and mortality rates, as other meta-analyses have shown. But Linden proved that psychosocial treatment adds a substantial dimension to these improved medical outcomes because, he argues, patients receiving psychosocial treatment experienced marked reductions in anxiety and depression. In Dusseldorp's analysis the interventions were not as uniformly directed toward, or successful at, alleviating psychological distress.

Underscoring this point is Frasure-Smith's intervention trial, the Montreal Heart Attack Readjustment Trial (M-HART). In a replication of a previous trial that yielded evidence of short-term success but only mixed long-term (five-year) success (Frasure-Smith and Prince 1985, 1989) she randomized 1,376 post-MI patients (men and women) to an intervention program ($N = 692$) or usual care ($N = 684$) and tracked them for one year (Frasure-Smith et al. 1997). The intervention involved nurses who had not been trained specifically as psychotherapists and who responded to patients on an "as-needed" basis. (The nurses contacted patients each month and assessed their stress levels, and if patients' stress levels were elevated, the nurses made home visits to provide supportive care.) The results were disappointing: the intervention had no impact on survival. There was no mortality difference among the men (cardiac mortality of 2.4% for those receiving intervention versus 2.5% for controls and 3.1% for all-cause mortality in both groups). And there was an unsettling finding among the women: higher cardiac mortality rates (9.4% versus 5%) and all-cause mortality rates (10.3 versus 5.4%) for those in the intervention groups. Importantly, the intervention led to minimal (insignificant) reductions in anxiety and depression for both men and women.

Frasure-Smith returned to her data to see whether a subset of patients who did benefit psychologically from the intervention also benefited medically. She and her colleagues evaluated 433 intervention patients (36% women) who received at least two home nursing visits after achieving a

136   high distress score (Cossette et al. 2001). Fifty-six percent of these patients showed significant improvements in distress scores within a two-month follow-up period. After one year these responding patients were less likely than nonresponding patients to die of cardiac causes ($p = .043$); marginally less likely to die of any cause ($p = .087$); less likely to be readmitted to the hospital for any reason ($p < .001$) and for cardiac reasons ($p < .001$); and less likely to have high levels of depression ($p < .001$) and anxiety ($p < .001$). Though the number of deaths was small, the difference in the number of hospital readmissions was highly significant. The results held for men and women, and they remained strong after controlling for all relevant demographic and medical variables. Frasure-Smith's conclusion was clearcut: individualized psychosocial treatments have the potential to improve medical outcomes if, and only if, they ameliorate psychological distress.

Based on Linden's and Dusseldorp's analyses, as well as on Frasure-Smith's findings, I would underscore this point even more forcefully: interventions without strong psychosocial components, trained mental health professionals, and treatments targeted to relieve depression will not be as successful in helping patients recover and survive.

There is virtually no evidence that cardiac rehabilitation programs are routinely expanding to include psychosocial treatments. One would expect that the data on depression and post-MI mortality would prompt a major effort to treat depression among patients who have suffered a heart attack. Approximately 1.1 million heart attacks occur each year in the United States (American Heart Association 2002), and more than 45 percent of the people who experience a coronary attack in a given year will die from it. Robert Carney and his colleagues at the Washington University in St. Louis point out that one in five post-MI patients (about 300,000, based on 1995 statistics; it would be somewhat less today) meet the criteria for major depression (Carney et al. 1990). (Other estimates put the figure closer to one in four, or higher [Dusseldorp 1999]). In their 1999 paper Carney and colleagues used Frasure-Smith's calculation of a fourfold relative risk of mortality among such patients to estimate that depression causes 75,000 deaths per year among patients discharged after a heart attack. The one-in-five figure does not include mild to moderate (but chronic) depressions that may also pose risks to MI patients, and it certainly does not encompass the hundreds of thousands of exhausted and/or depressed heart patients who might never experience a first heart attack if they had access to early psychosocial (as well as lifestyle) interventions after being diagnosed with CAD.

Given the bent of conservative biomedicine, the link between depression and post-MI outcomes might not, by itself, be expected to prompt broad implementation of psychosocial intervention programs. Only one form of evidence would suffice: intervention trials proving that the treatments actually improve medical prognosis. That such evidence now exists—based on Linden's and Dusseldorp's meta-analyses—has made no difference. A perfect example of the blind eye cast by biomedicine is apparent in the recent paper by Carney et al. (1999), "Can Treating Depression Reduce Mortality after an Acute Myocardial Infarction?"

Carney and colleagues frame the issue narrowly, seeking clinical trial evidence that "established" treatments for depression (by which they mean antidepressant medications, though they also mention cognitive-behavioral psychotherapy tailored for depression) help MI patients recover. By their standards, "there are not yet any published results from randomized, controlled clinical trials relating the treatment of depression to the subsequent risk of medical morbidity or mortality in post-MI patients" (Carney et al. 1999). I can only assume that Carney and colleagues ignored the several dozen studies in Linden's and Dusseldorp's meta-analyses because they did not meet their criteria for "treating depression." This is difficult to fathom. While many biological psychiatrists and cognitive therapists take their treatments to be the only legitimate therapies for depression, because (admittedly) there is more published evidence that they work, there is evidence that psychodynamic psychotherapy, group psychotherapy, supportive counseling, relaxation-based treatments, and stress management programs—which characterize the interventions evaluated by Linden and Dusseldorp—can also alleviate depression. Moreover, Linden's twenty-three studies, all randomized controlled trials, included a number with cognitive-behavioral components. Most importantly, Linden demonstrated that taken together, the treatments were successful both in reducing anxiety and depression and in reducing coronary morbidity and mortality.

Carney and his colleagues display a curious sort of myopia. Their paper focuses largely on the potential of selective serotonin reuptake inhibitor (SSRI) antidepressants to treat post-MI depression (the older tricyclic medications can be toxic to the heart). Such investigations are surely worthwhile, especially considering the track record of these medications for depression, including for CHD patients (Shores et al. 1998). While they also profess interest in cognitive-behavioral therapy, their view is so blinkered that they simply disregard the two dozen (at least) successful psychosocial intervention studies. They also tie the success of any treatment to its ability to increase heart rate variability, which they view as the single most important mechanism in MI outcome, and are dubious about whether this is possible. (Why they ignore the other critical mind-body mechanisms in CHD is not clear.) In sum, they repeatedly express skep-

138   ticism that even successful treatments for depression will prove to reduce cardiac morbidity and mortality. "Will treating depression in CHD patients reduce their mortality?" they ask in the conclusion of their paper. "The answer is still unknown, but some treatments for depression are very unlikely to improve the odds of survival" (Carney et al. 1999).

I single out Carney's paper because it sheds light on why there is no organized movement in medicine to institutionalize psychosocial programs for heart patients. The paper typifies a point of view that hinders progress, which may be summarized this way: If depression is a risk factor, we should, first and foremost, spend years and millions of dollars on clinical trials to test drug treatments that may or may not work, rather than turn to mind–body or psychological treatments already proven to work. Those treatments don't fit with our current view of what's best for depression, so we'll ignore the evidence supporting their efficacy for heart patients.

To their credit, Carney and colleagues make an essential point: "Regardless of whether treatment of depression can improve the prognosis of post–MI patients, comorbid depression can have devastating effects on functioning and quality-of-life; thus, it is a psychiatric disorder worthy of treatment in its own right." These clinician–researchers certainly want heart patients to get the treatment they need. But they recognize that broad implementation of treatment programs is more likely if patients' survival is proven to be enhanced, and by neglecting the existing positive evidence they make it less likely that heart attack patients will have ready access to psychosocial interventions any time soon. The neglect of the evidence also undercuts implementation of imaginative, broad-based psychosocial treatment programs for millions of patients with diagnosed CAD: if their hostility, fatigue, demoralization, or depression were treated, hundreds of thousands of initial heart attacks could conceivably be prevented.

WHAT PSYCHOSOCIAL INTERVENTIONS WILL BE MOST EFFECTIVE?

It is difficult to differentiate the "best" therapies for medical end points (progressive CAD, recurrent MI, fatal cardiac events) among the wide variety of psychosocial treatments that have been proven effective for heart patients. As noted, psychodynamic psychotherapy, supportive counseling, group psychotherapy, modification of Type A behavior, cognitive-behavioral approaches, stress management, relaxation techniques, breathing practices, and multimodal "packages" including several of these components have all been tried with some success. The only current marker of potential medical success may be psychological success, the capacity of a treatment to reduce depression and distress. By this measure, SSRI antidepressants would theoretically be among the most powerful treatments since they have exceptional track records for treating depression. Currently, a major multicenter clinical trial in progress, Sertraline Antidepressant Heart Attack Randomized Trial (SADHART), is evaluating the safety and efficacy of the SSRI sertraline (Zoloft) for depression (and recovery) in heart attack patients (Shapiro et al. 1999). Cognitive-behavioral psychotherapy targeted for depression has a similarly substantive track record, and the ongoing multicenter trial Enhancing Recovery in Coronary Heart Disease Patients (ENRICHD) "aims to investigate the effects of a psychosocial intervention that targets depression and/or low social support on survival and re-infarction among adult men and women who are at high risk for recurrent cardiac events because of psychosocial factors (depressive or social isolation)" (ENRICHD Investigators 2000). ENRICHD has recruited more than three thousand patients and will compare patients receiving tailored psychosocial interventions with control subjects. (Some depressed patients in ENRICHD will also receive sertraline.) Certainly the final results of SADHART and ENRICHD will reveal whether antidepressants and/or tailored psychological treatments influence medical end points and how they compare with psychosocial interventions already shown to be effective.

As research efforts continue, they should be guided not only by the generic assumption that what works for depression will work for heart disease but also by the more specific assumption that what works for depressed *heart patients* will work best for heart disease. Elise Dusseldorp and her colleagues elaborate this point: "Risk factor modification and reduction of emotional distress should be targeted in CHD patients to decrease their chances of a fatal or nonfatal recurrence of MI. The development of psycho-educational programs, however, has to be based on theory-driven research focusing on the relationship between specific components of interventions and changes in proximal and distal targets related directly to the needs of the individual patient" (Dusseldorp et al. 1999).

I wish to refine Dusseldorp's incisive argument about developing interventions based on theory-driven research. Knowledge of the natural history of mind-body relationships in the onset and progression of heart disease ought to shape psychosocial interventions. If we ask *why* heart patients often lapse into major depression, we recognize the arc from (1) hostile or anxious traits with latent depression or hopelessness to (2) chronic or acute stress leading to a breakdown in coping, triggering vital exhaustion and (3) subsequent (post-MI) depression. This process model is based on scores of studies, and it should be considered in the further design and testing of psychological treatments for heart patients.

140   Which leads me to assert that psychodynamic psychotherapy ought to be an essential component of these interventions since it can uniquely address maladaptive (hostile) coping and its developmental causes; the roots of anxiety; the unresolved grief, loss, or guilt that contributes to depression, whether the depression is latent or manifest; and the hopeless or helpless feelings that often arise after traumatic illness. On their own, antidepressants, relaxation techniques, breathing exercises, and even cognitive-behavioral treatments may not help patients delve into these dimensions. In the context of a multimodal program, however, each may work synergistically with psychodynamic therapy to promote more flexible coping, support seeking, emotional awareness, and psychospiritual revitalization. For instance, by easing depressive symptoms SSRIs may enable patients to sustain a course of psychotherapy with greater focus and less defensiveness. Mind-body techniques may ease anxiety and enhance body awareness, helping patients to explore inner terrain. By challenging negative thought constructs, cognitive-behavioral treatment may soften the specter of the judging mind, allowing patients in therapy to explore and express a range of emotion, resolve hidden grief, relinquish resentments, practice forgiveness, and reach beyond the confines of relative isolation to seek support. (In *The Type C Connection* Lydia Temoshok and I presented a model for integrating cognitive-behavioral and psychodynamic therapies [Temoshok and Dreher 1992].)

Heart patients may certainly improve with simpler treatments, and exploration of childhood conflicts or traumas may not be appropriate in the first weeks after a heart attack. But the breaking point represented by an MI can spur patients to introspection, so treatments that fail to help patients probe emotions and existential questions may short-circuit an emergent self-discovery that has the potential to promote healing. Demoralized and frightened heart attack patients may suddenly recognize long-held sorrows and disappointments and the thorny defenses they have used to defend against them. They may also become aware of a long-denied desire to change their methods of coping and their lifestyle, to regenerate embittered or estranged relationships. Within a few weeks of an attack such patients may benefit from a blend of psychodynamic and cognitive-behavioral treatment. In an interview I conducted years ago with Jack Morrison, a patient from the original RCPP study of Type A behavioral counseling, I was struck by the fact that counseling sessions twice a week over several years had enabled him to undergo just such a transformation.

Morrison was felled by a severe heart attack in 1977 while cleaning his boat. Had a passerby not noticed him lying on the deck and called 911, he likely would not have survived. After a difficult recovery he entered the

Type A behavioral-counseling program developed by Meyer Friedman,
joining a group led by Diane Ulmer, R.N., M.S. He came to recognize his
anxious, irritable, time-urgent behaviors and also his long neglect of family
and friendships. When I interviewed him in 1993, his candor was striking:
"If I dominated anybody, it was my children," he said. "Now we are much
closer than we would have been had I continued in that vein. . . . I'm less
impatient, kinder, and more thoughtful." Morrison's wife of forty years
confirmed her husband's assessment: "He's much more open, and the children are closer to their father than they ever were."

While Type A counseling as described by Friedman and Ulmer in their
book (1984) is primarily a blend of cognitive-behavioral and mind-body
techniques, Friedman increasingly encouraged patients to explore the
childhood roots and family dynamics behind their hostile, anxious, irritable, time-urgent, and hard-driving behaviors. In his multimodal lifestyle
intervention, the heart specialist Dean Ornish has also, increasingly, emphasized a therapeutic component that helps patients to open up emotionally and spiritually, to recognize their previous isolation and transcend
it (Ornish 1990). (Ornish's landmark 1990 study proved that a low-fat diet,
exercise, and mind-body program can reverse existing CAD [Ornish et al.
1990]. While it is not possible to calculate the healing contribution of the
mind-body component, Ornish believes it was essential.) Through group
therapy, imagery, and mindfulness-oriented meditations, Ornish has developed a practical model for delivering brief psychotherapy in a manner
that is profoundly supportive and appealing to the average heart patient.
In his popular book *Love and Survival* (1998) he makes a cogent argument:

> Some people believe that meditation, prayer, and related spiritual prac-
> tices can heal all problems, but I am not one of them. Many unresolved
> issues having to do with family, self-esteem, boundaries, developmen-
> tal issues, grief, intimacy, childhood abuse, addictions, neuroses, and
> so on are best addressed by a skilled psychotherapist. . . .
>
> Though supportive psychotherapy can be helpful in making it
> through a crisis, insight-oriented therapy helps you gain more aware-
> ness of the underlying patterns and causes that led to the problems. . . .
> Unfortunately, there is a growing trend for insurance companies to re-
> imburse short-term, drug-based supportive therapy rather than longer-
> term insight-oriented approaches.

Despite the current fashionable trends against psychoanalytic psychotherapy, I would argue that more rather than less emphasis on object
relations in the context of psychodynamic psychotherapy will have mind-
body healing effects on heart patients. Therapists trained in interpersonal,

142   relational, and self-psychology schools of psychoanalysis have long abandoned the Freudian model of the distant analyst, and they are uniquely
able to address the roots of maladaptive coping, to help patients peel off
layers of the proverbial onion of consciousness. Through this peeling
process may be found an authentic selfhood and a capacity for enriching
relationships that we know helps to heal the heart (Berkman et al. 1992).
In his eloquent book *Hope and Dread in Psychoanalysis* (1993) the late
Stephen Mitchell put it this way: "Whereas Freud could look to rationality as a natural bridge among individuals, reason itself can no longer serve
that function. The hope inspired by psychoanalysis in our time is
grounded in personal meaning, not rational consensus. The bridge supporting connections with others is not built out of rationality, superseding
fantasy and the imagination, but out of feelings experienced as real, authentic, generated from the inside rather than imposed externally."

Many contemporary psychoanalytic therapists abide by Mitchell's description of their calling: "If the goal of psychoanalysis in Freud's day was
rational understanding and control over fantasy-driven, conflictual impulses, the goal of psychoanalysis in our day is most often thought about
in terms of the establishment of a richer, more authentic sense of identity"
(Mitchell 1993). A call for the integration of psychoanalytic methods and
goals into the treatment of heart disease may seem both radical and fool-
hardy given today's inexorable managed-care march toward quick fixes and
medications for every ailment of heart and mind. But if we recognize that
many heart patients are indeed suffering from heartbreak, whether from
childhood losses, adult disappointments, the inability to establish an authentic identity, spiritual crisis, or some combination of each, the proposed
treatment should be designed to redress their suffering as it exists. How
such methods can be practically administered remains an open question,
but it is one that physicians, psychologists, and heart specialists should explore with an open mind.

REFERENCES

Adler NE, Boyce WT, Chesney MA, et al. 1994. Socioeconomic status and health:
the challenge of the gradient. *Am Psychol.* 49:15–24.

Akhtar S. 1995. Aggression: theories regarding its nature and origins. In: Moore BE,
Fine BD, eds. *Psychoanalysis: The Major Concepts.* New Haven, Conn: Yale University Press; 364–380.

Allgulander C, Lavori PW. 1991. Excess mortality among 3302 patients with "pure"
anxiety neurosis. *Arch Gen Psychiatry.* 48:599–602.

American Heart Association. 2002. Heart and Stroke Statistical Update, Dallas,

TX; 2002. Available online at http://www.americanheart.org/presenter.jhtml?identifier=1928. Accessed May 1, 2001.

Anda R, Williamson D, Jones D, et al. 1993. Depressed affect, hopelessness, and the risk of ischemic heart disease in a cohort of U.S. adults. *Epidemiology*. 4:285–294.

Angerer P, Siebert U, Kothny W, et al. 2000. Impact of social support, cynical hostility, and anger expression on progression of coronary atherosclerosis. *J Am Coll Cardiol*. 36:1781–1788.

Antonovsky A. 1994. A sociological critique of the "well-being" movement." *Advances*. 10:6–12.

Appels A. 1999. Inflammation and the mental state before an acute coronary event. *Ann Med*. 31(suppl 1):41–44.

Appels A, Bar FW, Bar J, Bruggeman C, de Baets M. 2000. Inflammation, depressive symptomatology, and coronary artery disease. *Psychosom Med*. 62:601–605.

Appels A, Golombeck B, Gorgels A, de Vreede J, van Breukelen G. 2000. Behavioral risk factors of sudden cardiac arrest. *J Psychosom Res*. 48:463–469.

Appels A, Kop W, Bar F, de Swart H, Mendes de Leon C. 1995. Vital exhaustion, extent of atherosclerosis, and the clinical course after successful percutaneous transluminal coronary angioplasty. *Eur Heart J*. 16:1880–1885.

Appels A, Mulder P. 1988. Excess fatigue as a precursor of myocardial infarction. *Eur Heart J*. 9:758–764.

Appels A, Otten F. 1992. Exhaustion as precursor of cardiac death. *Br J Clin Psychol*. 31(pt 3):351–356.

Ariyo AA, Haan M, Tangen CM, et al. 2000. Depressive symptoms and risks of coronary heart disease and mortality in elderly Americans. *Circulation*. 102:1773–1779.

Barefoot JC, Brummett BH, Helms MJ, Mark DB, Siegler IC, Williams RB. 2000. Repressive symptoms and survival of patients with coronary artery disease. *Psychosom Med*. 62:790–795.

Barefoot JC, Dahlstrom WG, Williams RB. 1983. Hostility, CHD incidence, and total mortality: a 25-year follow-up study of 255 physicians. *Psychosom Med*. 45:59–63.

Barefoot JC, Dodge KA, Peterson BL, et al. 1989. The Cook-Medley Hostility Scale: item content and ability to predict survival. *Psychosom Med*. 51:46–57.

Barefoot JC, Helms MJ, Mark DB. 1996. Depression and long-term mortality risk in patients with coronary artery disease. *Am J Cardiol*. 78:613–617.

Barefoot JC, Larsen S, Lieth L, Chroll M. 1995. Hostility, incidence of acute myocardial infarction, and mortality in a sample of older men and women. *Am J Epidemiol*. 142:477–484.

Barefoot JC, Peterson BL, Dahlstorm WG, et al. 1991. Hostility patterns and health implications: correlates of Cook-Medley scores in national survey. *Health Psychol*. 10:18–24.

Barefoot JC, Peterson BL, Harrell FE Jr, et al. 1989. Type A behavior and survival: a follow-up study of 1,467 patients with coronary artery disease. *Am J Cardiol*. 64:427–432.

Barefoot JC, Schroll M. 1996. Symptoms of depression, acute myocardial infarction, and total mortality in a community sample. *Circulation*. 93:1976–1980.

144 Berkman LF, Leo-Summers L, Horwitz RI. 1992. Emotional support and survival after myocardial infarction: a prospective, population-based study of the elderly. *Ann Intern Med.* 117:1003–1009.

Biasucci LM, Liuzzo G, Fantuzzi G, et al. 1999. Increasing levels of interleukin (IL)-1Ra and IL-6 during the first two days of hospitalization in unstable angina are associated with increased risk of in-hospital coronary events. *Circulation.* 99:2079–2084.

Bigger JT Jr, Fleiss JL, Steinman RC, Rolnitzky LM, Kleiger RE, Rottman JN. 1992. Frequency domain measures of heart period variability and mortality after myocardial infarction. *Circulation.* 85:164–171.

Blumenthal JA, Burg MM, Barefoot J, Williams RB, Haney T, Zimet G. 1987. Social support, type A behavior, and coronary artery disease. *Psychosom Med.* 49:331–340.

Blumenthal JA, Jiang W, Waugh RA, et al. 1995. Mental stress-induced ischemia in the laboratory and ambulatory ischemia during daily life: association and hemodynamic features. *Circulation.* 92:2102–2108.

Blumenthal JA, Williams RB Jr, Kong Y, et al. 1978. Type A behavior pattern and coronary atherosclerosis. *Circulation.* 58:634–639.

Bosma H, Peter R, Siegrist J, Marmot M. 1998. Two alternative job stress models and the risk of coronary heart disease. *Am J Public Health.* 88:68–74.

Brummett BH, Babyak MA, Barefoot JC, et al. 1998. Social support and hostility as predictors of depressive symptoms in cardiac patients one month after hospitalization: a prospective study. *Psychosom Med.* 60:707–713.

Bschor T. 2000. When the mind affects the body. Unmasking "masked" depression (in German). *MMW Fortschr Med.* 142:26–28.

Cain BS, Meldrum DR, Dinarello CA, et al. 1999. TNF-alpha and interleukin-1beta synergistically depress human myocardial function. *Crit Care Med.* 27:1309–1318.

Carney RM, Freedland KE, Jaffe AS. 1990. Insomnia and depression prior to myocardial infarction. *Psychosom Med.* 52:603–609.

Carney RM, Freedland KE, Rich MW, Jaffe AS. 1995. Depression as a risk factor for cardiac events in established coronary heart disease: a review of possible mechanisms. *Ann Behav Med.* 17:142–149.

Carney RM, Freedland KE, Veith RC, Jaffe AS. 1999. Can treating depression reduce mortality after an acute myocardial infarction? *Psychosom Med.* 61:666–675.

Carney RM, Saunders RD, Freedland KE, Stein P, Rich MW, Jaffe AS. 1995. Association of depression with reduced heart rate variability in coronary artery disease. *Am J Cardiol.* 76:562–564.

Case RB, Heller SS, Case NB, Moss AJ. 1985. Type A behavior and survival after acute myocardial infarction. *New Engl J Med.* 312:737–741.

Cobb S. 1974. Physiologic changes in men whose jobs were abolished. *J Psychosom Res.* 18:245–258.

Cohen HW, Madhavan S, Alderman MH. 2001. History of treatment for depression: risk factor for myocardial infarction in hypertensive patients. *Psychosom Med.* 63:203–209.

Cossette S, Frasure-Smith N, Lesperance F. 2001. Clinical implications of a reduction in psychological distress on cardiac prognosis in patients participating in a psychosocial intervention program. *Psychosom Med.* 63:257–266.

Dalack GW, Roose SP. 1990. Perspectives on the relationship between cardiovascular disease and affective disorder. *J Clin Psychiatry.* 51(suppl):4–9.

De Leon CFM, Kop WJ, de Swart HB, et al. 1996. Psychosocial characteristics and recurrent events after percutaneous transluminal coronary angioplasty. *Am J Cardiol.* 77:252–255.

Dembroski TM, MacDougall JM, Costa PT Jr, Grandits GA. 1989. Components of hostility as predictors of sudden death and myocardial infarction in the Multiple Risk Factor Intervention Trial. *Psychosom Med.* 51:514–522.

Dembroski TM, MacDougall JM, Williams RB, Haney TL, Blumenthal JA. 1985. Components of Type A, hostility, and anger-in: relationship to angiographic findings. *Psychosom Med.* 47:219–233.

Denollet J. 1998. Personality and risk of cancer in men with coronary heart disease. *Psychol Med.* 28:991–995.

Denollet J, Brutsaert DL. 1998. Personality, disease severity, and the risk of long-term cardiac events in patients with a decreased ejection fraction after myocardial infarction. *Circulation.* 97:167–173.

Denollet J, Sys SU, Brutsaert DL. 1995. Personality and mortality after myocardial infarction. *Psychosom Med.* 57:582–591.

Denollet J, Sys SU, Stroobant N, Rombouts H, Gillebert TC, Brutsaert DL. 1996. Personality as independent predictor of long-term mortality in patients with coronary heart disease. *Lancet.* 347:417–421.

Denollet J, Vaes J, Brutsaert DL. 2000. Inadequate response to treatment in coronary heart disease: adverse effects of type D personality and younger age on five-year prognosis and quality of life. *Circulation.* 102:630–635.

Dezube BJ, Pardee AB, Chapman B, et al. 1993. Pentoxifylline decreases tumor necrosis factor expression and serum triglycerides in people with AIDS. NIAID AIDS Clinical Trials Group. *J Acquir Immune Defic Syndr.* 6:787–794.

Dreher H. 1995a. *The Immune Power Personality: Seven Traits You Can Develop to Stay Healthy.* New York: Dutton.

Dreher H. 1995b. The Social Perspective in Mind-Body Studies: Missing in Action? *Adv Mind Body Med.* 11:39–54.

Dusseldorp E, van Elderen T, Maes S, Meulman J, Kraaij V. 1999. A meta-analysis of psychoeducational programs for coronary heart disease patients. *Health Psychol.* 18:506–519.

Eaker ED, Pinsky J, Castelli WP. 1992. Myocardial infarction and coronary death among women: psychosocial predictors from a twenty-year follow-up of women in the Framingham Study. *Am J Epidemiol.* 135:854–864.

ENRICHD Investigators. 2000. Enhancing recovery in coronary heart disease patients (ENRICHD): study design and methods. *Am Heart J.* 139:1–9.

Entman ML, Ballantyne CM. 1993. Inflammation in acute coronary syndromes. *Circulation.* 88:800–803.

Everson SA, Goldberg DE, Kaplan GA, et al. 1996. Hopelessness and risk of mor-

146   tality and incidence of myocardial infarction and cancer. *Psychosom Med.* 58:113–121.

Everson S, Kauhanen J, Kaplan G. 1997. Hostility, and increased risk of mortality and acute myocardial infarction: the mediating role of behavioral risk factors. *Am J Epidemiol.* 146:142–152.

Ferketich AK, Schwartzbaum JA, Frid DJ, Moeschberger ML. 2000. Depression as an antecedent to heart disease among women and men in the NHANES I study: National Health and Nutrition Examination Survey. *Arch Intern Med.* 160:1261–1268.

Folkman S, Lazarus RS. 1988. The relationship between coping and emotion: implications for theory and research. *Soc Sci Med.* 26:309–317.

Frank KA, Heller SS, Kornfeld DS, Sporn AA, Weiss MB. 1978. Type A behavior pattern and coronary angiographic findings. *JAMA.* 240:761–763.

Frasure-Smith N, Lesperance F. 2001. Long-term impact of continuing depression on post-MI prognosis [abstract]. *Psychosom Med.* 63:103. Abstract 1139.

Frasure-Smith N, Lesperance F, Gravel G, et al. 2000. Social support, depression, and mortality during the first year after myocardial infarction. *Circulation.* 101:1919–1924.

Frasure-Smith N, Lesperance F, Juneau M, Talajic M, Bourassa MG. 1999. Gender, depression, and one-year prognosis after myocardial infarction. *Psychosom Med.* 61:26–37.

Frasure-Smith N, Lesperance F, Prince RH, et al. 1997. Randomised trial of home-based psychosocial nursing intervention for patients recovering from myocardial infarction. *Lancet.* 350:473–479.

Frasure-Smith N, Lesperance F, Talajic M. 1993. Depression following myocardial infaction: impact on six-month survival. *JAMA.* 270:1819–1825.

Frasure-Smith N, Lesperance F, Talajic M. 1995. Depression and eighteen-month prognosis after myocardial infarction. *Circulation.* 91:999–1005.

Frasure-Smith N, Prince R. 1985. The Ischemic Heart Disease Life Stress Monitoring Program: impact on mortality. *Psychosom Med.* 47:431–445.

Frasure-Smith N, Prince R. 1989. Long-term follow-up of the Ischemic Heart Disease Life Stress Monitoring Program. *Psychosom Med.* 51:485–513.

Freedland KE, Lustman PJ, Carney RM, Hong BA. 1992. Underdiagnosis of depression in patients with coronary artery disease: the role of nonspecific symptoms. *Int J Psychiatry Med.* 22:221–229.

Freeman LJ, Nixon PGF, Sallabank P, Reaveley D. 1987. Psychological stress and silent myocardial ischemia. *Am Heart J.* 114:477–482.

Fricchione GL, Bilfinger TV, Hartman A, Liu Y, Stefano GB. 1996. Neuroimmunologic implications in coronary artery disease. *Adv Neuroimmunol.* 6:131–142.

Friedman M. 1974. *Type A Behavior and Your Heart.* New York: Fawcett Books.

Friedman M, Rosenman RH, Straus R, Wurm M, Kositchek R. 1968. The relationship of behavior pattern A to the state of the coronary vasculature: a study of fifty-one autopsy subjects. *Am J Med.* 44:525–537.

Friedman M, Thoresen CE, Gill J, et al. 1986. Alteration of type A behavior and its effect on cardiac recurrences in post-myocardial infarction patients: summary results of the recurrent coronary prevention project. *Am Heart J.* 112:653–665.

Friedman M, Ulmer D. 1984. *Treating Type A Behavior and Your Heart*. New York: Fawcett.

Gerin W, Pieper C, Levy R, Pickering TG. 1992. Social support in social interaction: a moderator of cardiovascular reactivity. *Psychosom Med.* 54:324–336.

Gold PW, Loriaux DL, Roy A, et al. 1986. Response to corticotropin releasing hormone in the hypercortisolism of depression and Cushing's disease [abstract]. *New Engl J Med.* 314:1329–1335.

Goodkin K, Appels A. 1997. Behavioral-neuroendocrine-immunologic interaction in myocardial infarction. *Med Hypotheses.* 48:209–214.

Gorman JM, Sloan RP. 2000. Heart rate variability in depressive and anxiety disorders. *Am Heart J.* 140:77–83.

Gottdiener, JS, Krantz DS, Howell RH, et al. 1994. Induction of silent myocardial ischemia with mental stress testing: relation to the triggers of ischemia during daily life activities and to ischemic functional severity. *J Am Coll Cardiol.* 24:1645–1651.

Grignani G, Soffiantino F, Zucchella M, et al. 1991. Platelet activation by emotional stress in patients with coronary artery disease. *Circulation.* 83(suppl 4):128–136.

Haines AP, Imeson JD, Meade TW. 1987. Phobic anxiety and ischemic heart disease. *BMJ.* 295:297–299.

Haney TL, Maynard KE, Houseworth SJ, Scherwitz LW, Williams RB, Barefoot JC. 1996. Interpersonal Hostility Assessment Technique: description and validation against the criterion of coronary artery disease. *J Pers Assess.* 66:386–401.

Hasdai D, Scheinowitz M, Leibovitz E, Sclarovsky S, Eldar M, Barak V. 1996. Increased serum concentrations of interleukin-1 beta in patients with coronary artery disease. *Heart.* 76:24–28.

Hecker MHL, Chesney MA, Blacks GW, Frautschi N. 1988. Coronary-prone behaviors in the Western Collaborative Group Study. *Psychosom Med.* 50:153–164.

Helmers KF, Krantz DS, Howell RH, Klein J, Bairey CN, Rozanski A. 1993. Hostility and myocardial ischemia in coronary artery disease patients: evaluation by gender and ischemic index. *Psychosom Med.* 55:29–36.

Hlatky MA, Lam LC, Lee KL, et al. 1995. Job strain and the prevalence and outcome of coronary artery disease. *Circulation.* 92:327–333.

Horsten M, Ericson M, Perski A, et al. 1999. Psychosocial factors and heart rate variability in women. *Psychosom Med.* 61:49–57.

Houston BK, Vavak CR. 1991. Cynical hostility: developmental factors, psychosocial correlates, and health behaviors. *Health Psychol.* 10:9–17.

Hughes JW, Stoney CM. 2000. Depressed mood is related to high-frequency heart rate variability during stressors. *Psychosom Med.* 62:796–803.

Iribarren C, Sidney S, Bild DE, et al. 2000. Association of hostility with coronary artery calcification in young adults: the CARDIA study. Coronary Artery Risk Development in Young Adults. *JAMA.* 283:2546–2551.

Ironson G, Taylor CB, Boltwood M, et al. 1992. Effects of anger on left ventricular ejection fraction in coronary artery disease. *Am J Cardiol.* 70:281–285.

Jamner LD, Schwartz GE, Leigh H. 1988. The relationship between repressive and defensive coping styles and monocyte, eosinophile, and serum glucose levels: support for the opioid peptide hypothesis of repression. *Psychosom Med.* 50:567–575.

148   Jenkins CD. 1978. A comparative review of the interview and questionnaire methods in the assessment of the coronary-prone behavior pattern. In: Dembroski TM, Weiss SM, Shields JL, et al., eds. *Coronary Prone Behavior.* New York: Springer-Verlag.

Jiang W, Babyak M, Krantz DS, et al. 1996. Mental stress—induced myocardial ischemia and cardiac events. *JAMA.* 275:1651–1656.

Johnson JV, Stewart W, Hall EM, Fredlund P, Theorell T. 1996. Long term psychosocial work environment and cardiovascular mortality among Swedish men. *Am J Public Health.* 86:324–331.

Kamarck T, Manuck S, Jennings JR. 1990. Social support reduces cardiovascular reactivity to psychological challenge: a laboratory model. *Psychosom Med.* 52:42–58.

Kaplan GA. 1995. Where do shared pathways lead? Some reflections on a research agenda. *Psychosom Med.* 57:208–212.

Kaplan GA, Keil JE. 1993. Socioeconomic factors and cardiovascular disease: a review of the literature. *Circulation.* 88(4 pt 1):1973–1998.

Karasek RA, Baker D, Marxer F, Ahlbom A, Theorell T. 1981. Job decision latitude, job demands, and cardiovascular disease: a prospective study of Swedish men. *Am J Public Health.* 71:694–705.

Kaufmann MW, Fitzgibbons JP, Sussman EJ, et al. 1999. Relation between myocardial infarction, depression, hostility, and death. *Am Heart J.* 138:549–554.

Kawachi I, Colditz GA, Ascherio A, et al. 1994. Prospective study of phobic anxiety and risk of coronary heart disease in men. *Circulation.* 89:1992–1997.

Kawachi I, Sparrow D, Vokonas PS, Weiss ST. 1994. Symptoms of anxiety and risk of coronary heart disease: the Normative Aging Study. *Circulation.* 90:2225–2229.

Kawachi I, Sparrow D, Vokonas PS, Weiss ST. 1995. Decreased heart rate variability in men with phobic anxiety (data from the Normative Aging Study). *Am J Cardiol.* 75:882–885.

Kawachi I, Sparrow D, Spiro A III, Vokonas P, Weiss ST. 1996. A prospective study of anger and coronary heart disease: the Normative Aging Study. *Circulation.* 94:2090–2095.

Kemeny ME, Cohen F, Zegans LS, Conant MA. 1989. Psychological and immunological predictors of genital herpes recurrence. *Psychosom Med.* 51:195–208.

Kennedy J, Shavelle R, Wang S, Budoff M, Detrano RC. 1998. Coronary calcium and standard risk factors in symptomatic patients referred for coronary angiography. *Am Heart J.* 135:696–702.

Kleiger RE, Miller JP, Bigger JT Jr, Moss AJ. 1987. Decreased heart rate variability and its association with increased mortality after acute myocardial infarction. *Am J Cardiol.* 59:256–262.

Kop WJ. 1997. Acute and chronic psychological risk factors for coronary syndromes: moderating effects of coronary artery disease severity. *J Psychosom Res.* 43:167–181.

Kop WJ. 1999. Chronic and acute psychological risk factors for clinical manifestations of coronary artery disease. *Psychosom Med.* 61:476–487.

Kop WJ, Appels AP, Mendes de Leon CF, Bar FW. 1996. The relationship between severity of coronary artery disease and vital exhaustion. *J Psychosom Res.* 40:397–405.

Kop WJ, Appels AP, Mendes de Leon CF, de Swart HB, Bar FW. 1994. Vital exhaustion predicts new cardiac events after successful coronary angioplasty. *Psychosom Med.* 56:281–287.

Kop WJ, Cohen N. 2001. Psychological risk factors and immune system involvement in cardiovascular disease. In: Ader R, Felten DL, Cohen N, eds. *Psychoneuroimmunolgy.* 3rd ed. Vol. 2. New York: Academic Press.

Kop WJ, Hamulyak K, Pernot C, Appels A. 1998. Relationship of blood coagulation and fibrinolysis to vital exhaustion. *Psychosom Med.* 60:352–358.

Koskenvuo M, Kaprio J, Rose RJ, et al. 1988. Hostility as a risk factor for mortality and ischemic heart disease in men. *Psychosom Med.* 50:330–340.

Krittayaphong R, Cascio WE, Light KC, et al. 1997. Heart rate variability in patients with coronary artery disease: differences in patients with higher and lower depression scores. *Psychosom Med.* 59:231–235.

Kubzansky LD, Kawachi I. 2000. Going to the heart of the matter: do negative emotions cause coronary heart disease? *J Psychosom Res.* 48:323–337.

Kubzansky LD, Kawachi I, Spiro A III, Weiss ST, Vokonas PT, Sparrow D. 1997. Is worrying bad for your heart? A prospective study of worry and coronary heart disease in the Normative Aging Study. *Circulation.* 95:818–824.

Kubzansky LD, Kawachi I, Weiss ST, Sparrow D. 1998. Anxiety and coronary heart disease: a synthesis of epidemiological, psychological, and experimental evidence. *Ann Behav Med.* 20:47–58.

Lahlou-Laforet K, Gelas MA, Pornin M, et al. 2001. Depression is associated with an impaired fibrinolytic capacity in coronary patients. *Psychosom Med.* 63:102. Abstract 1260.

Lane D, Carroll D, Ring C, Beevers DG, Lip GY. 2001. Mortality and quality of life twelve months after myocardial infarction: effects of depression and anxiety. *Psychosom Med.* 63:221–230.

Langeluddecke PM, Tennant CC. 1986. Psychological correlates of the type A behaviour pattern in coronary angiography patients. *Br J Med Psychol.* 59(pt 2):141–148.

Lazarus R, Folkman S. 1984. Coping and adaptation. In: Gentry WD, ed. *Handbook of Behavioral Medicine.* New York: Guilford Press.

Lesperance F, Frasure-Smith N, Talajic M, Bourassa MG. 2002. Five-year risk of cardiac mortality in relation to initial severity and one-year changes in depression symptoms after myocardial infarction. *Circulation.* 105:1049–1053.

Libby P, Hansson GK. 1991. Involvement of the immune system in human atherogenesis: current knowledge and unanswered questions. *Lab Invest.* 64:5–15.

Licinio J, Wong ML. 1999. The role of inflammatory mediators in the biology of major depression: central nervous system cytokines modulate the biological substrate of depressive symptoms, regulate stress-responsive systems, and contribute to neurotoxicity and neuroprotection. *Mol Psychiatry.* 4:317–327.

Linden W. 2000. Psychological treatments in cardiac rehabilitation: review of rationales and outcomes. *J Psychosom Res.* 48:443–454.

150   Linden W, Stossel C, Maurice J. 1996. Psychological interventions for patients with coronary artery disease: a metaanalysis. *Arch Intern Med.* 156:745–752.

Lowen A. 1988. *Love, Sex, and Your Heart.* New York: Macmillan.

Lowen A. 1993. *Depression and the Body: The Biological Basis of Faith and Reality.* New York: Viking Press.

Lown B, Verrier RL, Corbalan R. 1973. Psychologic stress and threshold for repetitive ventricular response. *Science.* 182:834–836.

Lown B, Verrier RL, Rabinowitz SH. 1977. Neural and psychologic mechanisms and the problem of sudden cardiac death. *Am J Cardiol.* 39:890–902.

Luecken LJ. 2000. Attachment and loss experiences during childhood are associated with adult hostility, depression, and social support. *J Psychosom Res.* 49:85–91.

Lynch J. 1977. *The Broken Heart: The Medical Consequences of Loneliness.* New York: Basic Books.

Lynch JW, Kaplan GA, Cohen RD, Tuomilehto J, Salonen JT. 1996. Do cardiovascular risk factors explain the relation between socioeconomic status, risk of all-cause mortality, cardiovascular mortality, and acute myocardial infarction? *Am J Epidemiol.* 144:934–942.

Maes M. 1995. Evidence for an immune response in major depression: a review and hypothesis. *Prog Neuropsychopharmacol Biol Psychiatry.* 19:11–38.

Marmot MG, Rose G, Shipley M, Hamilton PJ. 1978. Employment grade and coronary heart disease in British civil servants. *J Epidemiol Community Health.* 32:244–249.

Martin RL, Cloninger CR, Guze SB, Clayton PJ. 1985. Mortality in a follow-up of five hundred psychiatric outpatients. I. Total mortality. *Arch Gen Psychiatry.* 42:47–54.

May R. 1981. *Freedom and Destiny.* New York: W. W. Norton.

Mayou RA, Gill D, Thompson DR, et al. 2000. Depression and anxiety as predictors of outcome after myocardial infarction. *Psychosom Med.* 62:212–219.

Mendes de Leon CF, Kop WJ, de Swart HB, Bar FW, Appels AP. 1996. Psychosocial characteristics and recurrent events after percutaneous transluminal coronary angioplasty. *Am J Cardiol.* 77:252–255.

Miller TQ, Markides KS, Chiriboga DA, Ray LA. 1995. A test of the psychosocial vulnerability and health behavior models of hostility: results from an eleven-year follow-up study of Mexican Americans. *Psychosom Med.* 57:572–581.

Miller TQ, Smith TW, Turner CW, Guijarro ML, Hallet AJ. 1996. A meta-analytic review of research on hostility and physical health. *Psychol Bull.* 119:322–348.

Mitchell SA. 1993. *Hope and Dread in Psychoanalysis.* New York: Basic Books.

Mittleman MA, Maclure M, Sherwood JB, et al., for the Determinants of Myocardial Infarction Onset Study Investigators. 1995. Triggering of acute myocardial infarction onset by episodes of anger. *Circulation.* 92:1720–1725.

Myerburg RJ, Kessler KM, Mallon SM, et al. 1992. Life-threatening ventricular arrhythmias in patients with silent myocardial ischemia due to coronary-artery spasm. *New Engl J Med.* 326:1451–1455.

Nellison–de Vos YCM. 1994. Slaapklachten in de periode voorafgaande aan het hartinfaret. Ph.D. diss. University of Maastricht, Maastricht, The Netherlands.

Nemeroff CB, Widerlov E, Bissette G, et al. 1984. Elevated concentrations of CSF corticotropin releasing factor-like immunoreactivity in depressed patients. *Science.* 226:1342–1344.

Ornish D. 1990. *Dr. Dean Ornish's Program for Reversing Heart Disease.* New York: Random House.

Ornish D. 1998. *Love and Survival: The Scientific Basis for the Healing Power of Intimacy.* New York: HarperCollins.

Ornish D, Brown SE, Scherwitz LW, et al. 1990. Can lifestyle changes reverse coronary heart disease? The Lifestyle Heart Trial. *Lancet.* 336:129–133.

Parker G, Hadzi-Pavlovic D, Roussos J, et al. 1998. Non-melancholic depression: the contribution of personality, anxiety, and life events to subclassification. *Psychol Med.* 28:1209–1219.

Pennebaker JW, Susman JR. 1988. Disclosure of traumas and psychosomatic processes. *Soc Sci Med.* 26:327–332.

Penninx BW, Beekman AT, Honig A, et al. 2001. Depression and cardiac mortality: results from a community-based longitudinal study. *Arch Gen Psychiatry.* 58:221–227.

Pope ML, Smith TW. 1991. Cortisol excretion in high and low cynically hostile men. *Psychosom Med.* 53:386–392.

Posse M, Hallstrom T. 1998. Depressive disorders among somatizing patients in primary health care. *Acta Psychiatr Scand.* 98:187–192.

Pratt LA, Ford DE, Crum RM, Armenian HK, Gallo JJ, Eaton WW. 1996. Depression, psychotropic medication, and risk of myocardial infarction: prospective data from the Baltimore ECA follow-up. *Circulation.* 94:3123–3129.

Ragland DR, Brand RJ. 1988. Coronary heart disease mortality in the Western Collaborative Group Study: follow-up experience of twenty-two years. *Am J Epidemiol.* 127:462–475.

Rangell L. 1995. Affects. In: Moore BE, Fine BD, eds. *Psychoanalysis: The Major Concepts.* New Haven, Conn: Yale University Press; 381–391.

Rechlin T, Weis M, Spitzer A, Kaschka WP. 1994. Are affective disorders associated with alterations of heart rate variability? *J Affect Disord.* 32:271–275.

Rich MW, Saini J, Kleiger RE, Carney RM, TeVelde A, Freedland KE. 1988. Correlation of heart rate variability with clinical and angiographic variables and late mortality after coronary angiography. *Am J Cardiol.* 62:59–66.

Rosengren A, Orth-Gomer K, Wedel H, Wilhelmsen L. 1993. Stressful life events, social support, and mortality in men born in 1933. *BMJ.* 307:1102–1105.

Rosenman RH. 1975. Coronary heart disease in Western Collaborative Group Study: final follow-up experience of 8 1/2 years. *JAMA.* 233:872–877.

Rozanski A, Bairey CN, Krantz DS, et al. 1988. Mental stress and the induction of silent myocardial ischemia in patients with coronary artery disease. *New Engl J Med.* 318:1005–1012.

Rozanski A, Blumenthal JA, Kaplan J. 1999. Impact of psychological factors on the pathogenesis of cardiovascular disease and implications for therapy. *Circulation.* 99:2192–2217.

Saphier D, Welch JE, Chuluyan HE. 1993. Alpha-interferon inhibits adrenocortical secretion via mu 1–opioid receptors in the rat. *Eur J Pharmacol.* 236:183–191.

152   Scheier MF, Bridges MW. 1995. Person variables and health: personality predispositions and acute psychological states as shared determinants for disease. *Psychosom
Med.* 57:255–268.

Schnall PL, Pieper C, Schwartz JE, et al. 1990. The relationship between job strain,
work place diastolic blood pressure, and left ventricular mass index. *JAMA.*
263:1929–1935.

Schnall PL, Schwartz JE, Landsbergis PA, Warren K, Pickering TG. 1998. A longitudinal study of job strain and ambulatory blood pressure: results from a three-
year follow-up. *Psychosom Med.* 60:697–706.

Secci A, Wong N, Tang W, Wang S, Doherty T, Detrano R. 1997. Electron beam
computed tomographic coronary calcium as a predictor of coronary events: comparison of two protocols. *Circulation.* 96:1122–1129.

Seeman TE, Berkman LF, Blazer D, Rowe JW. 1994. Social ties and support and
neuroendocrine functions: the Macarthur studies of successful aging. *Ann Behav
Med.* 16:95–106.

Shah PK. 1998. Role of inflammation and metalloproteinases in plaque disruption
and thrombosis. *Vasc Med.* 3:199–206.

Shapiro PA, Lesperance F, Frasure-Smith N, et al. 1999. An open-label preliminary
trial of sertraline for treatment of major depression after acute myocardial infarction (the SADHAT Trial): Sertraline Anti-Depressant Heart Attack Trial. *Am
Heart J.* 137:1100–1106.

Shekelle RB, Hulley SB, Neaton JD, et al. 1985. The MRFIT Behavior Pattern
Study, II: type A behavior and incidence of coronary heart disease. *Am J Epidemiol.* 122:559–570.

Shekelle RB, Gale M, Ostfeld AM, Paul O. 1983. Hostility, risk of coronary heart
disease, and mortality. *Psychosom Med.* 45:109–114.

Shores MM, Pascualy M, Veith RC. 1998. Major depression and heart disease:
treatment trials. *Semin Clin Neuropsychiatry.* 3:87–101.

Siegrist J, Peter R, Junge A, Cremer P, Seidel D. 1990. Low status control, high effort at work, and ischemic heart disease: prospective evidence from blue-collar
men. *Soc Sci Med.* 31:1127–1134.

Simonsick EM, Wallace RB, Blazer DG, Berkman LF. 1995. Depressive symptomatology and hypertension-associated morbidity and mortality in older adults. *Psychosom Med.* 57:427–435.

Sinatra ST. 1996. *Heartbreak and Heart Disease: A Mind/Body Prescription for Healing the Heart.* New Canaan, Conn: Keats Publ.

Smith TW. 1994. Concepts and methods in the study of anger, hostility, and health.
In: Siegman AW, Smith TW, eds. *Anger, Hostility, and the Heart.* Hillsdale, NJ:
Erlbaum; 23–42.

Smith TW, Houston BK, Zurawski RM. 1983. The Framingham Type A Scale and
anxiety, irrational beliefs, and self-control. *J Human Stress.* 9:32–37.

Stoney CM. 1999. Plasma homocysteine levels increase in women during psychological stress. *Life Sci.* 64:2359–2365.

Stoney CM, Engebretson TO. 2000. Plasma homocysteine concentrations are positively associated with hostility and anger. *Life Sci.* 66:2267–2275.

Suarez EC, Blumenthal JA. 1991. Ambulatory blood pressure responses during daily life in high and low hostile patients with a recent myocardial infarction. *J Cardiopulm Rehabil.* 11:169–175.

Suarez EC, Shiller AD, Kuhn CM, Schanberg S, Williams RB Jr, Zimmermann EA. 1997. The relationship between hostility and beta adrenergic receptor physiology in healthy young males. *Psychosom Med.* 59:481–487.

Suarez EC, Williams RB Jr, Kuhn CM, Zimmerman EH, Schanberg SM. 1991. Biobehavioral basis of coronary-prone behavior in middle-age men. Part II: serum cholesterol, the Type A behavior pattern, and hostility as interactive modulators of physiological reactivity. *Psychosom Med.* 53:528–537.

Suls J, Wan CK. 1993. The relationship between trait hostility and cardiovascular reactivity: a quantitative analysis. *Psychophysiology.* 30:615–626.

Temoshok L. 1987. Personality, coping style, emotion, and cancer: towards an integrative model. *Cancer Surv.* 6:545–567.

Temoshok L, Dreher H. 1992. *The Type C Connection: The Behavioral Links to Cancer and Your Health.* New York: Random House.

Theorell T, Perski A, Akerstedt T, et al. 1988. Changes in job strain in relation to changes in physiological state. *Scan J Work Environ Health.* 14:189–196.

Unden AL, Orth-Gomer K, Elofsson S. 1991. Cardiovascular effects of social support in the work place: twenty-four-hour ECG monitoring of men and women. *Psychosom Med.* 53:53–60.

Vaishnav S, Stevenson R, Marchant B, Lagi K, Ranjadayalan K, Timmis AD. 1994. Relation between heart rate variability early after acute myocardial infarction and long-term mortality. *Am J Cardiol.* 73:653–657.

Verrier RL. 1987. Mechanisms of behaviorally induced arrhythmias. *Circulation.* 76(1 pt 2):148–156.

Verster GC, Gagiano CA. 1995. Masked depression (in Afrikaans). *S Afr Med J.* 85:759–762.

Vogt T, Pope C, Mullooly J, Hollis J. 1994. Mental health status as a predictor of morbidity and mortality: a fifteen-year follow-up of members of a health maintenance organization. *Am J Public Health.* 84:227–231.

Wassertheil-Smoller S, Applegate WB, Berge K, et al. 1996. Changes in depression as a precursor of cardiovascular events. *Arch Intern Med.* 156:553–561.

Watkins LL, Grossman P, Krishnan R, Sherwood A. 1998. Anxiety and vagal control of heart risk. *Psychosom Med.* 60:498–502.

Weinberger DA, Schwartz GE, Davidson RJ. 1979. Low-anxious, high-anxious, and repressive coping styles: psychometric patterns and behavioral and physiological responses to stress. *J Abnorm Psychol.* 88:369–380.

Welin C, Lappas G, Wilhelmsen L. 2000. Independent importance of psychosocial factors for prognosis after myocardial infarction. *J Intern Med.* 247:629–639.

Wheeler EO, White PD, Reed EW, Cohen ME. 1950. Neurocirculatory asthenia (anxiety neurosis, effort syndrome, neurasthenia): a twenty year follow-up study for one hundred and seventy-three patients. *JAMA.* 142:878–889.

Whiteman MC, Fowkes FG, Deary IJ, Lee AJ. 1997. Hostility, cigarette smoking, and alcohol consumption in the general population. *Soc Sci Med.* 44:1089–1096.

154 Williams RB Jr. 1987. Refining the type A hypothesis: emergence of the hostility complex. *Am J Cardiol.* 60:27J–32J.

Williams RB Jr. 1993. Hostility and the heart. In: Goleman D, Gurin J., eds. *Mind-Body Medicine: How to Use Your Mind for Better Health.* Yonkers, NY: Consumer Reports Books.

Williams RB. 1994. Neurobiology, cellular and molecular biology, and psychosomatic medicine. *Psychosom Med.* 56:308–315.

Williams RB. 1998. Lower socioeconomic status and increased mortality: early childhood roots and the potential for successful interventions. *JAMA.* 279:1745–1746.

Williams RB, Barefoot JC, Califf RM, et al. 1992. Prognostic importance of social and economic resources among medically treated patients with angiographically documented coronary artery disease. *JAMA.* 267:520–524.

Williams RB, Barefoot JC, Haney TL, et al. 1988. Type A behavior and angiographically documented coronary atherosclerosis in a sample of 2,289 patients. *Psychosom Med.* 50:139–152.

Williams RB, Littman AB. 1996. Psychosocial factors: role in cardiac risk and treatment. *Cardiol Clin.* 14:97–104.

Winkleby MA, Fortmann SP, Barrett DC. 1990. Social class disparities in risk factors of disease: eight year prevalence patterns by level of education. *Prev Med.* 19:1–12.

Yeith RC, Lewis L, Linares OA, et al. 1994. Sympathetic nervous system in major depression: basal and desipramine-induced alterations in plasma norepinephrine kinetics. *Arch Gen Psychiatry.* 51:411–422.

Yeung AC, Vekshtein VI, Krantz DS, et al. 1991. The effect of atherosclerosis on the vasomotor response of coronary arteries to mental stress. *New Engl J Med.* 325:1551–1556.

Yudkin JS, Kumari M, Humphries SE, Mohamed-Ali V. 2000. Inflammation, obesity, stress, and coronary heart disease: is interleukin-6 the link? *Atherosclerosis.* 148:209–214.

Zisook S, DeVaul R. 1985. Unresolved grief. *Am J Psychoanal.* 45:370–379.

Zyzanski SJ, Jenkins CD, Ryan TJ, Flessas A, Everist M. 1976. Psychological correlates of coronary angiographic findings. *Arch Intern Med.* 136:1234–1237.

Chapter 4

Cancer and the Mind:

An Integrative Investigation

The question whether psychosocial factors—stress, emotions, coping style, personality, and social support—influence the development or progression of cancer is arguably the most contentious in the allied fields of mind-body science and medicine. Most conventional oncologists and cancer specialists have long been skeptical of any assertion that the mind is involved in cancer, while mind-body scientists and clinicians hold differing views on the matter. Claims at either extreme seem unjustified: skeptics argue that no sound research has ever implicated psychological factors in cancer incidence or outcome, while uncritical adherents focus only on positive studies to support their belief that the mind is a determining factor in cancer risk and recovery. A reasonable interpretation of the research—and there are scores of such studies—should reject both extreme views. A review of the literature reveals a complex picture, one in which psychosocial factors may play a modest role in cancer risk and a somewhat stronger role in progression or recovery. Which factors are clinically most important remains an unresolved question, though a preponderance of research points to specific behavioral and coping patterns, not to stress per se.

The field of psychoneuroimmunology has provided ample evidence that psychological states and traits can cause deficits (or, conversely, enhancements) of portions of the immune system capable of recognizing and eliminating cancer cells (Turner-Cobbs et al. 2001). While the immune surveillance theory—which posits that the immune system is capable of detecting and eliminating microscopic cancer before it evolves into full-blown tumors—has been questioned, the field of cancer immunology has produced a wealth of findings in the past decade affirming that many types

156 of cancer can be resisted to varying degrees by immune defenses. Even metastatic tumors can be detected and vanquished by immune sentries in some cases. The rise of immunotherapies and biological therapies for treating cancer reinforces the notion that cancer can be opposed by the body's own arsenal of anticancer defenses. Moreover, these defenses are not limited to the immune system but include the regulation of gene expression, apoptosis (programmed cell suicide), DNA repair mechanisms, and the regulation of cell-signaling pathways. We are just beginning to see evidence that psychological factors can influence some of these other mechanisms as well, including gene expression and DNA repair (Glaser et al. 1990; Glaser et al. 1993; Kiecolt-Glaser et al. 1985; Wu et al. 1999).

In this chapter I present an overview of research on psychosocial factors in cancer incidence or etiology and then turn to research on the mind's role in cancer progression and survival, attempting to provide the clearest possible answer to the question, Do attitudes, coping styles, emotions, or personality traits influence the outcome for patients who have been diagnosed with cancer? I review the key studies in this area, paying special attention to one recent study on mental adjustment to cancer, an important paper by Margaret Watson and her colleagues that received much media attention and deserves special consideration (Watson et al. 1999). After reviewing the research findings I present a theoretical process model, as I did in chapter 3 for heart disease, to help interpret the disparate data, showing how psychosocial factors that influence cancer change over time. In this effort I draw upon the singular efforts of Lydia Temoshok, Ph.D., my coauthor for *The Type C Connection: The Behavioral Links to Cancer and Your Health* (1992), who first developed a process model for psychosocial factors in cancer in a 1987 paper. Before proceeding, however, I must address one of the thorniest issues in this area of research: the worry that any conclusive evidence of psychosocial factors in cancer risk or recovery "blames the victims" for their disease.

Blaming the Victim: An Inevitable Outgrowth of Mind-Cancer Research?

One of the chief complaints about mind-body-cancer research has been that any implication of thoughts, emotions, or traits in cancer blames the victim for his or her disease or decline. It is a legitimate concern that needs to be taken seriously. The issue goes to the heart of the philosophy and epistemology of mind-body science and medicine. From my perspective, blaming the victim is an outgrowth of a distorted conceptualization of mind-body interactions. If the mind influences a disease—any disease, not just cancer—why would an individual be to blame? The purported reasons would be that (1) people deliberately bring on pathology as an expression of a death wish or a lesson they need to learn; (2) people develop cancer, or their disease progresses, due to psychological or coping inadequacies; and (3) people's malignancies are the result of spiritual impoverishment. Many of these misplaced notions are expressions of "New Age guilt," an invidious popularization of mind-body ideas in which people are thought to cause an illness in themselves through psychospiritual self-neglect or a semiconscious effort to teach themselves a deeper lesson—in other words, illness as a metaphoric moral message.

These notions of mind-body interaction are baseless and also dangerous; they can cause enormous suffering on top of the grief and fear associated with a cancer diagnosis. Unfortunately, however, health professionals who are properly concerned about the psychological damage caused by such myths often throw out the baby with the bathwater, rejecting the notion that psychosocial factors can have *any* influence on disease processes for fear that patients (or their mind-body practitioners) will interpret the information in an emotionally damaging manner. The problem with this wholesale rejection is twofold: First, it is not scientifically founded. As I will show, there are sufficient sound data to support some psychological contribution to cancer recovery and perhaps even to cancer risk. Second, cancer patients who can be made aware of this contribution without moral judgments may take advantage of the information in ways that help them promote their own recovery process. While engaging the mind in an active, adaptive, emotionally healthy way in response to the trauma of a cancer diagnosis is no guarantee of improved survival, there is ample evidence that it improves quality of life and provisional evidence that it bolsters the odds of a more favorable medical outcome. (For data on this point, see chapter 6, on psychosocial interventions for cancer.)

How, then, do healthcare professionals of any stripe—from oncologists to nurses to psychotherapists—address the possible role of the mind in cancer without reinforcing illness as a metaphoric moral message? By debunking the invidious perspectives mentioned above (i.e., New Age guilt), and presenting the mind's role in a scientifically accurate, psychologically sensitive, and morally compassionate way. An appropriate philosophy and epistemology of mind-body interactions in cancer should lead to the following conclusions:

1. There is no evidence that putative psychological factors in cancer are consciously or deliberately brought on by the patient. The key factors implicated in cancer, including hopelessness, reflexive repression of negative

158   emotions, and an appeasing personality style, are not consciously willed
states or traits.

2. Dysfunctional coping styles or personality traits, which in some cases may
contribute to cancer risk or progression, are not consciously cultivated, nor
are they an expression of psychological inadequacy. A psychodynamic perspective reveals that such defenses are donned early in life in response to
trauma, stress, or familial pressures. Most frequently, in childhood these
defenses are adaptive, but they become automatic unconscious reflexes, and
if these defenses are too rigidly employed across developmental stages, they
can become maladaptive. For instance, repression of anger may be a survival mode for a child in a family system in which anger is harshly out-
lawed; in adulthood a complete inability to access or appropriately express
anger can be a hindrance. But in such instances the coping mechanism is
generally unconscious, and it is neither a sign nor a symbol of psychological inadequacy. Rather it represents a talent in early life that later became
a vulnerability, one that should be no source of shame or guilt. To the extent that genetic predisposition or biochemical perturbations are involved,
there is, of course, no rationale for blaming the victim. With compassionate therapeutic help such individuals can come to understand, even to
honor, the origins of their behavior and take positive steps on behalf of their
own psychological and physical well-being, to reorient their coping style.
A psychoanalytic or psychodynamic view of psychological (or psychiatric)
disorders passes no judgment on these vulnerabilities, no matter what the
diagnostic category, and the same should hold for anyone whose emotional
states or coping traits play a part in his or her illness.

Finally, the preponderance of evidence suggests that psychosocial factors are virtually never the sole contributor to disease etiology or progression; they are but one among many variables in a multifactoral model of
health and disease. To attribute a disease exclusively to psychosocial factors, over which we may have some control, ignores the many genetic, biochemical, and environmental factors over which we have little or no control. Understanding the embeddedness of psychosocial factors in a web of
other biological and environmental contributors can help patients recognize that any effort they make to transform their behavior or coping style
is no guarantee of recovery but an effort to modestly improve their odds—
no different, say, than the decision to embark on a low-fat diet, exercise,
and other lifestyle changes to improve overall health and possibly enhance
immune function. Healthcare professionals who put psychological and
lifestyle changes into this same proper context—they may improve your
odds but offer no guarantee—remove the onus of unrealistically high expectations (and the resulting guilt should the disease progress) from the

patient without robbing the patient of the sense of agency that comes from taking charge of his or her mind-body health.

3. The notion of cancer as spiritual impoverishment is an even more profound distortion, one that bespeaks self-loathing, introjection of damning cultural images and metaphors about cancer (Sontag 1978), and in some cases a mixing of negative self-images with extreme moral teachings of some organized religions (i.e., disease as a form of punishment by God). Though couched in a lexicon of good intentions, New Age simplifications of the mind's role in illness may also reinforce patients' feelings that their disease is a sign of moral or spiritual bankruptcy. In *Illness as Metaphor* Susan Sontag effectively demolished invidious cultural metaphors about cancer (e.g., cancer as the epitome of evil), although she asserted that any claim of psychological influence in cancer ipso facto blames the victim, an argument that I find unjustifiable. What is needed is rejection of illusory, unscientific, judgmental, condescending, simplistic, exaggerated, and condemnatory metaphors, as well as acceptance of scientifically founded, psychologically penetrating, balanced, thoughtful, and compassionate insights that help cancer patients to cope healthfully with the diagnosis and its aftermath.

The Mind's Role in Cancer Causation

In the second century A.D. Galen, the most respected physician of ancient Greece and a seminal figure in the history of medicine, noted that breast cancer occurred far more often in women with a "melancholic" temperament than it did in women with a "sanguine" temperament. It is the first recorded observation that emotional or mental factors might contribute to the development of cancer. In the modern medical era respected physicians and researchers have studied psychological patterns prevalent in cancer patients; these observations and retrospective analyses cannot identify causal links, but a certain consistency among them became the basis for later, more systematic studies. A brief sampling of these early observations, many compiled by the cancer psychotherapist and researcher Lawrence LeShan (1959), includes the following:

- In 1931 the French physician E. Foque published a paper in which he described his theory of the multiple causes of cancer. He found a clear pattern in many of his patients of "great crises, grave depressive afflictions, profound mourning, and all the sad emotions which have prolonged repercussions . . . you can see in the patients prolonged and silent sorrow without the release of sobs and tears" (LeShan 1959).
- In 1952 the researchers C. L. Bacon, R. Renneker, and M. Cutler reported

on the psychiatric histories of forty women with breast cancer. They observed that thirty-five of these patients exhibited "a masochistic character structure" and that thirty "had no techniques for discharging anger directly or in a sublimated fashion."

- In 1954 the researcher Eugene Blumberg and his colleagues published their study of cancer patients with a variety of tumors in the journal *Psychosomatic Medicine*. They described the majority of patients, and particularly those with rapid tumor growth, in these terms: "They were . . . consistently serious, over-cooperative, over-nice, over-anxious, painfully sensitive, passive, apologetic personalities and, as far as could be ascertained from family, friends, and previous records, they had suffered from this lack of self-expression and self-realization all their lives."

These early insights, among many others, set the stage for later research that met more stringent methodological criteria for studies identifying causal contributors to disease. The most reliable way to ferret out causality is the prospective study of large populations of healthy individuals in which "premorbid" psychological states and traits are measured years or preferably a decade or longer before cancer is diagnosed. Conventional biomedical wisdom has it that no such studies have been carried out, but that is not the case. Before discussing the prospective research, I will describe a series of studies that have uncovered associations between psychosocial factors and cancer development. These studies, using varying methods, are less conclusive than prospective studies but still worthy of consideration. One of the methods used is the so-called quasi-prospective study, in which patients undergoing biopsies are given psychological tests before either patients or physicians know who has a malignant disease. In 1975 the British psychiatrist Steven Greer and his colleague Tina Morris, then of King's College Hospital in London, published their study of 160 women with breast lumps, who were interviewed and tested prior to biopsy. Sixty-nine of these women were found to have cancer. In searching for differences between the groups, they found one key discriminator: the breast cancer patients were more likely to be extreme suppressors of anger (Greer and Morris 1975). Fully one-half of the cancer patients were found to be extreme suppressors (they "had never or not more than twice during their adult lives openly shown anger"), compared with only 15 percent of the patients without cancer. Over half of the breast cancer patients were also extreme suppressors of sadness and anxiety, compared with only 30 percent of the patients with benign lumps. Using judges' ratings of semistructured interviews to measure suppression of anger, Greer, Morris, and colleagues were able to replicate these findings (Morris et al. 1981).

Drs. A. H. Schmale and Howard Iker of the University of Rochester conducted a quasi-prospective study involving sixty-eight women undergoing biopsies for potential cervical cancer (Schmale and Iker 1971). Based on psychological analyses before biopsy results, Schmale and Iker were able to predict which patients would have malignancies with 73 percent accuracy. The single factor upon which they based their prediction was evidence that these women experienced hopelessness. Karl Goodkin and his colleagues at the University of Miami evaluated seventy-three women awaiting workup for an abnormal Pap smear. They discovered that patients with advanced disease had more life stress and had reacted to that stress with hopelessness (Goodkin et al. 1986). Two German studies, using methods similar to Greer and Morris's, also observed significant correlations between psychological factors and the presence of cancer among women receiving breast biopsies. Horst Scherg (1987) found that cancer patients expressed less anxiety, showed less Type A behavior, and were more committed to social and religious norms, "putting off their own wishes in favor of more socially desirable behavior." Michael Wirsching and colleagues (1982) reported that "adequate expression of emotions was not observed in any of the women with cancer." By contrast, among the women who did not have cancer fully half displayed to the researchers a healthy capacity for emotional expression.

While the studies evaluating patients undergoing biopsies were fairly consistent in finding that nonexpression of emotions is associated with cancer, one recent "quasi-prospective" study offers contradictory evidence. Investigators in the Department of Psychological Medicine at the University of Sydney measured coping and personality factors in 2,224 older women recalled for assessment after routine mammograms showed an abnormality. When the 298 women who were diagnosed with breast cancer were compared with controls with nonmalignant conditions, no significant psychological differences were detected (Price, Tennant, Smith, et al. 2001). (The measures included tests of "emotional expression-in" versus "emotional expression-out," as well as anxiety and depression.) But the same research team conducted a similar study with 514 women of varying ages, of whom 239 were discovered to have breast cancer, and found one stunningly significant result: women experiencing a stressful life event or problem objectively rated as highly threatening *and* who were without "intimate social support" had a ninefold increased risk of developing breast carcinoma (Price, Tennant, Butow, et al. 2001).

Though it has been conceptualized and measured in different ways, the most prominent finding in these mind-cancer studies has been a lack of emotional expression, variously categorized as "non-expression of emo-

162 tions," "emotional repression," "repressive coping," "anger suppression," and "Type C behavior." The Type C construct, developed independently by Steven Greer and the American psychologist Lydia Temoshok while she was at the University of California at San Francisco, centers around nonexpression of emotions (particularly anger, but other "negative" emotions as well) but also includes a tendency to be unassertive, appeasing, self-sacrificing, stoical, and compliant. Temoshok hypothesized that this behavior pattern was the polar opposite of the coronary-prone Type A pattern, which is characterized by hostility, aggressiveness, competitiveness, high anxiety, and controlling behavior.

To test her hypothesis, Temoshok conducted a case-control study comparing the behavior patterns of twenty patients with malignant melanoma with the behavior patterns of twenty patients with coronary heart disease (CHD) and those of twenty normal controls. The cancer patients displayed significantly more repressive coping (a combination of high physiological arousal and low self-report of upset in a stressful experimental procedure) than either of the comparison groups (Kneier and Temoshok 1984). Earlier case-control studies by David Kissen, a physician at the University of Glasgow, found that patients with lung cancer had "poorer outlets for emotional discharge" than controls and scored lower in neuroticism, often viewed as a sign of emotional expressiveness (Kissen 1966; Kissen et al. 1969). Like Temoshok, Claus and Marjorie Bahnson compared heart and cancer patients and found that the cancer patients scored significantly lower on hostility and social dominance—two Type A characteristics that would not be observed in so-called Type C individuals (Bahnson 1969).

More recently, G. A. Kune and his colleagues at the University of Melbourne, Australia, along with Claus Bahnson, conducted a case-control study as one arm of a large, population-based investigation of colorectal cancer (Kune et al. 1991). Patients and controls received structured psychosocial interviews; 637 histologically confirmed cases and 714 community controls matched by age and sex were compared. Self-reported childhood or adult life "unhappiness" was statistically significantly more common among the cancer cases. Moreover,

> questions which were formulated to test a particular personality profile as a cancer risk, and which included the elements of denial and repression of anger and of other negative emotions, a commitment to prevailing social norms resulting in the external appearance of a "nice" or "good" person, a suppression of reactions which may offend others and the avoidance of conflict, showed a statistically significant discrimination between cases and controls. The risk of colorectal cancer with re-

spect to this model was independent of the previously found risk factors of diet, beer intake, and family history of colorectal cancer, and was also independent of other potential confounding factors of socioeconomic level, marital status, religion and country of birth.

The researchers stated that while the results "must be interpreted with caution, the data are consistent with the hypothesis that this personality type may play a role in the clinical expression of colorectal cancer and merits further study." Such caution was warranted largely due to the design of the study, a case-control analysis that could not make firm conclusions about causality. Retrospective, quasi-prospective, and case-control studies can shed light on psychological factors in cancer development, but only prospective studies are considered acceptable signposts of causality. The following list describes the most prominent long-term prospective studies, in which psychological states and traits were evaluated in large healthy populations that were then followed for many years, enabling researchers to compare those who developed cancer to those who did not.

Study 1
Investigators: George Kaplan and Peggy Reynolds (1988)
Subjects: 6,848 healthy individuals taking part in the California Department of Health Services Study (Alameda County)
Years followed: 17
Findings: An increased risk for cancer incidence and death among individuals who were "socially isolated"

Study 2
Investigators: Ronald Grossarth-Maticek and colleagues (Grossarth-Maticek 1982; Grossarth-Maticek et al. 1983)
Subjects: 1,353 healthy inhabitants of a Yugoslav village
Years followed: 10
Findings: Subjects who contracted cancer had shown evidence of "rational and anti-emotional behavior." Grossarth-Maticek found similar patterns in two later studies conducted in Heidelberg, Germany. Some investigators have questioned the validity of Grossarth-Maticek's data, but his methods appear to have been sound.

Study 3
Investigators: Richard B. Shekelle and colleagues (1981)
Subjects: 2,010 middle-aged male workers at a Chicago Western Electric plant
Years followed: 17

Findings: The men who on original psychological tests were found to be depressed had a twofold increased risk of death from cancer.

Study 4
Investigators: Patrick J. Dattore and colleagues (1980)
Subjects: 200 disease-free veterans who had been psychologically tested upon entry into a VA hospital. Records of 75 who went on to contract cancer were compared with 125 who remained healthy or developed other diseases.
Years followed: 10
Findings: The cancer patients were far less depressed and evidenced significantly more emotional repression than control subjects.

Study 5
Investigators: Caroline B. Thomas, Pirkko Graves, John W. Shaffer, and colleagues (Thomas et al. 1979; Shaffer et al. 1982; Shaffer et al. 1987; Graves et al. 1991)
Subjects: 1,300 medical students at Johns Hopkins University
Years followed: Several intervals, up to 40 years
Findings: Thirty years after initial evaluation of students, Thomas found that the cancer patients were people who had reported a lack of closeness to their parents in childhood. They had also reported the least demonstrativeness—or open expression of love—in their families. Dr. Pirrko Graves analyzed the students' original Rorschach tests and found that of all members of the sick and healthy groups, the cancer patients had the poorest "relationship potential." This was defined as the capacity to accept negative and positive emotions in oneself and others in close relationships. In 1987 Graves and Shaffer reviewed the original personality tests for 972 of the students. Those who had been "loners" and who suppressed their emotions "beneath a bland exterior" had the highest risk of cancer. The "loners" were sixteen times more likely to develop cancer than those who "gave vent to their emotions."

Study 6
Investigators: Alan B. Zonderman and colleagues (Zonderman et al. 1989)
Subjects: 6,400 healthy adults in the National Health and Nutrition Examination Survey
Years followed: 10–15
Findings: Two brief depression scales, the Center for Epidemiologic Studies Depression Scale and the General Well-Being Schedule, were administered to all patients at the onset of the study. Neither measure of depressive symptoms was a significant risk for cancer morbidity or mortality.

Study 7

Investigators: E. M. Bleiker et al. (1996)

Subjects: 9,705 women involved in a population-based breast cancer screening program in the Dutch city of Nijmegen. Followed for incidence of breast cancer.

Years followed: 5

Findings: In this prospective analysis using a nested case-control design 131 women diagnosed with breast cancer during the follow-up period were compared with 771 age-matched controls (up to six per case). Only one psychological variable was significantly more prevalent among the breast cancer cases: a relatively high score on the personality scale of antiemotionality (versus a low score, odds ratio [OR] = 1.19). Although the finding was statistically significant, it may be considered a relatively weak discriminator.

Study 8

Investigators: Johan Denollet (1998)

Subjects: 246 men treated for CHD but free of cancer at baseline.

Years followed: 6–10

Findings: In this small prospective study of men with CHD, development of cancer was unrelated to cardiac pathology but was associated with pessimism, anxiety, and the so-called Type D (distressed) personality, which involves high negative affectivity coupled with high social inhibition. Denollet has characterized the Type D individual as nonexpressive of emotions. The cancer rate for Type D men was 13 percent, compared with 2 percent for non–Type D men; the cancer death rates were 10 percent and 2 percent, respectively. Among the psychological factors, regression analysis revealed Type D personality as the only independent prognostic factor for the development of cancer (OR = 7.2).

Study 9

Investigators: John R. Jacobs and Gregory B. Bovasso (2000)

Subjects: 1,213 women participating in the Baltimore Epidemiologic Catchment Area Study. Followed for incidence of breast cancer.

Years followed: 14

Findings: These subjects were initially assessed for depressive and anxious disorders, parental death in childhood and relatively recent adverse life events prior to cancer hospitalization. During the study period 29 women were hospitalized for breast cancer and 10 died of breast cancer. The psychosocial variables that predicted increased risk of breast cancer were maternal death in childhood (OR = 2.56; $p < .001$) and chronic depression with severe episodes (OR = 14.0; $p < .001$). Neither relatively recent life events nor other depressive and anxiety disorders were associated with increased risk. Maternal death and chronic depression with severe episodes were reported to have occurred at least twenty years prior to breast cancer hospitalization.

The prospective studies detailed here belie the commonly held belief among mainstream cancer specialists and some psycho-oncologists that there is no hard evidence of psychosocial factors—be they states or traits—associated with cancer development. But what can be made of this evidence? Only two of the nine studies, those led by Richard Shekelle and J. R. Jacobs, suggest that depression is a factor in cancer risk, and caveats are necessary in both instances. In the Shekelle analysis of the Western Electric study depression was found to be a risk factor, not for development of cancer, but rather for eventual death from cancer. In the Jacobs study depressive disorders in general were not associated with later cancer; however, "chronic depression with severe episodes" was associated with a fourteenfold greater risk of developing malignant disease. In sum, the evidence linking depression and cancer development can be characterized as weak. (Indeed, in one study, led by Patrick Dattore, the cancer patients were found to be *less* overtly depressed.) A meta-analysis of prospective studies of depression and cancer risk conducted by researchers at the University of Otago in New Zealand revealed "a small, but marginally statistically significant association between depression and the later development of cancer" (McGee 1994).

But the relationship between other psychological factors and cancer risk appears somewhat stronger. Nonexpression of emotions, classified variously as "anti-emotionality," "suppressing emotions," "repression," or "Type D," was significantly associated with increased risk in five of the nine prospective studies listed above (Grossarth-Maticek, Dattore, Graves, Blieker, Denollet). In one of these studies the association was weak (Blieker), but in the others it was considerably more robust. Three of the studies also identified social and familial factors and life events, namely, social isolation (Kaplan and Reynolds 1988), lack of closeness to parents or of parental expressions of love in childhood (Thomas), poor "relationship potential" (Graves), and maternal death in childhood (Jacobs). A meta-analysis by investigators at the University of Illinois included forty-six studies using different methodologies, some of them prospective, that specifically evaluated psychosocial factors in breast cancer. Among eight major construct categories three showed significant effect sizes: denial or repressive coping (.38), separation or loss experiences (.29), and stressful life events (.25) (McKenna et al. 1999); such effect sizes may be considered "moderate." Among the psychological complexes that did *not* show any significant effect were anxiety or depression and extraversion or intraversion. Given that denial or repressive coping had the strongest cancer association, this meta-analysis provides additional evidence that repressive defenses are more likely to be associated with cancer risk than depression per se. A recent review by Australian researchers focused on the same question—whether psychosocial factors influence development of breast cancer—and drew similar conclusions (Butow, Hiller, et al. 2000). Seven studies revealed that anger repression or "rationality/antiemotionality" predicted breast cancer risk, but there was no strong evidence that anxiety or depression presaged breast cancer.

In her process model Temoshok (1987) explained how these prospective findings (and the breast cancer meta-analysis and review) are generally consistent with her understanding of the putative Type C coping pattern. I detail this theory after presenting all the data, but the relevant point here is that the Type C individual is not likely to be manifestly depressed years before a cancer diagnosis. According to Temoshok's theory, the Type C coper often harbors an unconscious hopelessness or depression that would not be apparent to the person him- or herself; nor would it be measurable through standard psychological tests. This masked depression may well surface, however, when the individual's "fragile accommodation to the world" is strained by life stresses or by the cancer diagnosis itself. This explains why extant prospective studies have been less likely to detect depression years prior to a cancer diagnosis and more likely to find Type C behavior—nonexpression of emotions and an appeasing, self-sacrificing, nonassertive personality style—and some evidence, via self-reports, of early traumas (i.e., loss of a parent) or familial dysfunction.

The Mind's Role in Cancer Progression and Survival

There is now considerable evidence that psychological states and traits and social factors have an impact on cancer progression and even survival. While this evidence has been met by many scientists and physicians with a querulous or even dismissive attitude, it has been accumulating for over three decades and ought to be taken seriously.

The following list summarizes thirty-one prominent longitudinal studies of psychosocial factors in cancer prognosis, progression, and survival. It is based upon reviews of the literature and upon my own exhaustive search of publications in the National Library of Medicine's database, MEDLINE, publications from 1966 through 2001. Studies that appear to meet basic criteria for methodological soundness are included.

168   Stavraky et al. (1968)

Study: Longitudinal study of more than two hundred patients with mixed cancer types in search of psychosocial factors in survival time. The favorable-outcome group was compared with site-stage controls with average outcomes.

Results: The long survivors for particular cancer sites and stages showed evidence of being angrier or more hostile, but without loss of emotional control.

Weisman and Worden (1977)

Study: Patients with various tumor types were psychologically assessed and followed for differences between expected and observed survival time.

Results: Long survivors had closer personal relationships, were less distressed, and coped more effectively with stress than patients whose survival was briefer than expected.

Derogatis et al. (1979)

Study: Psychological testing of women with stage III and stage IV breast cancer (using a standard measure of distress, the SCL-90, a brief self-report inventory screening for a range of psychological problems), followed for differences between short- and long-term survivors (short-term = less than one year; long-term = more than one year).

Results: Long-term survivors expressed their distress more often and required more "adjustment" to having cancer; short-term survivors were more well adjusted and complained less.

Rogentine et al. (1979)

Study: Melanoma patients were followed for one year to differentiate those who had a recurrence from those who did not.

Results: Those patients who had recurrence required less adjustment to their disease and were less overtly distressed.

Greer et al. (Greer and Morris 1975; Greer et al. 1990)

Study: Sixty-nine breast cancer patients were assessed after at five, ten, and fifteen years to distinguish survivors from nonsurvivors in terms of mental adjustment to cancer measured three months after diagnosis.

Results: Those who responded to diagnosis with hopelessness or helplessness had the shortest survival time; those who were stoical in their adjustment also tended to have shorter survival. Those who survived longest exhibited "fighting spirit"; those who coped by denial (later reconceptualized as "positive avoidance") also fared relatively well.

Note: No baseline data were available on axillary nodes. In later analyses patients found to evidence "anxious preoccupation" had relatively poorer long-term survival. The study's findings were partially replicated by Di-Clemente and Temoshok (1985), who found that stoical and helpless or hopeless responses were associated with relapse or mortality.

Temoshok et al. (1985)
Study: Melanoma patients were assessed for personality and coping and evaluated for favorable versus unfavorable prognostic indicators (thicker, more invasive tumors).

Results: Unfavorable prognosis was significantly associated with a specific coping style: nonexpression of emotions, especially anger; compliance; self-sacrifice; passive responses to stress. This coping style was operationalized as the "Type C behavior pattern."

Temoshok (1985)
Study: A different group of melanoma patients were assessed through video-taped structured interviews evaluated by independent raters, as well as psychological tests, in search of correlations between emotional-expression variables and tumor thickness, as well as other biological prognostic indicators—tumor-cell mitotic rate and number of tumor-infiltrating lymphocytes.

Results: Less emotionally expressive patients had thicker tumors; tumor cells with a faster mitotic rate; and fewer lymphocytes invading the base of the tumor—all unfavorable prognostic indicators.

Cassileth et al. (1985)
Study: Using brief psychological scales, Cassileth and colleagues evaluated social ties, general life satisfaction, adjustment to illness, job satisfaction, and hopelessness or helplessness in cancer patients with stage IV (metastatic) disease (looking for factors in survival) and stage II breast cancer and melanoma (looking for factors in recurrence and survival).

Results: There was no correlation between the psychological factors measured and disease recurrence or survival.

Levy et al. (1985)
Study: Examination of psychological responses of breast cancer patients at time of diagnosis, in search of correlations with prognostic variables, including axillary node status and natural killer (NK) cell activity.

Results: A psychological state of apathy, fatigue, and a self-report of being more well "adjusted" correlated with lower NK cell activity and positive axillary nodes, the latter two being unfavorable prognostic indicators for

170   breast cancer. Levy characterized these individuals as displaying a passive
           response style.
           Note: Levy replicated these findings in a similar study in 1987 (Levy et al. 1987).

Holland et al. (1986)

Study: Using the SCL-90 distress scale, Holland and colleagues tested 346
women with stage II breast cancer after diagnosis to determine possible
correlations with survival.

Results: After 106 recurrences or deaths, there appeared to be no significant
correlation with psychosocial variables. The predominant predictors were
nodal status and, secondarily, estrogen-receptor status. Reanalysis after 137
recurrences or deaths did show a modest correlation with one psychosocial variable: a sense of alienation.

Jamison et al. (1987)

Study: Forty-nine women with metastatic breast cancer were given a variety
of psychological tests. By the time the data analysis was performed, all patients were deceased. They were evenly divided into "short" versus "long"
survivors.

Results: There were no consistent psychosocial differences between short and
long survivors.

Levy et al. (1988)

Study: Women with recurrent breast cancer were evaluated psychologically
and immunologically, then tracked for seven years.

Results: Two-thirds of the women had died when the seven-year follow-up
analysis was conducted. Those who survived had scored higher on one psychological variable at baseline: they had expressed more "joy" as measured
by the Affect Balance Scale. "Joy" was a more powerful predictor of survival than several biomedical indicators.

Stavraky et al. (1988)

Study: Newly diagnosed male and female lung cancer patients were given
structured interviews; information was obtained on biomedical, demographic, and psychosocial factors, including locus of control, social support, and personality traits. Survival analyses were conducted at one year.

Results: After controlling for stage and pathological diagnosis, several psychological variables increased the odds of death from lung cancer: a high
need for sympathy and devotion, coupled with a reserved personality, making a person less likely to reach out for support. (The adjusted odds ratio
for mortality among the reserved personalities was 3.9.)

Ramirez et al. (1989)

Study: Fifty women with operable breast cancer that recurred were matched with fifty comparable patients whose breast cancer had not recurred over equivalent follow-up times. Sociodemographic variables, including stressful life events, were evaluated.

Results: Severely threatening life events were significantly associated with a greater than fivefold increased risk (relative risk [RR] = 5.67) of recurrent breast cancer, and "severe difficulties" were similarly associated with increased risk (RR = 4.75).

Dean and Surtees (1989)

Study: One hundred twenty-two women with primary operable breast cancer were interviewed and psychologically tested before surgery and three months after surgery, then tracked for six to eight years.

Results: Women who had sufficient symptoms to meet the criteria for psychiatric illness (according to the Research Diagnostic Criteria and the General Health Questionnaire) before their operations were less likely to have a recurrence during follow-up. Those assessed three months after surgery as having employed denial as a coping strategy had a better chance of remaining recurrence-free than women who relied on other coping strategies.

Levy et al. (1991)

Study: Ninety women with recently diagnosed stage I or stage II breast cancer participating in a National Institutes of Health Clinical Center randomized trial were immunologically and psychosocially assessed at baseline (approximately five days after surgery) and again at three and fifteen months after surgery. All were followed for a minimum of five years; most were followed for seven years or longer.

Results: NK cell activity was a strong predictor of recurrence versus nonrecurrence. Psychosocial factors, namely, a passive, helpless response style, predicted faster time to disease progression among those who had recurrences.

Waxler-Morrison et al. (1991)

Study: One hundred thirty-three women were followed prospectively after an initial diagnosis of breast cancer. Data on social factors were obtained from a mailed questionnaire and hospital charts.

Results: Using multivariate method, researchers found the following to have significant and independent effects on survival: number of supportive friends; whether the patient worked; whether the patient was unmarried; extent of contact with friends; and size of social network.

172 **Andrykowski et al. (1994)**

Study: Forty-two patients undergoing allogeneic bone marrow transplant (BMT) for chronic or acute leukemia were biomedically and psychosocially assessed and followed for post-BMT survival.

Results: The quality of the bone marrow graft match was the only medical or demographic variable associated with survival. The addition of psychosocial variables to a multivariate model demonstrated that an attitude toward cancer of "anxious preoccupation" and a poorer functional quality of life were independently associated with shorter post-BMT survival time.

Maunsell et al. (1995)

Study: Two hundred twenty-four newly diagnosed patients with localized or regional breast cancer participated in home interviews (which focused on issues of social support) three months after surgery. Patients were followed for seven years.

Results: The seven-year survival rate for women who reported no close confidants was 56 percent; for those with one confidant, 66 percent; and for those with two or more confidants, 76 percent. The results remained significant after adjustment for demographic and medical variables, including lymph node status and adjuvant medical treatments.

Tross et al. (1996)

Study: Two hundred eighty women with stage II breast cancer were given the SCL-90; categorized as high-, medium-, or low-distress; and tracked prospectively for a minimum of twelve years.

Results: The degree of distress as measured by the SCL-90 did not predict the length of disease-free survival or overall survival.

Schulz et al. (1996)

Study: A total of 238 cancer patients receiving palliative radiation were followed for eight months, by which time seventy had died. Controlling for the site of the cancer and the level of symptomatology at baseline, the researchers studied the independent effects on mortality of pessimism, optimism, and depression.

Results: Among younger patients (aged 30–59), endorsing a pessimistic life orientation (including negative expectations about the future) was a significant risk factor for mortality.

Giraldi et al. (1997)

Study: A prospective investigation of psychosocial variables in ninety-five breast cancer patients evaluated within three months of diagnosis and followed for six years.

Results: A higher volume of primary tumor at surgery was shown among patients who had had stressful life events in the six months preceding cancer diagnosis. At follow-up, no relationship was found between psychosocial factors and disease course.

Faller et al. (1997)

Study: One hundred patients with lung cancer were psychosocially assessed and prospectively tracked for three to five years.

Results: After adjustment for biological risk factors, including disease stage, histology, and medical treatment, active coping and hope were associated with longer survival. Emotional distress, depression, and depressive coping were associated with shorter survival. The predictive effects of coping and distress were independent of the influence of somatic risk factors, and the best psychological predictor, an interviewer rating of active coping, was equal in its predictive power to the Karnovsky Performance Status measure.

De Boer et al. (1998)

Study: Head and neck cancer patients were included in a prospective study at pretreatment. Psychosocial variables, measured by self-reports, were evaluated at baseline.

Results: Patients who were physically self-efficacious (they had higher perceived physical abilities) had a better prognosis, and those who expressed intense psychosocial complaints prior to treatment had a better prognosis than those who did not express such negative feelings.

Kuderer et al. (1998)

Study: Seventy-nine breast cancer patients were given psychosocial inventories and prospectively followed for a median of 8.4 years.

Results: Emotional defensiveness and anger suppression were independent predictors of recurrence, while somatic symptoms of depression and habitual suppression of anger were independent predictors of mortality.

Walker et al. (1999)

Study: Ninety-six women with newly diagnosed large or locally advanced breast cancer participated in a prospective, randomized trial to evaluate the effects of relaxation training with guided imagery and L-arginine on response to primary chemotherapy. Before the first of six cycles of primary chemotherapy women were assessed for depression, anxiety, and personality traits.

174   Results: A high depression score was a significant independent predictor of poor
pathological response to chemotherapy. A high anxiety score was a significant independent predictor of poor clinical response. Results could not be
explained by tumor size, which was accounted for in the statistical analysis.

Butow et al. (1999)

Study: One hundred twenty-five patients with metastatic melanoma completed psychological questionnaires after diagnosis and, where possible,
every three months for the next two years.

Results: In a multivariate analysis that controlled for demographic and disease
predictors the psychological variables of perceived aim of treatment (to fully
recover), minimization (denying the threat potential of the illness), and
anger expression were independently predictive of survival. Patients who
were married and who reported a better quality of life also survived longer.

Watson et al. (1999)

Study: Five hundred seventy-eight breast cancer patients, assessed by means
of the Mental Adjustment to Cancer scale (MAC, used in Greer and Morris 1975 and in Greer et al. 1990) and other psychological measures of
mood, were followed for five years.

Results: After controlling for biomedical prognostic indicators (including
lymph node status), women who scored high in hopelessness/helplessness
on the MAC had a significantly increased risk of relapse or death than those
who scored low. Those who scored high on a standard measure of depression had an increased risk of death from all causes. The MAC measure
"fighting spirit" did not predict an improved medical outcome. Thus, this
study partially replicated the original findings of Greer and colleagues.

Butow et al. (2000)

Study: Ninety-nine patients with metastatic breast cancer completed psychological questionnaires approximately four months after diagnosis. Survival was measured from the date of study to the date of death, and data on
surviving patients were removed from the analysis on the date of their last
follow-up.

Results: Patients who minimized the impact of cancer survived significantly
longer (29.1 months) than others (23.9 months).

Weihs et al. (2000)

Study: Thirty-two patients with recurrent breast cancer, diagnosed six to
nineteen months earlier and receiving standard conventional therapies,
were evaluated at the outset of the study for negative affectivity and emo-

tional constraint. Cox regression survival analysis, including the initial severity of metastasis, was used to explore associations between psychological factors and survival.

Results: Patients with low reported anxiety who also had low emotional constraint had the longest survival (RR = 0.7; p = .007). However, patients with low anxiety but high constraint had higher mortality (RR = 3.7; p = .02). High chronic anxiety, with or without high constraint, and more intense emotional constraint also predicted earlier death.

Brown et al. 2000

Study: Four hundred twenty-six early-stage melanoma patients were evaluated every three months for two years. At follow-up 21 percent had relapsed and 14 percent had died.

Results: After controlling for known prognostic indicators, longer survivors (1) perceived cure to be the aim of their treatment; (2) did not use avoidance as a coping strategy; or (3) expressed concern about their disease. Those who had a shorter duration of survival (1) displayed a more positive mood; (2) used avoidance as a coping strategy; and (3) were less concerned about their disease though more concerned about the impact of their disease on family members than about the impact on themselves.

Twenty-six of the thirty-one studies showed a significant association between at least one psychosocial variable and disease progression or survival. A number of studies had limited psychosocial measures, focusing only on one narrow domain, such as social support or psychological distress, so they cannot be said to rule out other psychological or social variables. For example, Elizabeth Maunsell's positive study of social support and breast cancer survival did not evaluate psychological coping patterns or personality traits. Barrie Cassileth's negative study of psychological factors and cancer survival among cancer patients (most with metastatic disease) included only five psychosocial variables and did not measure personality traits, coping styles, or emotions other than hopelessness/helplessness. Leonard Derogatis's positive study and Jimmie Holland's and Susan Tross's negative studies used only the SCL-90 measure of distress; they did not investigate personality, coping, or other emotional indices. Such limitations must be carefully considered before studies are simplistically labeled as "proving" that the mind is or is not involved in cancer progression or survival.

Of the twenty-six positive studies fourteen showed results consistent with the hypothesis that nonexpression of negative emotions is associated with disease progression or poor survival or, conversely, that expression of

176 negative emotions is associated with slower progression or improved survival. (Again, this does not mean that the other twelve studies disproved this connection, since many of these other studies did not measure dimensions of emotional expression.) By seeming contradistinction, eight studies found that greater distress was a poor prognostic sign. In three of these studies distress was measured as depression and/or anxiety; in three it was measured as hopelessness or helplessness; and in one study it was measured as anxious preoccupation. But it should be noted that investigators in most of the fourteen studies linking distress to better outcomes characterized these patients as "expressors" of negative emotion, while the eight studies linking distress to poorer outcomes emphasized depression, anxious preoccupation, pessimism, and hopeless or helpless states rather than acknowledgment or ventilation of negative emotional states. Four studies evidenced better outcomes among patients who could be classified as "active copers," while three studies explicitly correlated positive emotional states ("fighting spirit," "joy," and "hope") with longer survival. Six studies associated a stoical or passive coping style with unfavorable medical outcomes, while four studies found that patients who used denial or minimization as coping strategies had more favorable outcomes (one study correlated minimization with a worse outcome). Finally, three studies found robust relationships between social support and improved survival for cancer patients. Only one study linked severely stressful life events or difficulties (other than the cancer diagnosis itself) as heralding a poor prognosis.

Taking a broad view of these studies, there is substantial support for the hypothesis that Type C coping—nonexpression of emotions, stoicism, and a passive coping style—is a risk factor for disease progression or less favorable survival outcomes among cancer patients. There is also evidence that hopeless depression is a poor prognostic indicator. Is this a contradiction? A careful interpretation of these studies suggests that severe, hopeless depression is distinct from expressing distress, complaining, or openly communicating fear or anger in the aftermath of a cancer diagnosis. The former may reflect a breakdown in coping capacities. The latter reflects an understandable situational response to the stress or trauma of a cancer diagnosis, a response that is frequently adaptive. (Patients who share their distress may be less self-deceptive, more direct, more active in their coping style, more willing to seek and accept social support, and more able in the medium and long term to work through negative emotional states.) At the same time, there is evidence that denial or minimization is associated with favorable outcomes for some patients; presumably, these

are coping mechanisms that enable these individuals to move forward from
the cancer diagnosis without lapsing into hopeless despair.

These overall results suggest, to some extent, that no one-size-fits-all
coping strategy favors better psychological and medical outcomes for all
patients. For instance, denial or minimization may be adaptive for some and
destructive for others. But several strong patterns across these studies suggest that emotional expression and social support, to name two prominent
variables, are generally associated with better outcomes. Still, the manner,
timing, and style of expressing emotions will differ markedly from one individual to the next. The same may be said for procuring social support:
for some cancer patients a large network of emotional and practical supporters will be salutary, while for others one close confidant will do.

One factor unexplored in these studies is whether the doctor's or clinician's interpersonal style influences patients' coping strategies and emotional states. This "clinician interaction" variable could certainly affect
psychological factors and outcomes in these sorts of psychosocial studies
and ought to be considered in future investigations.

The presence of a supportive social network and the capacity to make
use of that network appears to be an important factor in favorable outcomes. This may be due to instrumental factors: patients who have the
practical and emotional support of friends and loved ones are more able to
comply and cope with difficult medical treatments. But it may also be due
to internal, mind-body interactions: people who can confide in their
spouses, family members, and friends can more readily relieve their emotional turmoil, which would otherwise prove to be a psychobiological burden. (This theory has been confirmed in experimental studies of the psychological, immunological, and physical health benefits of disinhibition
[Pennebaker 1999].) As David Spiegel and others have argued, the ability
to express and cognitively process negative emotions ultimately reduces
distress and makes positive emotions—joy, hope, fighting spirit—more ac-
cessible (Turner-Cobbs et al. 2001). The studies on emotional expression
and those on social support may be seen to dovetail: expressors of negative emotion may be more likely to seek support; those who remain nonexpressive, stoical, passive, or self-sacrificing (Type C–like) may be less in-
clined to turn to their social networks, worrying more about others than
about themselves. While this response style is admirable, it may be physically and emotionally enervating and psychologically self-defeating if it disables patients from intimate connections during a time of personal crisis.

In many respects the fifteen-year prospective study led by Steven Greer
and colleagues remains the seminal piece of research in the field of psy-

178   chosocial factors in cancer survival. When first published in 1979, Greer's
work was a revelation because his coping categories—"fighting spirit,"
"denial," "stoic acceptance," and "helplessness/hopelessness"—were tai-
lor-made to reflect the experience of cancer patients: these four dimensions were true to life, capturing how people tend to respond to the devastating experience of receiving a cancer diagnosis. Importantly, a large
replication of the original study led by Greer's colleague Margaret Watson affirmed the negative prognostic effect of hopelessness but failed to
confirm the positive effect of fighting spirit. The ramifications of the original Greer study and the Watson replication are so important that they deserve special consideration here.

Beyond Fighting Spirit: Deeper into Psyche and Survival

An analysis of the prospective study of the effect of psychological coping
on survival in 578 early-stage breast cancer patients by Dr. Margaret Watson and her colleagues at the Royal Marsden Hospital in London is a
launchpad for a deeper exploration of the mind-body-cancer connection.*
The study is fascinating in its hypotheses and conclusions, but so was the
response to the study both by the researchers themselves and by the media.
What does this study says about mind-body-cancer relationships and the
social and cultural context of mind-body research?

"Influence of Psychological Response on Survival in Breast Cancer: A
Population-Based Cohort Study," by Watson et al., was published in October 1999 in the *Lancet* to some fanfare. It is a larger and more rigorous
replication of the seminal study by Greer and his colleagues (Greer et al.
1979; Pettingale et al. 1985; Greer et al. 1990), which demonstrated, over
fifteen years of follow-up, that breast cancer patients who evidenced "fighting spirit" were twice as likely to survive as those who were hopeless and
helpless in their coping response. "Fighting spirit" was one of several coping responses that Greer measured using his MAC scale. The other responses were "denial," "stoic acceptance," and "helplessness/hopelessness."
Greer has rightly been credited with helping to move mind-body-cancer
research to a new level of rigor, insight, and integrity.

Greer's initial study, launched in the early 1970s and copiously cited
since its publication, included fifty-seven patients, a relatively small number. In the aftermath of his five-, ten-, and fifteen-year follow-ups, all published in the *Lancet,* the most common criticisms of this otherwise well-

---

*This section on the replication study by Dr. Margaret Watson and colleagues, with three subsections,
is a revision of an article that first appeared in *Advances in Mind-Body Medicine* 16 (2000): 119–127.

designed study were that it involved a relatively small number of patients and that a key prognostic indicator in breast cancer—lymph node status—was not used. (Since few data were available on lymph nodes for the women in the study, Greer and his colleagues were unable to control for this highly significant variable.) Watson was able to overcome the deficits of the older study. She followed approximately ten times as many women, 578, and she controlled for lymph node status as well as other prognostic factors. She also used a MAC that had been slightly refined and updated over the years.

Watson's study, on which Greer was one of four coauthors, followed the 578 women for five years, at the end of which 395 were alive without relapse, 50 were alive with relapse, and 133 had died. Women who had high scores on the helpless/hopeless scale of the MAC had a significantly increased risk of relapse or death compared with those who had low scores in this category (Watson et al. 1999). Women who scored high on a scale of depression, the Hospital Anxiety and Depression Scale, or HAD, had a significantly increased risk of death from all causes. These significant associations remained after controlling for all key prognostic variables, including lymph node status. However, contrary to Greer's findings, the women who scored high on the fighting spirit category of the MAC scale did not have a significantly reduced risk of relapse or death.

What did the researchers make of these findings? I particularly want to focus on the finding that fighting spirit had no effect on relapse or death, which was perhaps the most startling of the results and the one that has drawn the most attention. After noting the significant linkages between, on the one hand, helplessness/hopelessness and depressed reactions to cancer and, on the other hand, a greater likelihood of progressive disease (findings that support the proposition that subjective factors can influence the course of cancer), the researchers come to the fighting spirit finding and make their assessment forcefully: "The idea that an attitude of fighting spirit, in relation to cancer, improves overall length of survival has been embraced with enthusiasm, especially by practitioners of alternative therapies. Fighting spirit (as assessed here on the MAC scale) was not associated with improved survival in this study; such claims should be far more cautious and circumspect. Our findings suggest that women can be relieved of the burden of guilt that occurs when they find it difficult to maintain a fighting spirit."

THE RUSH TO JUDGMENT ON FIGHTING SPIRIT

In the context of this study, the fighting spirit finding and the researchers' interpretation raise far more questions than they answer. Consider the

180   context: Hopelessness *does* increase the risk of relapse or death, but fighting spirit *does not* reduce that risk. The negative fighting spirit finding led Watson and colleagues to say, with a seeming sigh of relief, that patients need not feel scared or guilty if they cannot maintain a fighting spirit since it probably does not help them much anyway. However, they do not then apply this thinking to their statistically significant finding about helplessness or hopelessness. But if hopeless patients are indeed more likely to relapse or die, should patients with this response be scared and guilty?

The researchers were not alone in highlighting the supposed medical and social import of the lack of an association between fighting spirit (on the MAC scale) and both relapse and survival. The media also highlighted it. The headline of the 19 October 1999 story in the *New York Times,* which infrequently singles out mind-body studies for news stories, announced: "'Fighting Spirit' Little Help in Cancer Fight." The lead paragraph pointed out that "optimism and fighting spirit may help breast cancer patients cope with their illness, but positive thinking is unlikely to increase their chances of survival, according to a study by British researchers." The story went on to inform readers that hopelessness was linked to a greater risk of relapse or death, but it did not indicate the general importance of this finding until the last sentence, using a quote from David Spiegel, who was well known for his study showing that women with breast cancer who received group support lived longer on average than women who did not receive group support. Spiegel noted that the study supported "the idea that some mental attitudes have a predictive relationship to disease progression."

Had the researchers not been so quick to dismiss fighting spirit, and had not the media been so quick to follow the researchers' lead, the implications of the hopelessness finding for the possible value of fighting spirit might have been noted. The finding that helpless and hopeless patients were more likely to die or suffer relapse suggests that people who were not hopeless and not helpless were more likely to remain free of disease and survive longer. While none of the several types of coping responses measured by the MAC was statistically linked to survival, the strong possibility remains that some unmeasured dimension of "nonhopelessness" may have influenced survival. Simply put, fighting spirit, as measured by sixteen specific items on the MAC, may not have tapped that dimension. Thus, to proclaim fighting spirit a nonfactor may be technically accurate, but it is misleading because it is likely, given the connection of hopelessness or helplessness with relapse and death, that some aspect of nonhelpless, nonhopeless coping is associated with survival.

CULTURAL ATTITUDES AND COPING RESPONSES

But why did the Watson study fail to show an association between the MAC measure of fighting spirit and survival, when Greer's earlier study found a strong link? Why should this coping response seem suddenly to have no influence? Has it only to do with some of the weaknesses of the earlier study? I believe that the answer provides a precise explanation for the severe limitations of the MAC measure of fighting spirit.

The MAC offers statements about how one copes with cancer and asks subjects to rate the extent to which they agree with each statement. The coping categories in the MAC scale, slightly updated from the early 1970s, include fighting spirit, helplessness/hopelessness, anxious preoccupation, fatalism (formerly "stoic acceptance"), and avoidance (formerly "denial"). Statements about fighting spirit, which are roughly the same in the new as in the older MAC, include, "Since my cancer diagnosis I now realize how precious life is and I'm making the most of it," "I think my state of mind can make a lot of difference to my health," "I try to have a very positive attitude," "I count my blessings," and "I try to fight the illness."

I propose that these and similar items may have been good measures for a meaningful dimension of fighting spirit some twenty-five years ago in Britain—hence the positive association in Greer's 1970s study—but they no longer provide a sound basis for tapping fighting spirit. In the past ten to fifteen years the popular media—TV, magazines, books—have been saturated with stories about the presumably healing effects of "fighting spirit" and a "positive attitude," especially with regard to cancer. Bernie Siegel's books on love and positive coping have been bestsellers, as have Deepak Chopra's. This idea has permeated Western culture, making it difficult for some patients, I am certain, to resist the lure of a high rating next to items that read, "I try to have a very positive attitude" and "I try to fight the illness." Moreover, reams have been written about the tendency to give socially acceptable answers on psychosocial inventories, and several scales, including the Marlowe-Crowne Social Desirability Scale, have been designed to measure just this proclivity. Given the vast cultural shift in consciousness about mind-body interactions in health, it seems highly probable that the MAC items for fighting spirit may no longer capture a psychosocially and existentially meaningful dimension of a healthy (and health-promoting) response to a diagnosis of cancer.

A closer look at the data supports this proposition. As the researchers explain, patients were classified according to their predominant coping response. In Greer's initial study, in the early 1970s, 17 percent of the patients were classified as being "fighters" (Greer et al. 1979; Pettingale et al. 1985), compared with 29 percent in Watson's 1990s study (Watson et al. 1999), a marked increase. Easily the most prevalent coping response in 1975 was "stoic acceptance," which was embraced by fully 56 percent of the patients. The British "stiff upper lip," we may surmise, was a real cultural and characterological phenomenon. In Watson's study, however, Greer's category "stoic acceptance," renamed "fatalism" (fatalistic items include, "I've had a good life; what's left is a bonus," "I've left it all to my doctors," etc.), characterized only 17 percent of the women. In other words, the number of British women with cancer who acknowledge stoical or fatalistic reactions has likely dropped dramatically in the past several decades. (One caveat: I am comparing percentages from a relatively small cohort of 57 to a rather large one of 578.) If one considers cultural changes in Western Europe generally and Britain specifically over the past two decades, it is not hard to speculate that many people who once consciously acknowledged stoical or fatalistic reactions would feel compelled, based on prevailing social norms, to believe in and report their "positive attitude" today.

The deeper question is this: Have the cultural shifts in Britain (and elsewhere) induced real changes in coping and character or just a change in superficial attitudes about what people think their character should be? My guess would be some combination of both, but with a great deal of the latter—individuals' adopting cultural views of what is considered characterologically appropriate. (Cancer patients today are socially rewarded by family, friends, and doctors for their "positive attitude" in ways they were not as recently as twenty years ago.) Thus, it is conceivable that many study subjects raised to be stoical or fatalistic would today readily check the box next to statements like "I try to have a positive attitude" whether or not they are genuinely optimistic about their recovery. Clearly, this would make the response category "fighting spirit" less valid in a psychometric, psychosocial, and ontological sense than it was years ago.

The same cultural question can be raised with regard to another of Watson's findings, one that has not received much attention and that I have not yet mentioned. Watson and her colleagues, using the Courtauld Emotional Control Scale (CEC), which measures the tendency to suppress emotions, found no association between this tendency and relapse or death from cancer. Greer and Morris in their 1975 study had found such an association: using a measure similar to the CEC as part of their interviews with patients, they had found that patients with breast lumps who suppressed emotions were more likely to have cancer than benign breast disease.

To explain this divergence, we again must consider cultural factors over time. The CEC is a 21–item, self-rating scale with statements such as

"When I feel angry I smother my feelings," "When I feel anxious I bottle it up," "When I feel unhappy I hide my unhappiness," and so forth. In other words, the scale is tapping into the longtime British trait (certainly common elsewhere) of a stiff upper lip. It is clear, however, that cultural changes in Britain and other countries worldwide over the past twenty-five years have eased social pressures to maintain such a stance. Media commentators covering Princess Diana's funeral in 1997 noted that the histrionic outpouring of grief on such a large scale would have been unthinkable even a decade earlier. I would confidently surmise that fewer British people today either suppress or admit to suppressing emotions, which means they would not agree with such statements on the CEC as "When I feel miserable I refuse to say anything about it," or "When I feel unhappy I smother my feelings." I am arguing, in short, that, like the category "fighting spirit" on the MAC, the CEC is out of date because the culture has changed. In this case suppression itself has become something of an anachronism. To the extent that this is true, and to the extent that suppression contributes to cancer, then it follows that Watson would not in fact find a link between suppression and breast cancer among the study's British subjects.

Watson and colleagues' formulation of their finding raises another point. They correctly state that the CEC measures "the extent to which patients suppress negative emotions," but they go on to say that such suppression is "a focal variable of the suggested Type C cancer-prone personality." The implication is that there is no link at all between suppression and breast cancer and that any formulation that suggests there is a link is wrong.

As I have noted, the core of Type C behavior as elaborated by Lydia Temoshok is the nonexpression of emotions, which may encompass either suppression or repression (Temoshok and Dreher 1992). The difference, most researchers agree, is one of awareness: *suppression* refers to a conscious practice of emotional control, while *repression* refers to an unconscious practice in which the person is unaware of the emotions he or she keeps under wraps. Temoshok's basic argument was that either suppression or repression could compromise health and immune functions but that repression was more prevalent in American cancer patients during her mid-1980s research.

The CEC clearly measures suppression, not repression. Thus, we should be careful to recognize that while Watson's study found no link between breast cancer progression and emotional suppression, it remains possible that subjects in her study did indeed repress emotions. If fewer British citizens consciously control emotions and suppress them, it does

184   not follow that fewer use repression as a psychic defense, leaving aside the possibility, as psychodynamic theorists and therapists often maintain, that long-term suppression often gives way to unconscious repression. It would be a mistake to dismiss the link between emotional nonexpression and cancer on the basis of this limited finding with a narrowly gauged instrument.

Further, the pivotal mind-body issue with regard to emotions and cancer may require researchers to probe beneath the surface of public or even conscious behavior. That repressors may be unaware of their intrapsychic defense has been brilliantly addressed by the researchers Daniel Weinberger, Gary Schwartz, and Richard Davidson, who as early as 1979 recognized the need to develop cagier research tools in order to pick up a coping mechanism as covert and subtle as repression (Weinberger et al. 1979). They combined an anxiety scale, the Taylor Manifest Anxiety Scale, with the Marlowe-Crowne Social Desirability Scale in order to flush out repressors; for instance, people who claimed never to be anxious but who revealed a dyed-in-the-wool tendency to put a socially desirable face on everything could be deemed repressors. Before researchers claim no association between repression (the Type C pattern) and cancer progression, they need to be certain that their measures are sufficiently sensitive and accurate given the cultural, psychodynamic, and medical complexities at hand.

More generally, psychosocial researchers in the mind-body field and elsewhere need regularly to consider the effect of cultural transformations on their supposedly tried-and-true research tools. Comments like "It's been validated" and "It's generalizable" should be met with the respective questions "When?" and "To whom?"

A CLUE TO PSYCHE AND SURVIVAL: "NONE OF THE ABOVE"

The MAC scale may no longer be adequate to help researchers ferret out the facet or dimension of "nonhopelessness" that may be a boon to cancer survival. The question remains, however, What might this facet or dimension be? Does the Watson study contain any clues?

There is one intriguing, clandestine clue, one that hints at an understanding of an adaptive, life-affirming coping response to cancer that is more sophisticated than the view embodied in the fighting spirit category of the MAC. Watson and colleagues note, "Each patient was . . . assigned to the MAC subscale with the highest standardized score. Where no standardized score was greater than zero (i.e., the sample mean), the patient was classified as having no predominant response." In other words, some patients evidenced a number of coping styles (fighting spirit, fatalism, etc.), with no one style being statistically predominant. This group was categorized in Watson's data tables as "none," as in "none of the above."

The intriguing aspect of this "none" category is that while it was numerically small (only 50 of the 578 patients), patients in this category actually had a higher survival rate than patients in any other category of response. Seventy-four percent of the "none" group were alive at five years, compared with 70 percent of the "fighters," 65 percent of the "helpless/hopeless" group, and so forth. By a hair, the "none" group had the lowest percentage of deaths—20 percent at five years, compared with 21 percent of the fighters, 27 percent of the fatalists, and so on. The researchers, who did not comment on the "none" results, do not appear to have calculated whether the "none" group had a statistically significant edge over those in other coping categories, but they clearly did well, better, in fact, than any other group.

What can we make of this "none" finding? One possibility is that this group is made up of individuals who are coping in a particularly healthy, adaptive way that the MAC did not pick up because it did not operationalize the "X factor" of coping they possess. But another possibility is that there may be something specifically worth investigating about the fact that these individuals had *no predominant style*. Put differently, they may have varied their styles, including several of the five reactions in the MAC: fighting spirit, helpless/hopeless, anxious preoccupation, fatalism, avoidance. What could be healthy about such seeming vacillation?

In a superb, neglected book, *And a Time to Live: Toward Emotional Well-being during the Crisis of Cancer* (1978), the therapist Robert Chernin Cantor wrote compellingly of a natural shifting response to cancer that he called the "Resistance-Surrender Cycle." In a recent book about the healing themes found in the Book of Psalms, *For Thou Art with Me,* which I coauthored with Samuel Chiel (Chiel and Dreher 2000), we summed up Cantor's concept:

> There are times in the course of an illness when we want to give up the fight. We're tired of the tests, the fear, the treatments, the hospital food, the physical pain, the uncertainty about our prognosis. It's entirely understandable, and no sign of a character deficiency on our part, when we feel hopeless, exhausted, and resigned. But if we never cycle out of hopelessness, unable to reclaim our desire for life, our emotional and physical recovery becomes vastly more difficult. The research evidence is building that people with cancer, heart disease, and other diseases may have more trouble getting well—and staying well—once they lapse into chronic depression and despair.

The answer, according to health psychologists, is not to try to remain cheerful at all costs, planting a smile on our faces to please loved ones or to live up to a fantasized ideal about the mind-body road to health. The best approach is to allow ourselves to feel hopeless, but to share those feelings so they don't fester inside. When we work through vexing emotions, turning to others for solace and support, the feelings themselves change character. They shift and shuttle, back and forth, from despair to joie de vivre, from pessimism to optimism, from surrender to resistance. This "cycling" seems to be the most natural, even healthy, response to the painful vicissitudes of serious illness.

Perhaps we should redefine fighting spirit to encompass the resistance-surrender cycle so that we jettison the horribly simplistic and even punishing advice to cancer patients to buck up with a positive attitude. Yet to toss aside the notion that fighting spirit, better defined, may have an effect on survival—"'Fighting Spirit' Little Help in Cancer Fight"—may also be punishing, and it is probably inaccurate. It suggests that nothing we do on an emotional and an existential level contributes much to our physical recovery, that survival is strictly a matter of how aggressively we pursue treatment, the skill of our doctors, and the vagaries of our cellular response to chemotherapy and radiation.

Such a medically materialist approach may have the ring of logic, but the psychiatrist David Spiegel's landmark study showing that metastatic breast cancer patients who participated in his group therapy lived twice as long as those in a control group (Spiegel et al. 1989) suggests that psychosocial changes can indeed have an independent, beneficial effect on survival time. (This notion does not rest solely on Spiegel's study, but on at least four others as well. See chapter 6 for a review of evidence from psychosocial intervention trials.) Further, Spiegel's treatment was not "positive attitude therapy" but "supportive-expressive group therapy," to use his own term. Read any description or see any tape of Spiegel's clinical work, and it is clear that supportive-expressive group therapy encourages patients to experience and work through the gamut of emotional and coping reactions to cancer—terror, anger, sadness, joy, depression, determination, creative expression, turning inward, reaching out, and confronting the possibility of death. It has nothing to do with putting on a happy face.

I agree with Watson and colleagues when they write that women should be freed of the burden of guilt about "failing" to possess sufficient fighting spirit. But people with cancer can develop their own unique ways of coping in the hope that their efforts will contribute to their recovery, and with appropriate nonjudgmental support they should not have to experience a shred of shame over their efforts, regardless of the outcome. The resistance-surrender concept buttresses the hope inherent in the notion that our psychospiritual state matters not only to our psyche but also to our soma. It further suggests that we do not have to embrace an unrealistic, TV-movie-of-the-week definition of psychospiritual states that may promote healing—the heroic stance of an unrelenting fighting spirit. Resistance-surrender implies that there is a time for action and a time for rest, a time for anger and a time for acceptance, a time for conviction and a time for grief . . . and that our mind-body system can integrate them all, especially when we have strong social support and a resounding raison d'être. Resistance-surrender means that even hopelessness cannot harm us biologically unless we get caught in its relentless grip.

Now psychosocial cancer researchers only need a scale administered repeatedly over time that measures resistance-surrender in all its multilayered complexity. Perhaps "none of the above" is a start in that direction.

Temoshok's Model: An Integrative Timeline for the Mind-Body-Cancer Connection

Like the sprawling research on psychosocial factors in heart disease, studies on the mind's role in cancer would seem, on the surface, to present a laundry list of items in two different columns: column A for cancer risk, column B for cancer progression or survival. Some items occur on both lists, and some occur on only one, but they would seem to be a random inventory of emotional states, personality traits, behavior patterns, and social factors that do not cohere in any meaningful fashion. In some instances so-called negative emotions appear salutary, while in other instances they appear damaging. How do cancer patients, physicians, and mind-body clinicians interpret the seeming contradictions? I have already tipped my hand by distinguishing among the studies and by differentiating measurements of "negative emotions" into those that represent a coping collapse (i.e., hopelessness, severe depression) and those that reflect an adaptive expression of distress under circumstances of severe stress.

But a more comprehensive model is needed to make finer distinctions; to explain why the psychosocial variables involved in cancer risk among healthy individuals are different from those involved in cancer outcome among diagnosed patients; and to understand how stress, coping patterns, emotions, and personality interact to influence the development and course of cancer. In her 1987 paper "Personality, Coping Style, Emotion, and Cancer: Towards an Integrative Model" Lydia Temoshok developed just such a "process model." Her thesis is summarized here. In my view it remains the most penetrating theoretical effort to date. Moreover, studies listed in this chapter that have been published after 1987 tend to support the thesis she set forth fifteen years ago. (Before proceeding, I reiterate that I am biased here: I coauthored the 1992 book *The Type C Connection* with Temoshok.)

Temoshok uses the "Type C behavior pattern," the construct developed by her and independently posited by Steven Greer, as the centerpiece of her theory. Most of the mind-body-cancer research findings, she contends, can be viewed as coherent, both internally and with other studies, if they are placed in a context of understanding how the Type C individual develops this coping pattern and how it evolves over the course of a lifetime.

From childhood Temoshok's Type C individual learns first to suppress and later to repress strong emotions, primarily anger but also sadness, fear, and in some cases unbridled joy. (The change from suppression to repression means that holding back expression of emotions may at first be conscious but in time becomes an unconscious reflex, the definition of *repression*.) In early stages of development the nonexpression of emotions is adaptive; it is the child's accommodation to family dynamics and pressures, a way to maintain psychic integrity in the face of stress or loss. During later stages of development, through adolescence to adulthood, a rigid pattern of nonexpression can disable the person from healthy assertiveness, communication skills, the capacity to get one's needs met, and the development of a richly creative life rooted in authentic feelings. These deficits can cause suffering, but the Type C individual by definition has difficulty acknowledging his suffering. The Type C adult therefore harbors a latent hopelessness that is often wholly unconscious. (Simply put, it is a hopelessness about ever being fully whole, fully one's self. It may also represent the psychological effects of anger and grief that have not been integrated, a common cause of depression.) As a result, depression would not be explicit, and therefore would not be measurable, long before the development of cancer. It may only become apparent soon before or after a cancer diagnosis, when the hopeless-helpless complex breaks through into consciousness under the strain of severe stress. This would explain why depression is a weak or nonexistent risk factor in most long-term prospective studies, while Type C characteristics, namely, nonexpression of emotions and a "nice" social façade, are more detectable by psychological tests and interviews years before cancer is diagnosed.

According to Temoshok's theory, the Type C coping style can be effective for a prolonged period, enabling the person to maintain inner psychological balance, as well as balance with his or her environment (family, job, friendships, etc). But because rigid Type C coping disables the person from the full range of emotional expression and behavioral assertion, it is a "fragile accommodation to the world." Thus, an accumulation of stress ultimately leads to a breaking point, in which the person's capacity to cope falters and his or her unconscious hopelessness or helplessness begins to emerge. Often the cancer diagnosis itself is the breaking point (see fig. 4.1). Here is how Temoshok describes this phenomenon in her 1987 paper:

> The Type C coping style is a fragile accommodation to the world; homeostasis with the environment may be achieved to some degree, but psychological homeostasis is always precarious, while biological homeostasis is severely strained. At some point, it is believed that the Type C coping style will not be adequate to deal with the accumulated stressor load, or with an especially severe stressor. . . .
>
> The individual can no longer suppress needs, feelings, or disappointments in others or in life itself. It is increasingly difficult to "carry on" as before. There are hypothetically three denouements to this crisis: (a) the individual marshals resources and begins to develop a more stable and adequate coping style; (b) the Type C façade breaks down, exposing the chronic but hidden hopelessness, which now becomes conscious; or (c) the individual continues to cope, albeit with a great deal more strain on the system, using the same Type C style.
>
> Emotional expression is seen as contributing to the development of a more adequate coping style: the individual begins to express needs and feelings, recruits more genuine social support in this process and is believed to have a more positive health outcome as psychological and biological equilibrium is achieved. Psychological intervention may play a part at this point in helping the individual change longstanding behavioral and cognitive patterns. On the other hand, conscious hopelessness and learned helplessness are hypothesized to contribute to unfavorable health outcomes, as the individual gives up trying to achieve equilibrium in any area, and the previous state of biological disequilibrium is exacerbated.

Drawn from Temoshok's theories, this "process model" helps explain many of the seeming contradictions among study findings. Specifically:

- Since hopelessness and depression are not usually conscious until a "breaking point" of cumulative stress or a severe stressor, including a cancer diagnosis, is reached, hopelessness or depression would not show up strongly in prospective studies of cancer risk in which subjects are psychologically assessed many years or decades before diagnosis.
- Since Type C coping, whose core is nonexpression of negative emotions,

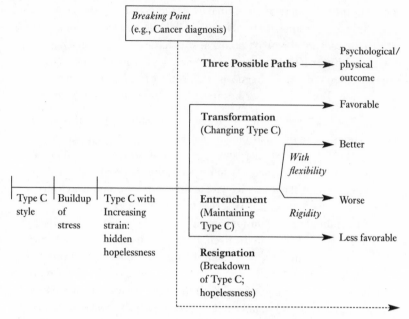

FIGURE 4.1 Lydia Temoshok's Process Model of Type C Behavior and Cancer. From Temoshok and Dreher 1992.

would be apparent early, it has been shown in some prospective studies to presage cancer years or decades before diagnosis.

- A cancer diagnosis may be preceded by a period of severe stress or by the gradual emergence of hidden hopelessness. Quasi-prospective studies that evaluated patients just prior to diagnosis (before a biopsy) have found evidence of hopelessness, as well as Type C nonexpression of emotions. (The individual still tries to cope by maintaining emotional repression, but this coping strategy has begun to founder.)

- As Temoshok maintains, once the Type C individual has been diagnosed with cancer (a "breaking point"), he may proceed in roughly three directions. Those who transform their Type C style by expressing emotion more readily, seeking support, becoming more active copers, and developing a healthy entitlement, are expected to have a more favorable prognosis. Studies of cancer patients who evidence "fighting spirit," "active coping," "emotional expression," or "social support" have shown positive results in terms of medical outcome.

- For the Type C individual whose latent hopelessness becomes conscious, an inability to transform Type C behavior may leave him or her without adequate coping capacities. When such individuals become chronically hopeless or helpless, their biological disequilibrium may worsen, and they are expected to have less favorable outcomes. Thus, studies of cancer patients who feel helpless, hopeless, or severely depressed have shown negative trends in terms of medical outcome.

- For the Type C individual who "hunkers down" by continuing his or her Type C style, there is, as Temoshok notes, "a great deal more strain on the system." While the medical outcome for such individuals may be expected to be unfavorable, Temoshok has found variance here. Individuals who show somewhat more flexibility in their expression of emotions, who seek support and "get on with their lives" with a degree of energy and purpose, may have a better prognosis. By contrast, those who are rigid in their continuing Type C style, who are stoical regardless of the stresses associated with their diagnosis, and who have difficulty acknowledging their need for support may have a less favorable prognosis. These insights are consistent with Steven Greer's findings. The flexible Type C individuals are similar to Greer's "deniers," who were later termed "positive avoiders" and who had a relatively favorable outcome. (Other studies listed above support the psychobiological value of denial or minimization among some patients.) The more rigid Type C individuals are similar to Greer's "stoic acceptors" and Levy's "passive copers," who on the surface remained calm and unfazed by the diagnosis and had a relatively unfavorable prognosis.

While Temoshok's integrative process model may not explain every study finding, the puzzle pieces generally fit, and it is consonant with the psychodynamics of depth psychology, as well as the mind-body dynamics of psychosomatic medicine, psychoneuroimmunology, neuroimmunomodulation, and psychoneuroendocrinology. It is a model rooted in the idea that stress per se is not the issue in the biological disequilibrium apparent in cancer. Rather, inadequate or maladaptive coping that leaves individuals in a state of psychological imbalance—hopeless, helpless, and unable to engage in positive assertion on behalf of the self—will lead to biological imbalances. These perturbations may include endocrine disruptions, deficits in neurotransmitter systems, and improper nervous system regulation of the immune system, leaving the person more susceptible to infectious or neoplastic diseases due to compromised immune defenses. In support of this idea, studies by Temoshok (1985) and Levy (Levy et al. 1985; Levy et al. 1987) correlated passive or nonexpressive coping styles with weakened immune defenses. Contrary to some critical commentaries that questioned the clinical importance of these immune decrements, the

192   immune components measured by Temoshok and Levy were specifically relevant to anticancer immunity: Temoshok measured tumor-infiltrating lymphocytes that had proven prognostic significance in melanoma (Temoshok 1985), while Levy measured NK cell activity that she and Ronald Herberman, the renowned immunologist at the University of Pittsburgh who discovered NK cells, demonstrated to have prognostic significance in breast cancer (Levy et al. 1985; Levy et al. 1991).

What the model clearly shows is that different psychosocial variables play different roles in successive stages of cancer initiation, promotion, progression, and metastases. The integrative timeline also shows that the person who may be susceptible to cancer due to psychological factors is a complex individual with a multilayered consciousness, including psychic defenses that are necessary and may be effective for a prolonged period. But like all of us, he or she changes over time, responds to stress and the flux of events with relatively more or less flexibility, and is vulnerable to mind-body disequilibrium when coping strategies that served his or her psychic sustenance no longer work, when his or her "fragile accommodation to the world" is challenged to the point of dissolution.

But the hope in Temoshok's model is as clear and resounding as the threat: coping responses can and do change; they do not have to remain static or collapse under pressure. The person can transform or replace Type C behaviors with novel, more authentic ways of being. That is why Temoshok does not refer to Type C as a personality. She insists on calling it a coping style or behavior pattern because it is a learned or adopted set of behaviors that do not represent the core of anyone's personality. While some shadings of the pattern may have genetic origins, and it could arguably be called a trait, an extreme pattern of emotional repression and appeasing behavior is best understood as a defensive style that evolves through developmental stages, not an intrinsic shard of a person's essential self. This distinction is important not only for scientific accuracy; it helps clinicians and patients alike to recognize that the patient's personality, the root of who the patient is, has not contributed to his or her disease. (This properly deflects the guilt or shame often associated with the so-called cancer personality.) The pattern can better be compared to a problematic habit, such as smoking or a high-fat diet, than to a personality trait: it is a reflexive stress manager that has a serious downside, and fortunately it can be changed.

While more clinical research is needed to determine whether the Type C pattern can readily be subject to therapeutic overhaul, there is no doubt that psychotherapists and mind-body clinicians have helped such patients to alter their style. David Spiegel's supportive-expressive group psychotherapy intervention, which was associated with a doubling of survival time in metastatic breast cancer patients (Spiegel et al. 1989), was specifically designed for, and has been proven effective in, helping patients to express difficult and troubling emotions—grief, abject fear, and anger—in the aftermath of a harrowing diagnosis. In *The Type C Connection* Temoshok reported her clinical experiences, which she claimed were successful in helping Type C cancer patients to modify longstanding and deeply ingrained patterns of emotional repression and self-sacrifice through intensive one-on-one counseling (Temoshok and Dreher 1992). As the cancer psychotherapist Lawrence LeShan has eloquently argued, cancer can be a turning point rather than a breaking point, and when the patient seeks the help of loved ones, as well as knowledgeable and compassionate clinicians, he or she may find the strength to transform one of life's most dreadful challenges into an enriching and life-affirming experience.

Cancer and the Mind: Closing Thoughts

While the overall evidence for a complex mind-body-cancer relationship appears stronger than most skeptics would acknowledge, it is also true that the contribution of psychological states and traits to cancer risk is probably modest, and their contribution to cancer progression or survival, while more robust, is often (though not always) less significant than that of established biological predictors. Recognizing that the mind is rarely the overriding factor in a person's disease or disease course is important for the sake of both scientific veracity and rejection of oversimplified beliefs—i.e., "I gave myself cancer and I can cure myself," "I create my own reality," and "I have cancer because I'm teaching myself a lesson"—that lead to self-blame and denigration.

Put simply, cancer-prone behaviors and coping styles probably play no role in many people's cancers, a minor role in some, and a significant role in others. This would explain why simple cause-and-effect relationships may never be uncovered in mind-cancer research but meaningful correlations will be. But this is no different from findings on the cancer-causing effects of various risk factors, from asbestos to high-fat diets to electromagnetic fields. The notion of psychological factors as one among many variables in cancer is based on a systems approach, also known as a multifactoral model of disease, and the specific breakdown of factors for any individual will be unique. In other words, every person who develops cancer has his or her own set of interacting contributors, including genes, diet, environment, and lifestyle behaviors, and psychosocial factors will amount

194   to one variably sized piece of the pie of cancer risk or recovery (Fox et al. 1989).

But the research cited here makes clear that for many individuals the mind's contribution to their illness or recovery matters. In a magazine interview in the late 1980s the transpersonal philosopher Ken Wilber highlighted this issue by telling the story of one hypothetical cancer patient. The patient's survival, he said, would be determined by many variables, including his genetic makeup and his diet, but his psychological coping style would also make a difference. Among the factors that would influence his recovery, psychological coping might contribute as much as 10 percent. Now, this patient has a common type and stage of cancer for which his prognosis for five-year survival is 50 percent. If his psychological handling of the stress of cancer had a 10 percent influence on his recovery, then it would be no small matter. "In a tight election," said Wilber, "ten percent can make all the difference in the world" (Wilber 1988).

Adherents who overstate the mind's contribution fall prey to the myth of mind-body omnipotence, while skeptics who claim that the mind has no influence on cancer risk or recovery fall prey to the myth of mind-body helplessness. With credible studies as a guide, it is fair to say that we are neither omnipotent nor helpless when it comes to the mind's role in resisting or surviving cancer. The middle ground—that we can *affect* but not *control* our fate when it comes to cancer—is scientifically grounded, ethically sound, and rationally balanced.

That said, it is difficult for many scientists, physicians, and patients to accept the idea that an aspect of our psychological selves is involved in such a painful disease. The very concept of a Type C pattern may seem pejorative, even when it is presented in a thoughtful, balanced, and compassionate way. To the extent that categorizing patients is experienced by them as stereotyping, the Type C label is unnecessary. But the fact that the Type C classification is hard for some to swallow may be a vestige of the cultural stigmatization associated with cancer. For instance, the coronary-prone Type A behavior pattern was popularized, became part of the cultural lexicon, and never took on a negative or stigmatizing connotation. Indeed, many people blithely describe themselves as Type As without a hint of shame. *Type A* was culturally accepted as a shorthand way to characterize a type of behavior believed to increase risk of heart disease. Arguably, this is because heart disease has never been a source of stigmatization in the way cancer has: the metaphors used for heart disease are not fraught with insinuations of characterological or spiritual inadequacy. If we managed to thoroughly expunge cancer stigma from our society, the notion of a Type C pattern might be considered as nonjudgmental and benign as the notion that stress can bring on a cold or that anxiety can trigger an asthma attack.

What is important, however, is not the label but what the label means. Lydia Temoshok's process model is not an indictment, it's a story: a collective narrative of individuals who are more susceptible to disease not because of their personal failures but because of their suffering; not because they lack spirit but because their spirit has been burdened; not because they cannot fight but because they have learned that to survive is to acquiesce; not because they are insensate but because they are exquisitely sensitive; not because they lack heart but because their hearts may have been broken. The deeper insights of mind-cancer research are profoundly compassionate, as far from blaming the victim as can be imagined. Proper interpretations of this research recognize that a person's passivity or non-expression is all surface, or to quote Rachel Naomi Remen, "Every victim is a survivor who doesn't know it yet" (Remen 1989).

Needed now are more mind-cancer studies with tighter methods, as well as measures designed to honor the complexity of the psyche, the cancer defense system, and the biological interface between them. Also needed is a fearless willingness to explore terrain that is as emotionally and socially complex as it is biologically complex, coupled with an abiding regard, in both the lab and the clinic, for the inner life of people whose diagnosis may be an earthshaking experience.

REFERENCES

Andrykowski MA, Brady MJ, Henslee-Downey PJ. 1994. Psychosocial factors predictive of survival after allogeneic bone marrow transplantation for leukemia. *Psychosom Med.* 56:432–439.

Bacon CL, Renneker R, Cutler M. 1952. A psychosomatic survey of cancer of the breast. *Psychosom Med.* 14:453–460.

Bahnson C. 1969. Psychophysiological complementarity in malignancies: past work and future vistas. *Ann NY Acad Sci.* 164:319–334.

Bleiker EM, van der Ploeg HM, Hendriks JH, Ader HJ. 1996. Personality factors and breast cancer development: a prospective longitudinal study. *J Natl Cancer Inst.* 88:1478–1482.

Blumberg EM, West PM, Ellis FW. 1954. A possible relationship between psychological factors and human cancer. *Psychosom Med.* 16:277–286.

Brown JE, Butow PN, Culjak G, Coates AS, Dunn SM. 2000. Psychosocial predictors of outcome: time to relapse and survival in patients with early stage melanoma. *Br J Cancer.* 83:1448–1453.

196   Butow PN, Coates AS, Dunn SM. 1999. Psychosocial predictors of survival in metastatic melanoma. *J Clin Oncol.* 17:2256–2263.

Butow PN, Coates AS, Dunn SM. 2000. Psychosocial predictors of survival: metastatic breast cancer. *Ann Oncol.* 11:469–474.

Butow PN, Hiller JE, Price MA, Thackway SV, Kricker A, Tennant CC. 2000. Epidemiological evidence for a relationship between life events, coping style, and personality factors in the development of breast cancer. *J Psychosom Res.* 49:169–181.

Cantor RC. 1978. *And a Time to Live: Toward Emotional Well-Being during the Crisis of Cancer.* New York: Harper & Row.

Casslieth BR, Lusk EJ, Miller DS, et al. 1985. Psychosocial correlates of survival in advanced malignant disease. *New Engl J Med.* 312:1551–1555.

Chiel S, Dreher H. 2000. *For Thou Art with Me: The Healing Power of Psalms.* Emmaus, Pa: Daybreak Press.

Dattore P, Shontz F, Coyne L. 1980. Premorbid personality differentiation of cancer and non-cancer groups. *J Consult Clin Psychol.* 48:388–394.

Dean C, Surtees PG. 1989. Do psychological factors predict survival in breast cancer? *J Psychosom Res.* 33:561–569.

De Boer MF, Van den Borne B, Pruyn JF, et al. 1998. Psychosocial and physical correlates of survival and recurrence in patients with head and neck carcinoma: results of a six-year longitudinal study. *Cancer.* 83:2567–2579.

Denollet J. 1998. Personality and risk of cancer in men with coronary heart disease. *Psychol Med.* 28:991–995.

Derogatis L, Abeloff M, Melisaratos N. 1979. Psychological coping mechanisms and survival time in metastatic breast cancer. *JAMA.* 242:1504–1508.

Faller H, Bulzebruck H, Schilling S, Drings P, Lang H. 1997. Do psychological factors modify survival of cancer patients? II: Results of an empirical study with bronchial carcinoma patients (in German). *Psychother Psychosom Med Psychol.* 47:206–218.

Fox B, Temoshok LR, Dreher H. 1989. Mind-body and behavior in cancer incidence. *Adv Mind Body Med.* 5:41–60.

Giraldi T, Rodani MG, Cartei G, Grassi L. 1997. Psychosocial factors and breast cancer: a six-year Italian follow-up study. *Psychother Psychosom.* 66:229–236.

Glaser R, Kennedy S, Lafuse WP, et al. 1990. Psychological stress-induced modulation of interleukin 2 receptor gene expression and interleukin 2 production in peripheral blood leukocytes. *Arch Gen Psychiatry.* 47:707–712.

Glaser R, Lafuse WP, Bonneau RH, Atkinson C, Kiecolt-Glaser JK. 1993. Stress-associated modulation of proto-oncogene expression in human peripheral blood leukocytes. *Behav Neurosci.* 107:525–529.

Goodkin K, Antoni M, Blaney P. 1986. Stress and hopelessness in the promotion of cervical intraepithelial neoplasia to invasive squamous cell carcinoma of the cervix. *J Psychosom Res.* 30:67–76.

Graves PL, Thomas CB, Mead LA. 1991. Familial and psychological predictors of cancer. *Cancer Detect Prev.* 15:59–64.

Greer S, Morris T. 1975. Psychological attributes of women who develop breast cancer: a controlled study. *J Psychosom Res.* 19:147–153.

Greer S, Morris T, Pettingale KW. 1979. Psychological response to breast cancer: effect on outcome. *Lancet.* 13:785–787.

Greer S, Morris T, Pettingale KW, Haybittle JL. 1990. Psychological response to breast cancer and fifteen-year outcome. *Lancet.* 335:49–50.

Grossarth-Maticek R. 1982. Interpersonal repression as a predictor of cancer. *Soc Sci Med.* 16:493–498.

Grossarth-Maticek R, Kanazir DT, Vetter H, Schmidt P. 1983. Psychosomatic factors involved in the process of cancerogenesis: preliminary results of the Yugoslav prospective study. *Psychother Psychosom.* 40:191–210.

Holland JC, Korzun AH, Tross S, et al. 1986. Psychological factors and disease-free survival in Stage II breast cancer. *Proc Am Soc Clin Onc.* 5:237. Abstract 928.

Jacobs JR, Bovasso GB. 2000. Early and chronic stress and their relation to breast cancer. *Psychol Med.* 30:669–678.

Jamison RN, Burish TG, Wallston KA. 1987. Psychogenic factors in predicting survival of breast cancer patients. *J Clin Oncol.* 5:768–772.

Jensen MR. 1987. Psychobiological factors predicting the course of breast cancer. *J Personality.* 55:317–342.

Kaplan GA, Reynolds P. 1988. Depression and cancer mortality and morbidity: prospective evidence from the Alameda County study. *J Behav Med.* 11:1–13.

Kiecolt-Glaser JK, Stephens RE, Lipetz PD, Speicher CE, Glaser R. 1985. Distress and DNA repair in human lymphocytes. *J Behav Med.* 8:311–320.

Kissen D. 1966. The significance of personality in lung cancer in men. *Ann NY Acad Sci.* 125:820–826.

Kissen DM, Brown RI, Kissen M. 1969. A further report on personality and psychosocial factors in lung cancer. *Ann NY Acad Sci.* 164:535–545.

Kneier AW, Temoshok L. 1984. Repressive coping reactions in patients with malignant melanoma as compared to cardiovascular disease patients. *J Psychosom Res.* 28:145–155.

Koopman C, Hermanson K, Diamond S, Angell K, Spiegel D. 1998. Social support, life stress, pain, and emotional adjustment to advanced breast cancer. *Psychooncology.* 7:101–111.

Kuderer NM, Krasner S, Spielberger CD, Lyman GH. 1998. Psychological measures and breast cancer survival. *Proc Ann Meet Am Soc Clin Oncol.* 15:A238.

Kune GA, Kune S, Watson LF, Bahnson CB. 1991. Personality as a risk factor in large bowel cancer: data from the Melbourne Colorectal Cancer Study. *Psychol Med.* 21:29–41.

LeShan L. 1959. Psychological states as factors in the development of malignant disease: a review. *J Natl Cancer Inst.* 22:1–18.

Levy SM, Herberman RB, Lippman M, d'Angelo T. 1987. Correlation of stress factors with sustained depression of natural killer cell activity and predicted prognosis in patients with breast cancer. *J Clin Oncol.* 5:344–353.

Levy SM, Herberman RB, Lippman M, d'Angelo T, Lee J. 1991. Immunological and psychosocial predictors of disease recurrence in patients with early-stage breast cancer. *Behav Med.* 17:67–75.

Levy SM, Herberman RB, Maluish A, Schlein B, Lippman M. 1985. Prognostic

198   risk assessment in primary breast cancer by behavioral and immunological parameters. *Health Psychol.* 4:99–113.

Levy SM, Lee J, Bagley C, et al. 1988. Survival hazards analysis in first recurrent breast cancer patients: seven-year follow-up. *Psychosom Med.* 50:520–528.

Maunsell E, Brisson J, Deschenes L. 1995. Social support and survival among women with breast cancer. *Cancer.* 76:631–637.

McGee R, Williams S, Elwood M. 1994. Depression and the development of cancer: a meta-analysis. *Soc Sci Med.* 38:187–192.

McKenna MC, Zevon MA, Corn B, Rounds J. 1999. Psychosocial factors and the development of breast cancer: a meta-analysis. *Health Psychol.* 18:520–531.

Morris T, Greer S, Pettingale KW, Watson M. 1981. Patterns of expression of anger and their psychological correlates in women with breast cancer. *J Psychosom Res.* 25:111–117.

Pennebaker JW. 1999. The effects of traumatic disclosure on physical and mental health: the values of writing and talking about upsetting events. *Int J Emerg Ment Health.* 1:9–18.

Pettingale KW, Morris T, Greer S, Haybittle JL. 1985. Mental attitudes to cancer: an additional prognostic factor. *Lancet.* 30:750.

Price MA, Tennant CC, Butow PN, et al. 2001. The role of psychosocial factors in the development of breast carcinoma: Part II. Life event stressors, social support, defense style, and emotional control and their interactions. *Cancer.* 91:686–697.

Price MA, Tennant CC, Smith RC, et al. 2001. The role of psychosocial factors in the development of breast carcinoma: Part I. The cancer prone personality. *Cancer.* 91:679–685.

Ramirez A, Craig T, Watson J, Fentiman J, North W, Rubens R. 1989. Stress and relapse of breast cancer. *BMJ.* 298:291–293.

Remen RN. 1989. The search for healing. In: Carlson K, Shields B, eds. *Healers on Healing.* Los Angeles: Jeremy P. Tarcher.

Rogentine G, Van Kammen D, Fox B, et al. 1979. Psychological factors in the prognosis of malignant melanoma: a prospective study. *Psychosom Med.* 41:647–655.

Scherg H. 1987. Psychosocial factors and disease bias in breast cancer patients. *Psychosom Med.* 49:302–312.

Schmale AH, Iker H. 1971. Hopelessness as a predictor of cervical cancer. *Soc Sci Med.* 5:95–100.

Schulz R, Bookwala J, Knapp JE, Scheier M, Williamson GM. 1996. Pessimism, age, and cancer mortality. *Psychol Aging.* 11:304–309.

Shaffer JW, Duszynski KR, Thomas CB. 1982. Family attitudes in youth as a possible precursor of cancer among physicians: a search for explanatory mechanisms. *J Behav Med.* 5:143–163.

Shaffer JW, Graves PL, Swank RT, Pearson TA. 1987. Clustering of personality traits in youth and the subsequent development of cancer among physicians. *J Behav Med.* 10:441–447.

Shekelle RB, Raynor WJ, Ostefoeld AM, et al. 1981. Psychological depression and seventeen-year risk of death from cancer. *Psychosom Med.* 43:117–125.

Sontag S. 1978. *Illness as Metaphor.* New York: Farrar, Straus, & Giroux.

Spiegel D, Bloom JR, Kraemer HC, Gottheil E. 1989. Effect of psychosocial treat-   199
ment on survival of patients with metastatic breast cancer. *Lancet.* 14:888–891.

Stavraky K, Buck C, Lott J, Wanklin J. 1968. Psychological factors in the outcome of
human cancer. *J Psychosom Res.* 12:251–259.

Stavraky KM, Donner AP, Kincade JE, Stewart MA. 1988. The effect of psychosocial factors on lung cancer mortality at one year. *J Clin Epidemiol.* 41:75–82.

Temoshok L. 1987. Personality, coping style, emotion, and cancer: towards an integrative model. *Cancer Surveys.* 6:545–567.

Temoshok L. 1985. Biopsychosocial studies on cutaneous malignant melanoma: psychosocial factors associated with prognostic indicators, progression, psychophysiology, and tumor-host response. *Soc Sci Med.* 20:833–840.

Temoshok L, Dreher H. 1992. *The Type C Connection: The Behavioral Links to Cancer and Your Health.* New York: Random House.

Temoshok L, Heller BW, Sagebiel RW, et al. 1985. The relationship of psychosocial
factors to prognostic indicators in cutaneous malignant melanoma. *J Psychosom
Res.* 29:139–153.

Thomas CB, Duszynski KR, Shaffer JW. 1979. Family attitudes reported in youth
as potential predictors of cancer. *Psychosom Med.* 41:287–482.

Tross S, Herndon J II, Korzun A, et al. 1996. Psychological symptoms and disease-
free and overall survival in women with stage II breast cancer: Cancer and
Leukemia Group B. *J Natl Cancer Inst.* 88:661–667.

Turner-Cobbs JM, Sephton SE, Spiegl D. 2001. Psychosocial effects on immune
function and disease progression in cancer: human studies. In: Ader R, Felten
DL, Cohen N, eds. *Psychoneuroimmunology.* 3rd ed. San Diego, Calif: Academic
Press.

Walker LG, Heys SD, Walker MB, et al. 1999. Psychological factors can predict the
response to primary chemotherapy in patients with locally advanced breast cancer. *Eur J Cancer.* 35:1783–1788.

Watson W, Greer S. 1983. Development of a questionnaire measure of emotional
control. *J Psychosom Res.* 27:299–305.

Watson M, Greer S, Young J, Inayat Q, Burgess C, Robertson B. 1988. Development of a questionnaire measure of adjustment to cancer: the MAC scale. *Psychol
Med.* 18:203–209.

Watson M, Haviland JS, Greer S, Davidson J, Bliss JM. 1999. Influence of psychological response on survival in breast cancer: a population-based cohort study.
Lancet. 354:1331–1336.

Waxler-Morrison N, Hislop TG, Mears B, Kan L. 1991. Effects of social relationships on survival for women with breast cancer: a prospective study. *Soc Sci Med.*
33:177–183.

Weihs KL, Enright TM, Simmens SJ, Reiss D. 2000. Negative affectivity, restric-
tion of emotions, and site of metastases predict mortality in recurrent breast cancer. *J Psychosom Res.* 49:59–68.

Weinberger DA, Schwartz GE, Davidson RJ. 1979. Low-anxious, high-anxious, and
repressive coping styles: psychometric patterns and behavioral and physiological
responses to stress. *J Abnorm Psychol.* 88:369–380.

200 Weisman AD, Worden JW. 1977. Psychological analysis of cancer deaths. *Omega: J Death Dying.* 6:61–75.

Wilber K. 1988. Do we make ourselves sick? *New Age Journal.* September–October.

Wirsching M, Stierlin H, Hoffmann F, Weber G, Wirsching B. 1982. Psychological identification of breast cancer patients before biopsy. *J Psychosom Res.* 26:1–10.

Wu H, Wang J, Cacioppo JT, Glaser R, Kiecolt-Glaser JK, Malarkey WB. 1999. Chronic stress associated with spousal caregiving of patients with Alzheimer's dementia is associated with downregulation of B-lymphocyte GH mRNA. *J Gerontol A Biol Sci Med Sci.* 54:M212–M215.

Zonderman AB, Costa PT Jr, McCrae RR. 1989. Depression as a risk for cancer morbidity and mortality in a nationally representative sample. *JAMA.* 262:1191–1195.

PART TWO

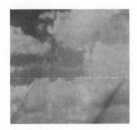

Clinical
Applications of
Mind-Body
Medicine

Chapter 5

Behavioral Medicine's New Marketplace

For about a decade, beginning in 1982, I had been writing about the studies and theoretical understandings that form the scientific basis of behavioral medicine, aspects of which are referred to colloquially as *mind-body medicine*. Over the years, I had formed the impression that practitioners, often on their own, were devising mind-body applications for a broad array of maladies and diseases, typically ones that contemporary biomedicine could not readily cure. Although mind-body techniques obviously had not swept the medical community, they appeared to be gaining in number, in use, and in popularity among a widening, if still selective, range of health-care professionals.

So when in 1991 I found in my mailbox the colorful, inviting brochure from the National Institute for the Clinical Application of Behavioral Medicine promoting its third annual conference, I thought it would be an opportunity to see firsthand just what was going on in the world of the practitioners who were developing and using new clinical applications of mind-body or behavioral medicine. I knew that some observers would consider it a waste of time to explore clinical applications that did not have a careful experimental basis. I said to myself, perhaps a bit rhetorically, "Whether or not there is a basic science foundation for every new clinical foray, there are patients out there getting sick, who believe in mind-body interactions and don't want to wait until medical science has come up with absolute empirical proof that a certain therapy works. They want what mind-body medicine has to offer now." Having imagined this response, I

Reprinted by permission, with changes, from *Advances in Mind-Body Medicine* 8 (1992): 46–69.

204 was led to another thought: that it would be useful to view the events of the conference not only from the perspective of a critical observer but from the perspective of a patient as well. I decided to try to do both.

Thankfully, I am not now a medical patient, but I have studied acting, and I recalled an approach of Stanislavsky, the great Russian theater director and the father of American "method" acting. The approach is known as *particularization*, which can be summed up by the phrase *as if.* When I attended a workshop on heart disease, then, it would be *as if* I were someone who had recently gone through the emotional upheaval of a heart attack. When I listened to a lecture on group therapy for cancer patients, it would be *as if* I were someone who had recently been told that he or she had cancer and had a fifty-fifty chance of living another five years.

I found that as a journalistic observer with a good knowledge of behavioral medicine I had one set of reactions to the conference, while as a "patient" with some awareness of mind-body interactions and a well-developed critical faculty I had a different though sometimes overlapping set of reactions. So that the reader will be clear about these differences, I use italics to present my reactions as a patient.

In the end, I left the conference feeling better informed and confused, ambivalent and optimistic—and somewhat rattled by my game of intrapsychic musical chairs. I hope this report fairly conveys the sources of my mixed reactions to the new marketplace of clinical applications now being offered by practitioners of behavioral medicine.

NICABM: A Buffet for the Mind-Body Practitioner

The National Institute for the Clinical Application of Behavioral Medicine was founded in 1987 by Ruth Buczynski, Ph.D., a private practitioner previously affiliated with the University of Connecticut, for the purpose of advancing knowledge among clinicians working in behavioral medicine and applying mind-body approaches to the prevention and treatment of illness. "We saw a need in behavioral medicine for more practitioner-oriented training opportunities," explained Dr. Buczynski in a telephone interview after the conference. To that end, the institute sponsors an annual conference for behavioral-medicine practitioners and will soon initiate specialized behavioral-medicine training programs around the country.

The institute's third national conference, "The Psychology of Health, Immunity, and Disease," was held in Orlando, Florida, on 4–7 December 1991. This "Practitioner's Conference on the Clinical Application of Psychoneuroimmunology and the Mind-Body Connection," as it was subtitled, covered an extraordinary range of topics, from quantum healing to anger management to group therapy for cancer patients, along with virtually every variety of behavioral-medicine approach in between. Present were well-known figures in the field—Bernie Siegel, Joan Borysenko, and Deepak Chopra, to name a few—as well as individuals working on a grassroots level in private clinics or academic settings. There were clinicians applying behavioral medicine with a relatively traditional bent ("Counseling Patients with Chronic Fatigue Syndrome") and others taking a seemingly more radical approach ("Unearthing the Emotional Roots of Physical Illness with Body-Centered Psychotherapy"). This diversity was one of the strengths of the conference.

Healthy Pleasures

The first day of the conference was devoted to lectures by several leading lights in behavioral medicine. David Sobel, M.D., coauthor with Robert Ornstein, Ph.D., of *Healthy Pleasures* (1989) and coauthor of many other books, gave a vibrant and funny talk on the health benefits of sensuality, optimism, and altruism. Sobel referred repeatedly to the health benefits of feeling good and decried what he called the "medical terrorism" inflicted on us by doctors and the media, who, Sobel argued, have stirred up so much fear about our diets and environments that many of us have become anxiety-ridden, pleasureless, compulsive health nuts. He showed a cartoon of a doctor sitting with a befuddled patient, whose caption read, "Well, there's no improvement, Henry. Are you sure you've given up *everything* you enjoy?"

Sobel's message was that we should stop worrying so much about grams of fat in our diet, an alcoholic drink or two a day, and too much chocolate. Instead of punishing ourselves with self-blame every time we indulge in one of these guilty pleasures, we should start concentrating on fundamental issues relevant to health, such as how much joy we experience in our daily lives.

It has been clear for some time that attitudes, beliefs, and moods can affect certain health behaviors (e.g., the anxious person who smokes to reduce anxiety), which in turn affect health outcomes (the person develops heart disease). Sobel claimed that evidence is mounting that attitudes, beliefs, and moods affect health outcomes *apart* from their affect on health behaviors. In other words, an anxious man may develop heart disease even if his anxiety does not cause him to smoke; his anxiety may directly influence blood pressure or atherosclerosis through internal, mind-body mechanisms.

But Sobel's primary emphasis was on positive behaviors that engen-

206   der positive outcomes, the pleasurable, sensual activities that he believes
stimulate our immune defenses or otherwise create an inner psychobiological climate that is hostile to disease agents and resistant to cardiovascular damage. He mentioned studies on the salutary, health-promoting
benefits of sensual pleasures involving the visual, tactile, auditory, or ol-
factory realms. "Looking at fish in a fish tank," he said, "might produce
the same [health] benefits without requiring the learning of sometimes
threatening or difficult disciplines, like meditation and guided imagery."
He contended that we overlook the small, simple pleasures—hugging a
child, smelling the roses, taking in scenes of nature.

According to Sobel, one of the major causes of our pessimistic, pleas-
ure-denying outlook, which leads to ill health, is the negative stories we
tell ourselves when we try to interpret our own experience. The only
people who face reality squarely, he said, are the clinically depressed. Some
denial is necessary if we are to restructure and reshape our cognitions in
order to take a more positive view of ourselves and our prospects for meaning, fulfillment, and joy in the face of real-world obstacles. We will never
be optimists, he said, if we do not work hard to challenge the relentlessly
negative stories we tell ourselves about ourselves and the world.

*Dr. Sobel is genuinely charming, funny, and very reassuring. He had a light
touch, and none of his humor seemed forced. Rehearsed, but not forced. Why
am I focusing on how he presented rather than on what he presented? In the
state I'm in, having been recently diagnosed with cancer, I find that I respond
to much more than words when trying to evaluate the information being con-
veyed to me about how to get well. Whether it's a medical doctor, an oncologist,
a mind-body therapist, a psychiatrist, a nurse, or a shaman speaking, I react
with head, heart, and gut. I believe strongly that I must fuse thoughts, feelings,
and intuitions if I am to follow the path that's right for me. Throughout this
conference, I'll be looking at both content and form: what the clinician says he
or she has to offer in terms of practice and how he or she presents.*

*In terms of presentation Sobel was a winner. But I had some problems with
his content. By the end of his talk I felt there was an element of Dr. Feelgood
in his approach (or, "How I learned to stop worrying and love my life"). Yes,
he talked about "selfless pleasures,"the gratification we derive from helping others, but his primary message was that many of us have lost our health because
we've lost the small, simple, daily pleasures. If we could only recapture our in-
nocence, our joy, our capacity for sensual receptivity, we'd begin to regain our
health. I like the message, but it seemed too Pollyanna for me at this moment.
I know Sobel wasn't saying that if someone like me just went out and smelled
the roses, my cancer would melt away, but still his approach sounded too easy.*

Is it because I have too little faith in simple, joyful experience? Perhaps. Or maybe it's because I feel that there's so much blocking my path to simple, joyful experience.

Especially since my diagnosis, I've been depressed a lot, and it's gotten in the way of my capacity to enjoy nature, to appreciate sex, to feel openhearted pleasure. Have I talked myself into these difficulties with my negative inner dialogue, as Sobel and some of the cognitive therapists suggest? Can I talk myself out of my fear and sadness by telling myself more optimistic stories about my health, my relationships, my recovery? I doubt it. My gut tells me that I actually need to go deeper into that despair—something very hard for me to do— if I'm ever to get out of it.

Maybe I'm not being fair to Dr. Sobel. Perhaps he was really talking about preventing illnesses rather than about curing them. Perhaps I'm trying to make everything he said apply to me. I wound up with this thought: I like his vision of where I should go, but I don't think he's provided me with a sufficiently detailed road map to get there.

The Arduous Path to a Healthy Heart

In 1990 Dean Ornish and his colleagues published in the British medical journal *Lancet* their now famous study demonstrating that a comprehensive program of lifestyle changes could reverse heart disease in patients who had already suffered heart attacks (Ornish et al. 1990). A strict regimen of exercise, yoga, vegetarian diet, stress management, and group support enabled Ornish's patients to reduce their cholesterol levels, improve the symptoms of their heart disease, and actually reverse their coronary artery blockage. It was the first time a nondrug approach had been shown to produce such effects. The second speaker at the conference was Larry Scherwitz, Ph.D., one of Ornish's key collaborators on the study, who fully described the "Open Your Heart" program.

While Ornish's findings have been publicized, discussed, and debated extensively, hearing them presented again by Scherwitz confirmed how remarkable the effects of this program were. Eighty-two percent of the participants in Ornish's intervention showed overall regression of coronary artery disease; 53 percent of the controls showed overall *progression*. PET scans, the state-of-the-art technology for assessing blood flow to the coronary muscle, demonstrated marked improvements in most patients in the program, while a reduction in blood flow was noted in most nonparticipants. The frequency and severity of angina attacks went down drastically in the experimental group; it went up dramatically in the controls. A 37 percent drop in cholesterol occurred without drugs—according to

208   Scherwitz the most significant reduction ever seen in any such trial. Scherwitz showed the now famous before-and-after arteriograms demonstrating the literal opening of the arteries in patients; they were graphic, dramatic testimony of the reversal of heart disease achieved.

Scherwitz emphasized the tight "dose-response" effect in this trial, meaning that the more assiduously a patient adhered to the program, the more marked the reversal of heart disease. This finding highlights an oft-expressed concern regarding Ornish's lifestyle-change program: it is too hard to stick with. The diet is strictly vegetarian, with the percentage of fat from calories at 10 percent or less; the exercise program involves three hours a week; the stress-management techniques, which include yoga, meditation, and visualization, must be maintained. The physical benefits (reversal of coronary artery blockage, reduced cholesterol, less angina, etc.) depend entirely on whether the patient can adhere to the program, and the degree of benefit depends on the degree of adherence.

The aspects of Ornish's program involving the least self-denial were the stress-management and group support sessions. Scherwitz convincingly argued that without stress management and without group support to "break the sense of isolation," the other lifestyle changes might not have been possible. Why? Although Scherwitz did not say so explicitly, the message I received was this: the discipline required to eschew poor eating habits—which are often compulsive behaviors based on stress and anxiety—depends upon the capacity to relax; and the discipline needed to take on a rigorous daily-exercise and visualization program depends on a passionate desire for life and health, a desire stoked by human connectedness and spiritual development.

Now I'm really confused. I had a heart attack two years ago, and I was thrilled listening to Larry Scherwitz talk about these dramatic reversals in coronary artery blockage produced by the Dean Ornish program. I know it's a tough regimen, but the mere fact that there's something I can do, without drugs, to open up those arteries gives me real hope. So why am I confused? Because I also sat through David Sobel's talk, which I really liked, and he said that we should stop obsessively micromanaging our diets and punishing ourselves for not being perfect health-mavens. (Ornish's program surely requires that we micromanage our diets.) We should allow ourselves those guilty pleasures and quit worrying so much—it's the constant worrying that's making us sick with heart disease and other such maladies.

It's a tough call, but I must resolve this ambivalence. If you believe Scherwitz—and I do—then there's no middle ground. You stick with the program and get the benefits or you allow yourself indulgences and pretty much forget .

about those beautiful little canals opening up in your arteries. As sympathetic as I am to Sobel's philosophy, as a person who's had a brush with death I feel I must choose the Ornish/Scherwitz path of vegetarianism and disciplined practice.

Of course, now I must actually begin. That's the hard part. Scherwitz showed a slide of a vegetarian meal (I think it was vegetable chili, but it was such an amorphous mass I couldn't tell for sure) to show how appetizing the food could be, and all I thought about were guilty pleasures like linguine bolognese and steak tartar.

The part of Ornish's program about which I had no qualms was the stress management and group support. I know that I have always had trouble relaxing. I can barely sit still much of the day. More importantly, I have a terribly difficult time opening up to others—even to close friends—when I'm stressed out, frightened, or angry. The idea that an emotionally blocked heart can lead to a physically blocked heart, therefore, strikes a chord with me. I imagine that participating in such a group would be difficult, but I can also imagine it as a liberating experience. It's hard for me to understand, intellectually, how that aspect of Ornish's program actually contributes to opening those beautiful little canals, but my heart tells me it could be so.

Informed Choice in Cancer Treatment

Today's cancer patients find themselves in a high-tech medical obstacle course. It begins with a hair-raising waiting game (for test results, diagnoses, etc.), moves on to a quick series of meetings with doctors out of which life-and-death decisions must be made in a short time frame, and leads to medical treatments that range from merely unpleasant to painful to traumatic. Patients often feel shuttled though this obstacle course, led by authoritarian coaches—the doctors—who often don't have the time to help patients make conscious, deliberate, and autonomous choices regarding their medical care.

Michael Lerner, Ph.D., presently of Commonweal, an organization devoted to service and research in health and human ecology, and the founder of the Commonweal Cancer Help Program, was a keynote speaker who addressed issues of choice in cancer treatment. Lerner has been an outspoken voice in the cancer support movement and is perhaps the country's leading authority on complementary and alternative cancer therapies. (He was the special consultant to the U.S. Office of Technology Assessment [OTA] in preparing its major report *Unconventional Cancer Treatments* [U.S. OTA 1990].)

Lerner addressed the question of informed choice in five areas: healing, conventional cancer therapies, complementary and alternative cancer therapies, pain control, and dying. He did not discuss the latter two points fully, but he did cogently argue that cancer patients and cancer caregivers should not shy away from dealing with questions of death and dying. Since all of us must eventually face issues of death and dying, we might as well train ourselves to face them more openly and fully. These issues should be part of the "curriculum for the second half of our lives." We can detoxify these subjects, Lerner said, by taking the fear out of them.

How Lerner became involved in researching unconventional cancer therapies revealed much about the humanistic underpinnings of his approach to the field and to cancer patients. He began his investigation of complementary and alternative cancer therapies ten years earlier, spurred on initially by hopes of finding treatments for his father, who had been stricken with two different types of cancer that "unquestionably should have killed him in a short period of time." (His father is Max Lerner, the renowned writer, who wrote a fine book about his experiences in healing, *Wrestling with the Angel* [1990].) Lerner devoted a decade of his life to this pursuit, helped to write the OTA's definitive report (at that time) on unconventional therapies, and wrote a remarkable book on the subject, *Healing Choices: Integrating the Best of Conventional and Complementary Approaches to Cancer* (1994). In the meantime his father recovered from his supposedly terminal cancer.

"Here's the most interesting fact of all," said Lerner. "In the ten years I put into this, he never used a single one of the complementary cancer therapies that I researched. To me there's great beauty in that fact, because it reveals the real truth—there's no single right way [to go about healing]. What he grasped was that the right way for him was simply to find his own way. And his way was to bury himself in work that he loved, and to continue his incredible fight to keep this very fragile boat of his afloat. I approach complementary therapies in that spirit."

Healing and curing are two different things, Lerner argued, and the distinction is critical. Healing is not only a physiological phenomenon; it is also psychological, emotional, and, to those for whom the term has meaning, spiritual. It is a mind–body state that can endure whether or not the physical body is in the process of recovery. Healing can occur even when a cancer spreads or death is near, a realization that should allow cancer patients to transcend the limited, sometimes dangerous view that if they are not getting well, they must not be healing. (That mistake, taken to its logical extreme, carries the invidious implication that the patient who is not healing physically must be doing something terribly wrong.) By the same token, the multileveled phenomenon of healing may indeed enhance the prospect of survival. "Healing seems to me to be a psychophysiologic response that opens every gate to reserves of energy or to ways of reordering priorities; and so it opens every gate to physical recovery, if such a thing is possible," said Lerner.

Choice in healing, then, means that the patient treks his or her own path, which often involves finding more outlets for emotional and creative expression. The cancer psychotherapist and psycho-oncology pioneer Lawrence LeShan saw a "foiled creative fire" in many of his patients (LeShan 1977); and the researcher Lydia Temoshok found that cancer patients were unable to express either negative or positive emotions (Temoshok and Dreher 1992). Whether a patient chooses meditation, visualization, psychotherapy, group support, all of the above, or none of the above, he or she must follow the dictates of his or her needs, feelings, dreams, images, or creative impulses.

Complementary cancer therapies are treatments used alongside conventional cancer treatment (surgery, chemotherapy, radiation). Lerner developed the following categories for such approaches: spiritual, psychological, nutritional, physical, pharmacologic, traditional Chinese medical, electromagnetic, and esoteric. After his decade-long investigation, which took him to many parts of the world, Lerner has come to the following strong conclusions: (1) he has not found any cure for cancer among the unconventional methods he examined; (2) he has found little scientific evidence to answer the question whether any of these approaches extend life above and beyond what can be achieved with conventional methods; (3) he has accumulated powerful anecdotal evidence that many such therapies greatly enhance quality of life; and (4) the stereotypic notion that patients who pursue unconventional cancer therapies are blindly ignorant and that the practitioners of such methods are by definition quacks or hucksters is false. (The latter point has been conclusively demonstrated by medical sociologist Barrie Cassileth [Cassileth et al. 1984].) In fact, consumers of nontraditional cancer treatments are among the best-informed patients, and the majority of nontraditional cancer therapists are primarily licensed practitioners who charge reasonable fees—doctors with integrity who believe that their work genuinely improves the outcome for their patients.

To Lerner, the ongoing argument between the self-proclaimed quackbusters of the establishment, who believe that all unconventional practitioners are charlatans, and the extreme advocates of nontraditional therapies, who believe that all mainstream treatments are evil variants of the cut, burn, and poison school of medicine, is "an utterly boring, trivial, stupid debate" that has no value for cancer patients. What has value for cancer patients is an integration of the best of mainstream Western medicine and

212   alternative medicine. After making this point, Lerner provided a detailed description of the wide variety of complementary therapies, from mind-body approaches to nutritional programs to agents that stimulate the immune system.

A strange lack of common sense seems to have pervaded the medical establishment's approach to the powerful evidence that mind-body interactions can be a significant factor in cancer recovery. Lerner tore through the thin tissue of logic used by conservative critics to defend the credo that mind-body factors are irrelevant to cancer survival by making the following two points:

- Doctors have known for a long time—and it has been scientifically documented—that "functional status," an index of overall mental and physical well-being and the capacity to function effectively from day to day, is one reliable predictor of survival in cancer patients. Why, then, he asked, does it not make sense to actively pursue any and all approaches (nutritional, psychological, spiritual) that improve overall health and functional status? Why are these not considered legitimate means to enhance the prospects for recovery or at least better medical outcomes?

- Dr. David Spiegel's remarkable finding that patients with metastatic breast cancer survived twice as long when they participated in a program of group support (Spiegel et al. 1989) provided substantial scientific support for what mind-body advocates and practitioners have been claiming for decades. "Had this been a new chemotherapy," said Lerner, "do you want to guess how big the headlines would have been and how much National Cancer Institute money would have been poured into the replication of that study?"

Lerner's talk amounted to an eloquent call for rationality and compassion on all sides of the debate over complementary therapies for cancer. His balanced approach to unconventional medicine was credible because he had directly researched alternative treatments so extensively. At the same time, there was no lack of passion in his argument for an informed blending of traditional and nontraditional treatments that meet the unique needs of every individual cancer patient.

Lerner's presentation impressed me greatly. No slides, no tired anecdotes, no self-congratulation. I had the sense that his remarks were made extemporaneously, even though he was clearly prepared and had given something like this talk before. Ergo, he spoke from the heart. His commitment stemmed originally from wanting to help his father; that he so gracefully accepted the fact that his father never used a single one of the therapies he researched told me that Lerner practices what he preaches. Rather than grinding an axe and finding himself frustrated or hurt when his father declined to accept his advice, he was open to learning a truth that revealed itself through experience: what his father needed most was to find his own way.

This told me that if I went to Lerner's Commonweal Cancer Help Program, the last thing I would get was dogma. The first thing I would get, I'm certain, is a feeling of utter respect for the process I would have to go through to make my own choices. What a relief!

I was heartened by these words: "Let me say that I am no advocate of alternative therapies. My goal in this field has been to raise the level of dialogue about unconventional cancer treatments, and about the process of informed choice in integrating the best of mainstream and complementary therapies for the people with cancer." That meant I would get from Lerner no speeches, no pleading, no mindless advocacy. If I went to Commonweal, which he said provides group support, nutritional guidance, meditation, and yoga, I would be counseled about my medical options—traditional and nontraditional—in an objective way. That's what I want. I've come to believe that an important aspect of healing is the sense of control, which means that the choices are mine. I won't do anything simply because someone tells me that's what I should do, no matter how charismatic or brilliant or committed they may be. What I wish for most is someone I respect who can lay out the choices for me—and that's what Lerner seemed to represent. Then, upon making my own decisions, I can be fully committed to my treatment program, because my sense of hope and belief will be the product of my own intellectual, psychological, and spiritual process—not someone else's.

His emphasis on combining the best of conventional and unconventional approaches also touched a deep chord in me. The angry strains of rhetoric I've heard floating through the polarized discourse between true believers on both sides of this argument have alienated me. It's always struck me as a symptom of black or white, either-or thinking I've come to believe is a convenient way of bypassing the truth, whether it's in politics, philosophy, or medicine. To me, it simply makes common sense to combine these approaches. When I'm honest with myself, I have serious qualms that nutrition and psychotherapy alone (two paths I am pursuing) will produce an immune-boosting effect powerful enough to vanquish my tumor. I believe I need surgery and chemotherapy—despite my qualms about chemo—to eliminate enough of the tumor to then allow natural mechanisms to wipe out any remaining tumor cells. I also believe that nutrition, psychotherapy, and acupuncture will help me better withstand the rigors of chemo and keep whatever damage it causes to my immune system to a minimum.

When Lerner talked about "detoxifying death," it was one of the few times I have found myself not recoiling from the mere mention of the subject. Hard

214   *as it may be, I want to be able to look at it, face it, and talk to my friends and family about it. I don't want the subject to fester in some inner closet, where I know it will turn into the monster I most fear and spring out at me when am least prepared to deal with it. Lerner gave me hope that I could begin now to open the closet door without becoming overwhelmed, without losing my bearings and lapsing into a full-scale depression. In this regard his discussion of shamanism helped the most. As he explained:*

> Shamanism is based on a bedrock of human experience and that fact means that even today, among cancer patients everywhere, there are people who are literally having that ancient shamanic experience of facing life-threatening illness and trying against all odds to find their way back from the edge. The idea is that the shaman did try to help you recover physically, but that was not his primary priority. His primary priority was to safeguard the passage of the soul. Whether the soul was meant to move back to life or through death, he was there to safeguard it.

When I began to think about my struggle with cancer not as a struggle against death but as a search for ways to safeguard my own soul—through death or back to life—I began to experience a sense of peace about the future.

Truth or Dare: The Health Effects of Opening Up

Many psychologists and mind-body scientists have long believed that inhibiting strong emotions—negative or positive—can have long-term damaging effects on both psychological well-being and physical health. James W. Pennebaker, Ph.D., a psychologist at Southern Methodist University, is a leading expert on the psychophysical aspects of inhibition versus confession. In his keynote address Pennebaker described his fascinating experimental studies on the health effects of disclosure.

One of the early experiences that got Pennebaker interested in inhibition and confession was a series of talks he had with polygraph instructors. Pennebaker learned of a peculiar but telling sequence of events that typically occurred when individuals guilty of a crime were given a polygraph test. When people are initially hooked up to psychophysiological equipment in preparation for a polygraph—whether guilty or not—their autonomic nervous systems are racing, with elevated heart rate, breathing rate, blood pressure, and skin conductance. The polygraph expert is trained not only in reading results but also in inducing confessions. When a confession is induced, the suspect is booked and readied to go to jail, but in most instances he or she is required to take one more polygraph to ensure that the confession was truthful, and it is here that the peculiarity occurs. Although at that very moment the person's life is in shambles, re- markably he or she is often found to be physiologically very relaxed. The person's heart rate has slowed, breathing has slowed, skin conductance has normalized, and blood pressure has lowered. Often the suspect warmly thanks the polygraph instructor before he or she is carted off to jail.

This was Pennebaker's first and strongest clue to the physiological ef- fects of confession. He began developing a model of inhibition and dis- closure that posited that psychological traumas, to which we are all sub- ject, call upon a range of coping strategies. One of those strategies is inhibition, or holding back the thoughts and feelings associated with the trauma. The crux of Pennebaker's theory is that inhibition requires a great deal of physiological work; hence the increases in autonomic nervous sys- tem parameters. This work is by itself a cumulative, low-level, chronic stressor. Confession, whether through talking or writing, represents a re- lease from this difficult work, as well as a means for organizing and struc- turing thoughts and feelings about the trauma so that it is better under- stood and ultimately resolved.

His theory was not far afield from theories long advanced by researchers in psychodynamics, constructs that have explained the integrative psy- chological effects of psychotherapy. What was new was Pennebaker's em- phasis on the physiological work associated with inhibition and its rami- fications in terms of health. If confession relieves the person of this chronic psychobiological stressor, are the effects measurable? More specifically, do these effects, which presumably involve reduced strain on the autonomic nervous, cardiovascular, and immune systems, really result in better health?

To answer these questions, Pennebaker initiated a series of experimen- tal studies in which the vehicle for confession was writing (Pennebaker and Beall 1986). A group of students were asked to spend fifteen to twenty minutes a day for five consecutive days writing about the most traumatic experience they could remember. A control group was asked to write about insignificant experiences, such as their plans for the day. Pennebaker dis- covered that most of the students in the experimental group—all from Southern Methodist University—were surprisingly willing to write about terrible traumas in their lives, ranging from freak accidents to family fights to physical and sexual abuse. In the initial days of writing these students reported feeling sad, anxious, guilty, or angry immediately after complet- ing the exercise. By the final day of writing they felt as undisturbed as the control group. Confession, it seems, increases inner distress for a short pe- riod until the thoughts and feelings elicited are gradually integrated, after which time relaxation ensues. Indeed, in psychophysical tests of people talking about traumas, Pennebaker found that once the confessions were completed, blood pressure, heart rate, and skin conductance levels went down, often to below baseline and indicative of a state of relaxation. The subjects in Pennebaker's study were then followed for six months to determine health outcomes. Those who wrote about traumas made significantly fewer visits to the doctor than they had before the writing exercise and significantly fewer than members of the control group.

Pennebaker has since replicated this study many times, always turning up the same finding: writing about traumas in one's life reduces physical symptoms and illnesses over a period of months. One of his replications had particular relevance to psychoimmunology research. In collaboration with the psychologist Ronald Glaser, Pennebaker conducted a study in which blood samples were taken before, immediately after, and six weeks subsequent to the writing experiment (Pennebaker et al. 1988). Those who wrote about traumas, unlike those in control groups, showed significant increases in immune function (namely, in T-cell responsivity to substances that stimulate cell division, CON-A and PHA) after both the five-day exercise and six weeks later. These same subjects also made fewer visits to the doctor during the following six months than did members of the control group. This is the kind of study psychoimmunologists dream about. Not only did it show the long-term health benefits of a psychosocial intervention but it revealed that a psychobiological mechanism was probably mediating this effect. One critical aspect of immune function had been enhanced.

Pennebaker has observed and documented the health benefits of confession among a group of university staff members (unpublished), among Holocaust survivors (Pennebaker et al. 1989), and among a group of senior corporate executives who had recently been traumatized by the loss of their jobs (Spera et al. 1994). Based on this research, he concluded that the salutary effects of writing and confession occur whether the trauma is ongoing or a distant memory.

The study of unemployed executives had a special resonance both because of its health implications and because of its relevance to our times. The one hundred laid-off white-collar workers were randomized to one of three groups: the first group wrote about their deepest feelings about the loss of their jobs; the second group participated in a "time-management exercise" wherein they wrote a careful record of what they were doing daily to procure a job; the third group wrote about trivial subjects. After four months Pennebaker had to call off the experiment: 35 percent of the people who wrote about their feelings had gotten jobs, compared with 5 percent of the control group and none of the "time-management" group. (This situation is comparable to studies in which a drug performs so much better than a placebo in ameliorating illness that the trial is called off and everyone gets the drug.)

According to Pennebaker, the subjects who had confided their feelings had not developed greater motivation to get a job; rather, they had worked through their anger and bitterness and developed a balanced perspective on their loss. They were able to move on in their lives, unlike the "time-management" subjects, whose exercise, which Pennebaker likened to "obsessiveness-training," seemed to keep them stuck in anger and anxiety.

The value of confession, whether through writing or talking, centers on the uniquely human function of putting thoughts and emotions into words. According to Pennebaker, the key is not catharsis, the venting of negative emotions through dramatic expression. Emotional expression and sharing may certainly be one component of these exercises, but the key component, as Pennebaker sees it, is the structuring and organizing of feelings and cognitions, the opportunity to put back together the pieces of a fragmented psychic puzzle left scattered after the experience of a disintegrating trauma. Not only does one experience a sense of release and relief, he argues, but one develops greater insight into one's behavior patterns, more self-understanding and acceptance, and a greater feeling of coherence and psychic integrity.

Now I'm confused again. Sobel had said that optimistic copers are able to exercise healthy denial, and the result is better health. They don't become overwhelmed by traumas or unpleasant experiences because they are able to interpret them positively or tuck them away on the shelf of the unconscious. Pennebaker is saying that we're invariably better off when we face our traumas, talk about them or write about them, deal directly with our concomitant thoughts and feelings, and get on with our lives. Isn't that another contradiction?

Sobel introduced Pennebaker and in recognition of the differences between them acknowledged that denial is not always the best coping strategy when major traumas exert a chronic negative effect on mind and body. Does that mean that denial is useful for minor insults but not major ones?

I came to a somewhat different conclusion. I know from personal experience that it is impossible to face pain and trouble all the time, that I need denial or repression to put aside sadness or anger associated with stressful events—at least until I can get enough distance to work them through. Whether the stressful event was minor or major, I need to shelve my rougher emotions until I can find the time and space to explore them. Invariably, I shift back and forth between coping strategies of inhibition and confession, though resolution is not achieved until I put my thoughts and feelings into words. Pennebaker's way, it

218   *seems to me, is the desirable coping strategy because it is the culmination of a
process that must unfold in order for me to finish my unfinished business. It does
seem important to recognize that we imperfect humans can't always willfully
shift into confession mode. We may need to wait until we're ready. I'm thinking of the extreme example of Pennebaker's Holocaust survivors. Could they
have been expected to sit down and write about their traumas within weeks of
being released from concentration camps?*

*I have suffered from chronic health symptoms for many years. I've had ten-
sion headaches, heart palpitations, and asthma that comes and goes. I rarely
find that I am completely healthy. It's as if there's an inner caravan of pain
that sets up camp in one bodily region until it is driven away by medical interventions (aspirin, beta-blockers, or bronchodilators, respectively), after which
it relocates in another bodily region. What is this caravan of pain? My instinct
tells me that it's primarily a cluster of still-reverberating memories and emotions associated with painful past experiences.*

*After listening to Pennebaker I was left with the strong impression that I
need to do more work on those old memories and emotions if I am to rid myself
of the caravan. To me, that means journal writing and psychotherapy.*

*While Pennebaker is not a behavioral-medicine clinician, I think his ideas
ought to find their way into more behavioral-medicine applications. His concepts were so clear and clean, and their ramifications are inescapable. He struck
me as a consummate scientist who allowed his human instincts to be a coequal
guide along with his rational, empirical thinking in the development of his theories. After hearing Pennebaker I became more convinced that the "positive attitude" approach, so familiar to me from my readings on mind-body interactions,
has severe limitations, especially if it is used to buttress a pattern of long-term
denial. In my experience, my efforts to "rise above" my pain have actually kept
me in a more vulnerable mind-body state.*

Hope, Healing, and Controversy

Bernie Siegel, one-time Yale surgeon, author of *Love, Medicine, and Miracles* (1986) and *Peace, Love, and Healing* (1989), and developer of the EcaP
program (Exceptional Cancer Patients), spoke about his approach to healing in patients with cancer and other life-threatening illnesses. He told
jokes, delivered numerous anecdotes of patients who survived terminal
cancer, and philosophized about mind-body healing. Much of the time, he
seemed to be directly or indirectly answering critics who have accused him
either of simplifying mind-body interactions or of causing some patients
to feel guilty for getting sick or for not getting well.

While Siegel defended himself against his critics' charges, he also appeared to have taken some of the criticism to heart. The toughest charge against him has been that patients who use his approach and do not get well are made to feel like failures. Siegel went out of his way to say that death is not a failure, that psychospiritual healing can occur for patients approaching death as well as for survivors. He also stressed that cancer patients should embark on any healing endeavor in order to live life to the fullest, not to conquer death. "Don't do things to not die," he proclaimed. "It doesn't work."

Siegel's whiz-bang style of delivering stories, quotes, and homilies made it sometimes difficult to follow his train of thought. He reminded me of Robin Williams in the way his quick one-liners and stories sometimes hit their mark and sometimes did not. He was most effective in critiquing the disturbing lack of training that doctors receive in how to deal with patients' emotions and how to involve patients in the decision-making process. He spoke movingly of the human dilemma of the doctor faced with so much fear and pain and of how badly doctors need preparation and education to handle their own and their patients' anguish. Siegel argued that doctors suffer *more* by anesthetizing themselves to their patients' psychic and physical pain.

Though much of his talk was persuasive, Siegel could not completely dispel the notion that some patients who accept his views wholeheartedly might feel guilty if they do not fully recover. "I don't make anybody feel guilty," said Siegel defensively. "If I create guilt in you, then I'd say you've got to look at your life and what's happened in it to make you feel so vulnerable." The problem of some cancer patients' blaming themselves for their illness or decline may well be traceable to a psychological predisposition to feelings of guilt, shame, or worthlessness. However, Siegel wishes to abdicate any responsibility on his part, or on the part of mind-body advocates, for triggering guilt feelings in cancer patients. He has not considered that the induction of guilt becomes more likely when psychologically vulnerable patients are *also* exposed to such oversimplified ideas about healing as "you are totally responsible for your own recovery." (We are not: too many factors are out of our control.) Perhaps if Siegel acknowledged that he *does* have the power to trigger (not cause) some guilt feelings, he would be even more sensitive to the problem and less subject to unfair criticism.

That said, Siegel *is* more sensitive than he once was (as evidenced by media appearances in years past) regarding the issue of guilt, and he is still subject to some unfair criticism. The criticism comes from both mind-body scientists and members of the medical establishment. Although the problematic aspects of Siegel's writings and lectures should not be ignored or discounted, neither should his important contributions. He has disseminated knowledge of mind-body interactions to a broad audience, and he has offered hope to tens of thousands, if not hundreds of thousands, of patients with life-threatening diseases.

It is easy to take potshots at Bernie Siegel because he has not conducted his own research and because his image is ubiquitous. With his high profile and unapologetic political stance, Siegel has become a lightning rod for anger from all sides. He is, in this respect, the Bill Clinton of mind-body healing: his ideas are mostly sound, and his heart certainly seems to be in the right place, even if he sometimes undermines his own best instincts.

I have lung cancer, and I've been told I have a 10 percent chance of living five years. I read Bernie Siegel's book Love, Medicine, and Miracles. *I saw him on* The Oprah Winfrey Show. *I read an article on him in* New York Magazine *[Schwartz 1989] that was highly critical. While all this has made me ambivalent about Siegel, I still believe in his basic message, and I appreciated his keynote address. His message of hope is something I can't get enough of.*

I understand that he's been accused of making patients feel guilty and of fudging research findings to make points in his books or on TV. While this concerns me, it doesn't make me think he's a charlatan. After all, he's not selling snake oil. He's selling hope and the idea that psychological and spiritual development can help people like me live longer—simple truths I accept without reservation.

But I don't know if I would get into one of Siegel's groups. He never described what he does in his EcaP groups to my satisfaction. During his lecture I was alternately uplifted and let down. He makes one believe with his rat-a-tat-tat of inspirational anecdotes, and he does so with authority and a comforting paternalism. (He's the paterfamilias of mind-body healing.) For someone who's sick like me, that's powerful stuff. But he spoke quickly and never stuck with any one subject long enough. I wanted longer stories, more reflection, and less defensiveness. And I wanted more specifics on what he does with patients, besides telling them the same anecdotes he told all eight hundred of us in the audience.

When I saw Siegel on The Oprah Winfrey Show *a few years ago I thought he was an angry person. (A paradox, I thought, since the man has become a symbol for peace and love.) He attacked a patient who criticized him. I forgave him with the following thought: Bernie's a warrior on the front lines of a fight I deeply believe in, a fight for more humanism in medicine. Moreover, I suspected that patients responded as much to his anger—at doctors, at medical institutions, at patients who give up—as they did to his love. Still, the anger worried me. For every patient who was spurred on by his fire, were there others who were burned by it?*

My concerns were lessened at the conference. My impression of Siegel, both in his talk and over the whole four days, was that he seemed less angry. His tone of voice was softer than I remembered it. He was readily approachable, and when I spoke with him personally, he was warm and direct. Nothing about his manner was forced or phony. He showed up at workshops and asked questions that demonstrated a true interest in what others were thinking and doing. He was at James Spira's workshop on group therapy for cancer patients (Spira is an associate of David Spiegel, the psychiatrist who had shown that breast cancer patients in group therapy survived twice as long as patients without therapy and who recently was sarcastic about Bernie Siegel in the pages of Advances *in* Mind-Body Medicine *[Siegel 1992; Spiegel 1991, 1992]) and asked Spira how he deals with the problem of guilt. All of which led me to believe that Siegel is humble enough to want to learn. These impressions may mean nothing to the scientists who criticize Siegel, but they told me something I wanted to know.*

A very close friend of mine has leukemia. She met Siegel at one of his workshops, and he spoke with her for an hour. He made her feel uplifted and left her with a greater sense of empowerment. I wondered: Should she have ignored those positive feelings because he tends to overinterpret mind-body research findings? Should she forget the hope he engendered for her because his critics think he's facile? Obviously not. Therein, I thought, lies the importance of Bernie Siegel.

Psychosocial Interventions for Cancer Patients

Two days of the conference were devoted to workshops, most of which were led by doctors, psychotherapists, nurses, or medical specialists who are applying behavioral medicine in their own practices, clinics, or hospitals. A few of the workshop leaders were originators of or participants in behavioral-medicine programs or ongoing clinical studies that have received much attention in academic circles and in the mass media. But most workshop leaders were clinicians who have developed their own behavioral-medicine approaches without publishing many (or any) academic papers on their work and without any media fanfare.

More than sixty workshops were offered; it was possible to attend only six. Many workshops were devoted to psychosocial interventions for patients with cancer and AIDS, such as "How to Lead a Cancer Support Group," "Enhancing Hope in the Chronically and Terminally Ill," and "A Practical Model for Empowering Cancer Patients." I attended two others in this area: "Group Psychotherapy for Advanced Stage Cancer/AIDS Patients," led by James L. Spira, Ph.D., and "Psychoneuroimmunology and Relational Aspects of Cancer: Relationship, Psychotherapy, and Deep Healing," led by Diane Perlman, Ph.D.

Spira was one of the workshop leaders involved in a highly publicized endeavor. A fellow in the Department of Psychiatry at the Stanford University School of Medicine, Spira collaborates with David Spiegel, M.D., the psychiatrist who showed in the landmark 1989 study that advanced breast cancer patients survived twice as long when they participated in a group therapy program (Spiegel at al. 1989). They are currently replicating their earlier study on women with metastatic breast cancer and have added new components, one of which will answer a critical psychoimmunological question: If group therapy patients survive longer, is it because their immune systems are augmented?

In his first workshop Spira lectured on the results of the initial study, but I attended his second workshop, in which he described the specific principles and techniques used in his (and Spiegel's) group therapy for patients with cancer and HIV/AIDS. (This is the workshop that Bernie Siegel attended.) Was there something particular about their therapeutic methods that explained Spiegel's remarkable survival effects?

Spira spent ninety minutes laying out in methodical terms precisely how he and Spiegel conduct their group therapy, which he called "supportive-expressive group therapy." Patients with primary breast cancer or HIV infection are asked to participate in sixteen once-a-week sessions. By contrast, patients with metastatic or recurrent breast cancer or full-blown AIDS are asked to commit to a one-year program of weekly sessions. Spira stressed the need for the homogeneity of these groups. He explained that a person with, say, asymptomatic HIV infection might feel disinclined to share his distress in a group that included dying AIDS patients for fear that his problems might be considered trivial by comparison.

Since many patients have a difficult time with doctors and oncologists, the groups aim at enabling participants to share their anger and sense of isolation regarding doctors and medical institutions. Group leaders impart techniques for establishing improved communication and partnership. Altered and stressed family and social relationships are a key topic, as are life values, religious and philosophical perspectives, illness-related coping skills, group-interaction issues, and issues of death and dying. Much time is devoted to helping patients "work through" their grief over the loss of others in the group, which is another way to help patients confront and accept their own mortality.

Patients receive support and give support, relieving their feelings of isolation, hopelessness, and helplessness. Group support not only helps patients accept their condition, it helps them face upcoming crises in their struggle with life-threatening illness (recurrences, opportunistic infections, failure of treatment, etc.). Unlike patients in conventional group treatments, participants in these groups are also encouraged to maintain ties with one another outside the group, to visit one another in the hospital, and to attend social events and funerals together. These ties enhance the sense of connectedness and of commitment to the group.

A cliché in group therapy is that it "encourages expression of emotion." Most impressive in Spira's presentation was his highly specific description of what it means to express emotions, which expressions are therapeutic and which are not, and how group leaders are able to stimulate healthy expression. Spira stressed that patients are not pushed to acknowledge or express more anger, fear, or grief than they are prepared to accept and integrate. "Pushing a patient too hard to express feelings is a bit like Rolfing," said Spira, acknowledging that excessive pressure can leave a person exhausted, overwhelmed, and more hurt than before. When patients already prone to repressing emotion in the face of stress find themselves in an overly confrontative group, they are likely to think, "Aha! I was right to shut down."

Patients in Spira's group are encouraged to move from external, or general, expression of feelings to personal, or specific, expressions, for example, from "All men are bastards" to "I wish my husband would be more supportive when I am undergoing chemotherapy treatments." It is common for patients to lose themselves in solipsistic expressions of despair ("Why me?"), which can keep them locked into a pattern of isolation. Through gentle prodding, patients can be helped to connect and empathize more, a process that expands their emotional repertoire and deepens their sense of compassion for themselves and others.

Spiegel and Spira's model for group treatment appeared not to miss a single theme relevant to people with life-threatening illnesses. From death and dying to practical questions of finances to existential issues of selfhood, these groups appear to provide a structured experience for cancer and HIV/AIDS patients that acknowledges the complexity of their experience and addresses their multileveled psychological, spiritual, and physical needs.

No wonder David Spiegel was the first to demonstrate the survival effects of group therapy for cancer patients. As described by Spira, the therapy groups for cancer patients sounded so supportive, so carefully structured, so finely tuned to everyone's needs. Spira was soft-spoken but articulate, deliberate, and painstaking in his descriptions of these groups. I have gone to several talks on this subject, and I have usually left wondering, "What really goes on in these groups?" Spira left me with no doubts.

I have cancer, and my only question is this: Where do I sign up? Spira stressed simple things that for me would make a difference. From the first day of the group he wants to know who's in attendance. Every group begins this way, so patients get the message that the therapist and the other participants care what happens to them. A commitment is required; it's not OK to drop in and out as you please. Spira explained that casual participation can be worse than no participation because you get enough exposure to feel distressed by the reality of others' pain and mortality but not enough involvement to work through your feelings of sadness and fear and to establish close ties with others, ties that would facilitate your healing process. All of this demonstrated to me the utmost in compassion and care.

I don't want to be pushed to express my feelings. I want to be encouraged by the support of others; to know that it's safe to get upset and equally safe not to. That strikes me as a healing environment, and that's exactly what Spira described.

Diane Perlman, Ph.D., is a clinical psychologist in private practice who deals with individuals, couples, and families. In her work with cancer patients she has integrated methods from family systems theory, Jungian analysis, and applied psychoimmunology in order to enhance psychological and immunological well-being. She addressed head-on the controversy regarding the role of personality and psychosocial factors in cancer onset and progression. In Perlman's view, there is a cancer "personality," but the construct has been badly misunderstood and misinterpreted. Some patients who accept the idea of a cancer personality, Perlman maintains, have suffered "New Age guilt," particularly when this notion is presented without proper contextualization. "People are no more responsible for cancer than they are for being abused or for developing allergies, multiple sclerosis, or any other disease," she said. Moreover, the term *personality* contains the Jungian term *persona*, which refers to the social mask, not the fixed structures of personality. Perlman argued that New Age guilt should be diminished when we view the psychological contribution to cancer as stemming not from an individual's fixed personality but rather from his or her shifting and changeable persona.

Research has uncovered certain behavior patterns or personality styles in cancer development, most notably: stoicism; nonexpression of negative emotions; self-sacrificing behavior; harmonizing, "nice guy" behavior; and helpless or hopeless coping patterns. Perlman believes that cancer patients can transform and transcend these patterns in psychotherapy both as a form of self-actualization and as a way to strengthen and stimulate the anticancer arms of immunity. To support her view she cited psychoneuroimmunological research on the link between psychosocial factors or psychosocial interventions and natural killer cell activity. While Perlman's review of psychoneuroimmunological research was incomplete and therefore unconvincing, her presentation of a theoretical framework to enrich our understanding of the development of cancer-prone patterns and to support a therapeutic model of change and health promotion was more successful.

Over the past decade the so-called relational schools of psychoanalytic theory have become more prominent. Perlman drew on relational theory to piece together a developmental model of the cancer personality and seemed to draw on the "life energy" theories of the radical psychoanalyst Wilhelm Reich as well. She followed the stages of development from the infant's initial bonding and attachment to the mother through the earliest stages of individuation. With each new phase of separation and exploration the person's sense of security—based on the quality of the initial connection to parents—enables him or her to move out into the world while retaining his or her "eros" or "life force." When that security is lacking, exploration and individuation is tentative, and the person gets stuck in a stage of conformity. He or she is unable to break the bonds, fearing a loss of contact or confirmation, and thus maintains behavior designed strictly to hold the attention or approval of the parents. The person's individuality is blocked, Perlman argued, and stays that way through later stages of development.

If I understood Perlman's theory correctly, the relational basis of the development of the cancer personality means that healing must involve transformations in relationships. According to Perlman, the role of relationships in healing "is often neglected in the popular culture, which gives more attention to inner states and deals primarily with relaxation, imagery, visualization, positive attitude, and meditation." Perlman agrees that these techniques can be powerful but feels that "relationship is a critical factor that is missing in the mind-body-spirit triad. A person's relationship system, both family of origin and current family as well as vocational system, plays an important role both in etiology and in healing." For this reason, Perlman advocates a multifaceted approach to psychotherapy for cancer patients, one that emphasizes changes in relationships and family systems. The development of greater autonomy and authenticity in all of one's relationships appeared to be Perlman's primary goal.

Pieces of the puzzle are fitting together. Perlman's notion that the role of relationships in cancer development and healing has been neglected, while private activities and techniques like meditation and imagery have gotten all the press, made sense to me. Maybe that's why David Spiegel hit the jackpot, as it were.

226   *I believe in meditation and imagery, and I practice them, but in all my reading it seems that no bona fide studies have yet proven the life-extending benefits of meditation or imagery. Yet Spiegel was able to demonstrate life-extending
benefits with group therapy—to the surprise of many, including Spiegel, who
did not expect the results he found. Group therapy is about relationships—about
developing honesty in the group, about coming to terms with the meaning of
old relationships, about more authentic relationships with family and friends and
partners in the here and now. Perlman's point about dealing more with relationships in mind-body therapies could not be better underscored than by Spiegel's surprising findings about the medical benefits of his psychosocial treatment.*

   *Am I a cancer personality? Perhaps. I certainly relate to many of the char-
acteristics Perlman mentioned. I have trouble expressing anger. I tend to keep
up a good front for family and friends, not saying when I'm troubled, especially
by them or by their behavior. I want to enter a therapy program where I can
explore these patterns and change them. I found it difficult to judge whether I
would enter therapy with Perlman, mainly because her focus was primarily
theoretical, with little practical information about how she works clinically with
patients. But I was impressed by her attempt to understand the origins of the
cancer personality and the compassion she demonstrated in dealing with issues that
I feel are both delicate and crucial, like New Age guilt. I particularly appreciated her comment that we should focus on the persona within personality so as not
to make the mistake of believing that who we are can make us sick or die.*

   *I also liked Perlman's opening touch. We walked into her workshop to the
loud strains of "Smile (When Your Heart Is Breaking),"a song I've always
associated with the Jerry Lewis telethon. Participants flashed befuddled looks
at one another as if to ask, What's this about? Then Perlman began her talk
and explained to us that people prone to cancer and immune dysfunction often
do just that—smile when their hearts are breaking.*

The Power of Negative Emotions

In 1989, at the age of forty-four, Bonnie K. Schindler, R.N., Ph.D., was
diagnosed with multiple sclerosis. After three months of temporary blind-
ness, double vision, severe vertigo, and depression, she made life changes
that she believes explain her complete recovery. Since her recovery
Schindler, a professional counselor and clinical hypnotherapist, has
opened a new counseling endeavor called the Mind-Body Connection, in
which she assists physically ill patients in using the same techniques she
employed to get well.

   In Schindler's workshop, "The Power of Negative Emotions," she emphasized changing the negative self-talk that makes us feel helpless and

hopeless in the face of stress or illness. These negative messages and feelings are "toxic to our bodies," she claimed, and need to be challenged and dislodged. Using language familiar from cognitive reframing, neurolinguistic programming, and popular books on healing, Schindler spoke about substituting positive affirmations for the negative thoughts, feelings, and memories that drag us down. It is entirely possible to "replace old programming with new programming," she explained. The positive affirmations—statements such as "I am precious, unique, one of a kind," "I deserve love," and "I release the past"—are repeated to one's self and reinforced.

Schindler's own story of healing was more illuminating than her prescription for others. With a passion born of hard-won experience Schindler explained how she used self-hypnosis, relaxation, imagery, affirmations, forgiveness, and a take-charge attitude of accepting responsibility, all in order to reverse her debilitating and frightening condition. Over the course of many months she maintained her steadfast commitment to wellness until she achieved her goals.

Schindler's program for herself was a package of behavioral medicine and popular healing techniques; now she applies the same program to clients who have chronic physical conditions. One of her strongest themes was the need to teach patients to resist the role of victim or sick person. However, there was some confusion in her views about negative emotions. One moment Schindler would advocate expressing and resolving negative emotions, and the next moment she would advocate replacing and overcoming them with positive affirmations. This contradiction, apparent in so many holistic and behavioral healing approaches today, was not adequately addressed and left me with two irreconcilable prescriptions for psychological and physical well-being—express and resolve or replace and overcome.

I'm glad I heard Pennebaker and Lerner yesterday because otherwise I would have a harder time ferreting out the contradictions in Bonnie Schindler's talk "The Power of Negative Emotions on Disease."I have an incapacitating case of rheumatoid arthritis. I'm often angry and sad about my condition and the myriad ways in which it limits my activities. Positive affirmations are fine, and I'd like to use them, but I don't think they can erase my anger and sadness. Experience tells me that I need to gently explore and express these feelings and find new ways of coping. If I tried to talk myself out of them, I'd be running a treadmill. If I tried to cover them with positive affirmations, I'd be repressing the feelings—the very problem that may have contributed to my arthritis or made it worse. In my view, affirmations should come later, after I've allowed myself to feel bad. Otherwise I'd be engaging in one more form of self-tyranny.

228   *I don't for one second begrudge Bonnie Schindler her remarkable recovery or the usefulness of her techniques—for her. That's the point. It worked for her; I don't think it would work for me.*

An example of my problem with Schindler's approach was her mixed messages about anger. She told a funny and touching story about how she would release anger during her arduous recovery. She'd drive around her block a dozen times, screaming and cursing so loudly that her neighbor became alarmed. Months later the neighbor would smile and wave as Schindler drove by and cursed, so inured to her bizarre behavior that it had become an accepted routine. Schindler lit up when she told the story, as if the mobilization of energy and emotion was actually a pleasurable memory for her. Why, then, did Schindler later counsel us to "let go" of anger (as in "give up," not "express") whenever it arises? Not that I want to "hold on" to anger; I simply want to accept, resolve, and transcend it.

I know Schindler didn't mean it that way, but I'm not a computer that can "override old programming" and replace it with "new programming." The New Age concept of human software concerns me deeply.

I asked Schindler how she would advise a client who said he had legitimate anger toward someone in the present. She suggested writing down the feelings, self-hypnosis, and hitting pillows. I thought that was an interesting answer because I had so specifically used the terms legitimate *and* present. *Why wouldn't she advise this client to express his anger in some appropriate way to the person who had affronted him? If his boss had been abusing him daily, what good would it do him to hit pillows?*

Heartbreak and Heart Disease

The prevailing concept of biobehavioral factors in heart disease centers on the influence of Type A behavior and hostility. Research in this area has been largely devoted to refining the Type A construct, and the latest conclusion of investigators is that the *hostility* component of Type A behavior is the true contributor to excess risk of atherosclerosis, heart attack, and death from heart disease.

In something of a challenge to this mind-body orthodoxy, the cardiologist Stephen T. Sinatra, M.D., ran a workshop in which he asserted that Type A behavior and hostility were both symptoms of a fundamental problem in coronary-prone individuals. According to Sinatra, the core contributor to increased coronary risk is the unmet needs of early childhood that lead to heartbreak. To Sinatra, heartbreak is more than a metaphor: it is a psychophysical reality. To protect himself or herself the individual builds a wall of muscular and character armor around the heart and is thus unable to give or receive love. The hostility of the Type A individual, Sinatra maintains, is a powerful *reaction*, both to the early heartbreak and to the later frustration in relationships stemming from the person's unwitting but nevertheless self-imposed isolationism.

The originators of the Type A construct, the cardiologists Meyer Friedman and Ray Rosenman (1974), dabbled in such speculation but never fully developed a research methodology or a theory to explicate such underlying psychodynamics. Stephen Sinatra drew only from clinical experience to form his theory, but it was a more clearly articulated and fleshed-out concept of etiology than can be found in Friedman and Rosenman. The question arises, How could the influence of childhood frustrations and a mind-state as largely unconscious and deeply embedded in a person's character as *heartbreak* be scientifically studied as contributors to heart disease? For now the probable answer is that they cannot. However, the difficulty in evaluating such questions empirically should not exclude clinicians like Sinatra from investigating them. If biobehavioral science were entirely delimited to what can be readily measured or seen, it would arguably be a much poorer science.

Sinatra is an experienced cardiologist who heads the New England Heart Center in Manchester, Connecticut, where he practices "nontraditional cardiology," which includes, along with weight loss and exercise, bioenergetic therapy techniques designed to help the patient contact and express emotions and to explore the childhood conflicts that drive his or her Type A behavior. Sinatra believes that not only anger but also fear and sadness are blocked in the coronary-prone individual, so much so that he or she often has little feeling from the neck down. Type A men cannot cry, he said, and then admitted that he himself had been unable to cry until he entered therapy and went through a series of life-transforming experiences. Sinatra also claimed that most coronary-prone people have unsatisfying sex lives because their emotional energies are so bound up that releasing them pleasurably in sex becomes difficult.

Sinatra's insights into his patients were a by-product of his insights into himself. In a surprisingly confessional portion of the workshop Sinatra spoke of his own childhood frustration and heartbreak and the resulting blocks to emotional expression and creativity that dogged him throughout adulthood. The turning point for him came when he entered therapy with Alexander Lowen, a psychiatrist and founder of bioenergetic therapy. In treatment with Lowen, Sinatra, as he explains, was able to soften his muscular and character armor, release energy and emotion, and discover the origins of his childhood pain. Later on, stressful events, including a divorce and the death of his father, put him more deeply in touch with his sorrow. Interestingly, he saw these painful experiences as a gift, enabling him to "find his heart."

Sinatra said that his pent-up patients do not breathe fully, so he helps them breathe. Stuck in anxiety and anger, they cannot allow themselves the lightness of play, so he helps them play. He talks to them about otherwise taboo subjects, such as how satisfied they are with their sex lives. And he uses bioenergetic physical exercises to eliminate muscular blocks in the head, neck, chest, and abdomen. Combining these elements with traditional cardiac care and nutritional counseling, Sinatra believes he has developed a program of treatment and prevention for heart patients that is genuinely holistic.

Sinatra's workshop was for me a pleasurable experience. But it didn't start that way. I walked in two minutes late, having just made my second trip in two days to the rent-a-car office, once again returning a defective car. That's a total of three cars since I've been here. The first car had a steering wheel with a mind of its own; the second car was apparently manufactured without shock absorbers. I told them car number three had better be all right. Again I had to wait in line, again I had to wait for the paperwork to be completely redone, all the time checking my watch, wondering whether I'd make it to the heartbreak workshop on time. The irony was not lost on me. Yes indeed, my heart was pounding from frustration, anger, and anxiety.

I walked in and tried to compose myself. I knew enough to try to breathe. I'm not sure how successful I was, but I think I got my breath going down a few inches below my neckline. Then I tried focusing on Sinatra. Here was this forty-something man speaking extemporaneously while moving freely around the room, talking about heartbreak and heart disease. There was something streetwise and straight-shooting about his manner, which I found appealing. It took me a while to realize how radical his approach to heart disease was.

I have a family history of heart disease (both my parents died from it) and hypertension. I'm easily stressed out, and in certain circumstances I'm fully capable of exploding irrationally. I almost did at the car-rental office. I've long considered my background and behavior as risk factors, and wondered how I could change my Type A characteristics. Sinatra's emphasis on underlying heartbreak and the emotional, energetic aspects of this behavior pattern was new. Everyone has heartbreak, he said, and the heart always remembers your history. Is there heartbreak in my early history? Nothing so obvious as losing a parent or being abandoned, but yes, I know there's heartbreak in my history. I don't know if that's the reason why situations like three rent-a-cars drive me up the wall, but I'm willing to make the exploration. My intuition tells me he may be right.

My intuition also tells me I would benefit greatly from the kind of therapy Sinatra uses and advocates. I think the energetic component is often ignored by Western mind-body practitioners because it's hard, if not impossible, to study. But when Sinatra talked about opening up blocks in the throat, chest, and abdomen, I had a strong reaction: that would be a boon to my health. I cry, but not easily. I'm sure I could release a great deal of tension if I could cry more easily. Sinatra's admission of his own inability to cry was refreshing. Instead of "You people are all emotionally blocked!" we got "I've been emotionally blocked. I changed, you can too." He also confided sources of heartbreak in his own life and demonstrated how we can use traumas in our lives, not as opportunities to paste positive meaning over them, but rather as opportunities to open our emotional windows to the whole range of human experience, both "negative" and "positive."

Is Healing Quantum?

A recent spate of books have contended that physical healing is dependent on processes of consciousness that are nonlocal and nonmaterial. Among the leading spokesmen for this point of view is Deepak Chopra, M.D., author of such books as *Quantum Healing* (1989) and *Unconditional Life* (1991). Chopra has been a practicing endocrinologist, but now he is president of the Maharishi Ayur-Veda Health Center in Lancaster, Massachusetts. Many of his books are bestsellers, and his concept of quantum healing appears to have great popular appeal.

Chopra's keynote address was an unbroken stream of ideas, facts, and case examples rushing toward an inevitable conclusion: consciousness, a nonmaterial phenomenon that cannot be reductively tied to molecular or even atomic events, is the prime etiologic factor in illness and the prime mover of healing. In order to drive this home he began with a sweeping critique of Western mechanistic science and medicine: "Behind our backs is a radically ambiguous, ceaselessly flowing quantum soup, and in the act of perception we take that quantum soup which is in potentiality a field of infinite possibilities, and freeze it in the moment of attention into a fixed perceptual reality. And if we happen to agree about it, we call that science. Science is just a way of exploring our reality map."

Mechanistic science, Chopra said, has always viewed consciousness as an epiphenomenon of materialistic events, namely, the "dance" of atoms and molecules that are the basis of our biochemistry. Chopra turned this paradigm on its head, asserting that consciousness is the phenomenon, and matter the epiphenomenon. Put simply, molecules do not produce thought: thought produces molecules. (He cited as supportive evidence

232   the neuroscientist Candace Pert's work on the neuropeptides as mediators of thoughts, feelings, and immunological responses.) Moreover, the boundaries we draw between our bodymind and our universe may themselves be arbitrary and artificial, while the overlooked concept of a "nonlocal" mind may have importance for spiritual and physical healing. (This argument was also made cogently by Larry Dossey in his book *Recovering the Soul* [1989].) The implication Chopra drew was that changes in awareness, whether stemming from our local or our nonlocal ("cosmic") mind, undoubtedly affect physiological changes in our bodies and should be the starting point of the healing endeavor.

What an amazing showman Chopra is. Here is this fit, attractive, charismatic doctor reeling off facts, figures, and theoretical challenges at a clip so rapid that I could barely follow his train of thought. I never knew that I remake my skin every month, my liver every six weeks, my skeleton every three months. I never knew that 90 percent of the atoms in my body are replaced every year and that I have atoms in me that have gone through the body of every living being who ever existed on the planet, including Gandhi, Buddha, Christ, and Saddam Hussein. I never knew that when I walk into a room and feel tense, it's because people are releasing pheromones into the atmosphere and I've picked them up and interpreted them. I never realized that my body only appears to be solid, that in fact it is just a field of transformations in the frequencies of my own consciousness. The universe and our own bodies are nonstuff, nonmatter. They are just plain empty.

Strangely, though, I left his talk feeling a bit empty. While Chopra was nothing short of dazzling, I had to wonder: What did all this add up to? On the one hand, his questioning of nearly all our assumptions about our bodies, our minds, and our medical practices was provocative. On the other hand, he never made the leap to clinical applications, which was the point of the conference. While his intellectually acute observations and clever ripostes were stimulating, they were never translated into practices specific enough to be helpful to me in terms of my healing.

I have cancer, and the most pointed advice he gave that I could use was, "Healing requires a shift in awareness." I wanted to know what kind of shift stimulates healing. Is it the mere idea that consciousness is the moving force behind physiology that is healing? If so, that's not enough for me. I'm certain that Chopra, an expert in Ayur-Veda medicine, does a lot for his patients, but I wish he had revealed more about what he does and what Ayur-Veda medicine is all about.

As a cancer patient, I had another difficulty with Chopra. "In order to restructure these patterns we must learn to become silent witnesses of these pat-

terns and then change them by mere intention," he wrote in his description of his workshop. "I [can] reinterpret my body as a field of changing patterns that, in fact, I control." Is he implying that if I really figured out how to shift my awareness, I could, through sheer intention, change the configurations of matter that constitute my tumor or my body's immune response to it and hence rid myself of cancer? I don't know if that's what he means, but the implication is troubling.

Here we come back to that grubby little local-mind problem of guilt. If I create my own reality, then by inference I should be able to get rid of my cancer. I just have to find that level of control and exercise quantum healing. There are two problems. First, I don't believe we create our own reality. Perhaps that's why I have a problem with the idea of matter as an epiphenomenon of mind—the same problem I have with mind as an epiphenomenon of matter. I think mind and matter are so dialectically interconnected that we shouldn't view either as a product of the other. If we view matter as secondary to mind, then we totally create our own reality, and I don't believe that. I believe there are factors entirely out of our control, just as there are factors in our control. If I breathe in asbestos particles, have I somehow issued them an invitation?

My second problem is the lack of direction given concerning the shifts in awareness we must make. Perhaps Chopra believes that his radical critique of our mechanistic, lifeless, and obfuscating model of physics and medicine should, by itself, produce a shift in awareness that leads us toward wellness. When we simply open our eyes and stop confusing our constricted, delimited "reality map" as reality itself, our emotional and perceptual field will open to the "infinite possibilities" for creative and healing responses to life. He may be right, and my tendency to operate in a region of "local mind" may be one of my problems. But I'm afraid that this otherwise nimble and even brilliant mind has unintentionally limited his own field of awareness regarding the needs of people like me.

Joan Borysenko, Ph.D., a former cell biologist who previously directed the Mind/Body Clinic at the Beth Israel Deaconess Hospital in Boston and now heads her own organization, Mind/Body Health Sciences, had a view of healing not dissimilar from Chopra's, but in terms of clinical application she filled in many of the gaps he left open. She began by relating a story of her own childhood "descent into madness" when she was about the age of ten, when she completely withdrew from her family and retreated into a world of fantasy and ritual. When her obsessive-compulsive rituals were interrupted for any reason, she would begin to hallucinate that snakes and scorpions were attacking and killing her parents. She was taken to a psychiatrist and had to drop out of school. Borysenko reported that just when it seemed as if her descent had become irreversible,

234 a "voice" relayed to her a choice: she could continue to be crazy, or she could recover. A comforting poem came to her, one that she repeated whenever she stopped her rituals and her hallucinations threatened to take over. Soon thereafter she was able to stop her compulsive behavior and return to a non–obsessive existence free of bizarre ideation.

As an adult she has been able to interpret her experience, one she described as comparable to the development of multiple-personality disorder. In her view, an early trauma had caused a split in her personality that propelled her into that world of ritual self-protection. While she did not reveal the actual trauma(s) that brought on her inner split, she did identify the source of her healing. The "voice" was her innate "inner self-helper," a construct used in research on multiple-personality disorder to explain the personality that can emerge during a process of healing to integrate the fractured selves and provide a sense of intrapsychic protection. According to Borysenko, the inner self-helper is our essence, and as such it is a "conduit for divine wisdom."

Finding our "core," our "inner self-helper," our "connection to others and a larger whole" was the focus of Borysenko's healing prescriptions. She cited studies and anecdotes from her own and others' clinical practices to support this point of view. Like Chopra, she spoke of the false separations we make between ourselves and others and between ourselves and the world. A fundamental question we must ask ourselves is, Is the universe a friendly place or not? If we see the universe as hostile, we cut ourselves off and solidify our deep fear of being eternally separated from the divine. Though she wants "friendly" to be the answer to her question about the universe, she did not sugarcoat her cosmic perspective. "The world is crazy, it isn't safe. Children fall down wells, and people get cancer. Yet at some level, there is an intrinsic perfection."

While she spoke movingly about the need for unconditional love, human connectedness, and recognition of the divine in ourselves, Borysenko was far from being Pollyannaish about the power of psychospiritual healing to eradicate disease. She was extremely sensitive to the potential of patients with life-threatening illness to blame themselves unjustly for their illness or decline. (Her book *Guilt Is the Teacher, Love Is the Lesson* [1990] addressed these issues in great depth.) "Sometimes these [psychospiritual] changes lead to physiologic changes, and sometimes not," she said. "The more I learn, the more I recognize how much I don't know. Some people who have achieved inner peace still get cancer and die."

Borysenko's address felt like a corrective to Chopra's talk. Here was the compassion and perspective I felt somewhat lacking before. On the one hand, her paradigm was wide open—to the interactive influence of mind, body, relationships, culture, cosmos, and spiritual essence. At the same time, she eschewed the notion that we have conscious or even unconscious control over all our bodily processes all of the time. Her candor about her childhood experiences made it easier to relate to her message.

As a cancer patient, I experienced her approach to the guilt problem as liberating. "Even great mystics and saints have gotten cancer and died," she said. A mere comment like that means a great deal to me. Right away, I feel freed from that insidious stigma associated with "cancer"—the stigma handed down to us from generations past, when the word was not to be spoken, and revived by some New Age acolytes today in the question, "Why did you give yourself this cancer?"

I want to explore the ways in which my behavior patterns or emotions or childhood traumas might have contributed to my illness. I don't think that means I am to blame or that cancer is a by-product of a character flaw, an insufficient connection to the Divine, a circumscribed reality map, or a bad choice I made at some critical turning point in my past. Borysenko provides a context within which I can take this journey sans unhealthy guilt.

I couldn't completely relate to the spiritual side of Borysenko's talk, and she mixed science and religion a bit too liberally for my taste. That may be due to my unresolved feelings about spirituality in general. My internal division of church and (mind-body) state is, perhaps, too rigid, but I approach spirituality as honestly as I can, trying not to create for myself an external godhead separate from me (whatever "me" is), as the Buddhists teach. The role of spirituality in healing is a difficult subject for behavioral medicine. It isn't quantifiable, and it runs totally counter to the biomedical model. Borysenko's contribution has been to open up this area for discussion and, despite my reservations, I thank her for it.

The Broad Scope of Behavioral Medicine

There were many other workshops beyond those I attended. They are hard to characterize easily. Hearteningly, one group of workshops dealt with the application of family therapy to medical conditions. Two examples: "Practitioners, Caregivers, and HIV Infection: A Family Systems Approach" and "Family Therapy and Chronic Illness." These workshops properly recognized that physical illness, like mental illness, not only is a product of family systems but also has an impact on them. Healing itself may thus depend, at least in part, on transformations of family systems. Other workshops dealt with chronic pain, chronic fatigue syndrome, imagery for allergies, art therapy for dying children, and smoking cessation. A number

236 of workshops, in addition to Sinatra's, explored different psychosocial interventions for heart patients, for example, "New Ways to Provide Crisis Intervention to Heart Surgery Patients" and "Modifying the Destructive Hurry Sickness of the Type A Behavior Pattern."

Is there an explosion in the clinical application of behavioral medicine? For a journalist/observer immersed in four days of lectures and workshops, hearing about a range of new potential treatments for often untreatable diseases, it seems so. The question remains, How many of these applications can consistently deliver the results they promise?

I enjoyed this conference immensely. I was at times exhilarated by it. Now, I want to apply these concepts and practices in my own life. I've come away with renewed hope that psychotherapy and group support will contribute to my healing—regardless of whether I am able to recover fully. While meditation and visualization are practices I will apply and still believe to be crucial, I left the conference more convinced than ever that I must deal with psychological issues directly and make changes in my relationships with family and friends. I am also certain that I must not talk myself out of "negative emotions" in the name of positive attitude, or even in the name of hope. I want hope, but I don't believe I can conjure hope magically or willfully. Hope, for me, is a state of mind that must be cultivated with the utmost respect for all the facets of my character, not just the "good" ones that my judging mind deems worthy of divine acceptance.

REFERENCES

Borysenko J. 1990. *Guilt Is the Teacher, Love Is the Lesson.* New York: Warner Books.

Cassileth BR, Lusk EJ, Strouse TB, Bodenmer BJ. 1984. Contemporary unorthodox treatments in cancer medicine: a study of patients, treatments, and practitioners. *Ann Intern Med.* 10:105–112.

Chopra D. 1989. *Quantum Healing.* New York: Bantam Books.

Chopra D. 1991. *Unconditional Life: Mastering the Forces That Shape Personal Reality.* New York: Bantam Books.

Dossey L. 1989. *Recovering the Soul.* New York: Bantam Books.

Friedman M, Rosenman RH. 1974. *Type A Behavior and Your Heart.* New York: Ballantine Books.

Lerner M. 1990. *Wrestling with the Angel.* New York: W. W. Norton.

Lerner M. 1994. *Healing Choices: Integrating the Best of Conventional and Complementary Approaches to Cancer.* Cambridge, Mass: MIT Press.

LeShan L. 1977. *You Can Fight for Your Life.* New York: M. Evans.

Ornish D, Brown SE, Scherwitz LW, et al. 1990. Can lifestyle changes reverse coronary heart disease? *Lancet.* 2:888–891.

Ornstein R, Sobel D. 1989. *Healthy Pleasures.* Reading, Mass: Addison-Wesley.

Pennebaker JW, Barger SD, Tiebout J. 1989. Disclosure of traumas and health among Holocaust survivors. *Psychosom Med.* 51:577–589.

Pennebaker JW, Beall SK. 1986. Confronting a traumatic event: toward an understanding of inhibition and disease. *J Abnorm Psychol.* 95:274–281.

Pennebaker JW, Kiecolt-Glaser JK, Glaser R. 1988. Disclosure of traumas and immune function: health implications for psychotherapy. *J Consult Clin Psychol.* 56:239–245.

Schwartz T. 1989. Dr. Love. *New York Magazine,* 12 June, 40–49.

Siegel B. 1986. *Love, Medicine, and Miracles.* New York: Harper & Row.

Siegel B. 1989. *Peace, Love, and Healing.* New York: Harper & Row.

Siegel B. 1992. Letters. *Adv Mind Body Med.* 8:2–3.

Spera SP, Buhrfeind ED, Pennebaker JW. 1994. Expressive writing and coping with job loss. *Academy of Management Journal.* 37:722–733.

Spiegel D. 1991. A psychosocial intervention and survival time of patients with metastatic breast cancer. *Adv Mind Body Med.* 7:10–19.

Spiegel D. 1992. Letters. *Adv Mind Body Med.* 8:3–4.

Spiegel D, Bloom J, Kraemer HC, Gottheil E. 1989. Effect of psychosocial treatment on survival of patients with metastatic breast cancer. *Lancet.* 2:888–891.

Temoshok L, Dreher H. 1992. *The Type C Connection: The Behavioral Links to Cancer and Your Health.* New York: Random House.

U.S. Congress, Office of Technology Assessment (U.S. OTA). 1990. *Unconventional Cancer Treatments.* OTA-H-405. Washington, D.C.: U.S. Government Printing Office.

Chapter 6

The Scientific and Moral Imperative of
Psychosocial Interventions for Cancer

The 1990s ushered in a flush of excitement about the role of mind-body interventions in the treatment of cancer. Two highly publicized studies suggest that not only do group psychosocial interventions help cancer patients to cope more effectively but they may also help them to live longer. One study was conducted by the Stanford University psychiatrist David Spiegel with breast cancer patients (Spiegel et al. 1989), and the other by the UCLA psychiatrist Fawzy I. Fawzy with malignant melanoma patients (Fawzy et al. 1993). A third, less-publicized study, led by Jean Richardson of the University of Southern California, showed that a supportive educational program conferred a survival advantage among patients with leukemias and lymphomas (Richardson et al. 1990).* These studies generated a rush of enthusiasm and the beginnings of a push for broad application. But now that energy seems trapped like steam in a covered cauldron; not much has leaked out into the world.

David Spiegel initiated his research in the early 1980s. He had designed a group psychotherapy program for metastatic breast cancer patients who had a grim prognosis. In Spiegel's program the patients shared their emo-

Reprinted by permission, with changes, from *Advances in Mind-Body Medicine* 13 (1997): 38–49.

* The intervention trial of Jean Richardson and colleagues at the University of Southern California is not always included in these discussions, largely because the intervention—a brief, supportive educational program designed to enhance medical compliance—was so different from the other, more explicitly psychological treatments. The researchers did not expect a survival difference independent of the program's effects on compliance with medical treatments, but that is just what they found. Richardson and colleagues hypothesized that their intervention may have yielded a survival advantage by virtue of "the greater amounts of time and attention paid by the health care providers to intervention group patients" and the resulting increase in social support, self-care, and sense of control.

tional distress, supported one another, and confronted the existential issues that inevitably arise with life-threatening illness. Patients were also taught mind-body skills, primarily self-hypnosis as a relaxation method. Spiegel's supportive-expressive group therapy was rooted in established traditions of group psychotherapy, but it was carefully tailored to the needs of people with cancer. The study included eighty-six patients, who were randomized to either the psychotherapy group or a control group; both groups received the same standard medical treatments. He tracked these patients for years to determine whether they experienced improved quality of life and reduced distress. He would also conduct a survival analysis.

Spiegel has been candid about his initial biases. He expected his psychotherapy patients to become less distressed, more expressive, better able to procure social support, and better able to confront the reality of their disease. But he had been irked by advocates of mind-body medicine for cancer, whom he felt made extravagant claims, and he admitted that he did not expect his therapy patients to live longer than controls. A decade later, after tabulating the results, Spiegel discovered to his evident surprise that the metastatic breast cancer patients who participated in his therapy had lived twice as long as the nonparticipants, a median of thirty-eight months for the treatment group compared with nineteen months for controls (Spiegel et al. 1989). His study was published in the British medical journal *Lancet,* and even avowed skeptics found his methods unassailable.

In the early 1990s Fawzy I. Fawzy published his study of group therapy for melanoma patients. He randomized sixty-eight patients into a treatment group and a control group, and after six years of follow-up he found that group members had one-third the mortality rate and roughly one-half the recurrence rate of controls (Fawzy et al. 1993). Fawzy's treatment included relaxation techniques, cognitive therapy to cultivate active coping, and psychological support. In the USC study led by Jean Richardson, hematologic cancer patients who participated in a brief, supportive educational program lived significantly longer than nonparticipants, and their improved recovery could not be explained by greater medical compliance (Richardson et al. 1990).

Two studies in the literature have had negative results, however. Linn and colleagues randomly assigned 120 men with "end-stage cancer" to an experimental group and a control group and found no differences in survival between the two groups (Linn et al. 1982). But the experimental subjects were only "seen regularly by a counselor," and this description falls far short of the structured psychological support groups, run by trained therapists who also teach mind-body techniques, used in the Spiegel and Fawzy studies. Ilnyckyj and colleagues randomized breast cancer patients

240   into a treatment group and a control group, and while no survival benefit was found, there were also no documented psychological benefits (Ilnyckyj et al. 1994). When an intervention fails to help patients improve in psychological indices, it may not be expected to aid their recovery. Thus, both these studies appear flawed with regard to the interventions themselves.

The finding that well-designed psychosocial interventions yield a survival advantage has stimulated a few follow-up studies, as I will shortly detail. But it has prompted no large-scale research effort and no institutional call for wide implementation of psychosocial interventions in hospitals and cancer treatment centers. According to a review by Fawzy and his colleagues at UCLA (1995), 60 percent of cancer patients probably have no access to psychosocial interventions of any kind, much less the structured psychological approaches applied in the breakthrough studies. The question is, Do the studies of Fawzy, Spiegel, and Richardson constitute a sufficient basis for a broad-based effort in both research and clinical application? With regard to psychosocial interventions for cancer patients, where are we now and where should we be?

In previous writings I contended that these three studies constituted a sufficient basis for broad-based applications (Dreher 1996). In developing my case, I made an analogy between the findings of Spiegel and Fawzy and similarly positive findings from chemotherapy studies. I noted that the chemotherapy findings would instantly stimulate clinical applications or even, in some cases, streamlined passage from the lab to the clinic. The Spiegel and Fawzy studies, I maintained, should do the same. My comments prompted one commentator (Stuart Roath, M.D., in a letter to *Advances in Mind-Body Medicine*) to question my analogy between data from chemotherapy trials and data from psychosocial intervention trials. Roath argued that fewer sound clinical trials have been conducted of psychosocial interventions than are usually carried out for chemotherapy drugs before such drugs enter mainstream practice and, more specifically, that fewer research subjects have been involved in psychosocial intervention trials to date. Shortly, I will respond to this criticism with a detailed exploration of the chemotherapy analogy.

Even setting aside the issue of survival benefits, I believe that group psychotherapy and other supportive mind-body interventions should be made available in hospitals and cancer treatment centers nationwide— right now, without delay. Currently there is voluminous, unassailable evidence that such interventions have pronounced psychological and quality-of-life benefits. As a debate rages in academic quarters about whether these interventions lengthen life, cancer patients should not be denied the

The Scientific and Moral Imperative

psychological sustenance these programs provide. As David Spiegel re-   241
cently wrote, "The oldest adage of medicine is to 'cure rarely, to relieve
suffering often, and to comfort always.' In this century, we seem to have
inverted this job description, acting as though our job were to 'cure always,
relieve suffering if there is time, and let someone else do the comforting'"
(Spiegel 1995). In a healthcare system that could more accurately be called
a health cure system, quality-of-life outcomes are unwittingly overlooked.

At the same time, I will not cloak my contention that such treatments
have potential survival benefits in the more circumspect language of quality of life. Quality of life is an "end point" with every bit as much validity
as length of life, but in all candor, most cancer patients are desperately concerned about the length of their lives, and so are responsible healthcare
professionals. Moreover, I believe that evidence to date regarding the survival effects of psychosocial interventions has cleared several hurdles that
constitute credible scientific evidence. (See the final section of this chapter, "Update 2002," for the most recent study findings.) I also recognize
that it has not passed enough hurdles to satisfy many biomedical and behavioral scientists, including some who are doing the research themselves
and many who are kindly disposed to these efforts.

The point here is to suggest not that the jury has reached a final verdict
on this issue but that biomedicine's criteria shift depending on the nature
of the treatment being judged. Drugs such as Taxol for ovarian cancer have
been quickly shuttled through the pipeline from clinical trials to broad-
based applications with evidence that is roughly similar to that produced
by Spiegel in his breast cancer study. Moreover, a recent Food and Drug
Administration (FDA) directive to shorten the pipeline for chemotherapy
agents lowered the beam for expensive drugs, while an inexpensive, nontoxic "agent" such as group psychotherapy was being provided no such
largesse. More to the point, the issue is so far from the radar screen of biomedical attention that, to my knowledge, no single individual or institu-
tion within the biomedical establishment has even *addressed* the issue in
these terms.

I also believe that the chemotherapy analogy is politically useful since
it offers biomedical scientists and policymakers the opportunity to consider nonpharmacologic "agents" in the same light that they routinely
consider pharmacologic ones. If the positive effects on recovering cancer
patients are indeed comparable, or even close, is there not a medical and
moral imperative to provide broad access?

Chemotherapy and Psychosocial Intervention Trials:
A Fair Comparison?

Let me examine in more detail the chemotherapy comparison. In my initial comments I compared the psychotherapy data with evidence that led the drug Taxol to be approved as the first-line chemotherapy for patients with advanced ovarian cancer. In his critique, Dr. Stuart Roath noted that the experience with Taxol has involved many more studies and subjects over the past seventeen years than have psychosocial intervention cancer studies. (He claimed that 960 patients had participated in recent Taxol trials, comparing this with a total of 154 in the Spiegel and Fawzy studies.) But my comparison referred specifically to research that justified Taxol's move from a second-line therapy (after relapse on other drugs) to a first-line therapy, making it the drug of choice for this disease. Taxol's ascendance was, to my knowledge, based on a single study led by McGuire and colleagues (1996). That study involved 216 women with measurable disease, and it showed a significantly longer survival time for those taking Taxol and cisplatin (38 months) than for those taking cyclophosphamide and cisplatin, the previous first-line treatment (24 months). Dr. Roath's figure of 960 patients included patients who received second-line therapy or, as it is called, salvage therapy with Taxol—a different matter altogether. In short, Taxol was elevated to the first line of treatment on the basis of one study of 216 evaluable patients that demonstrated fourteen months' life extension for women with advanced ovarian cancer.

While the Spiegel and Fawzy study totaled 154 subjects, if the 96 subjects from the often overlooked Jean Richardson study are included, the total number of patients in published psychosocial intervention studies with positive results is 250. One can readily compare the fourteen months' life extension of the Taxol studies to the nineteen months' life extension for breast cancer patients in the Spiegel study, the only one of the psychosocial intervention trials to use length of survival as its principal survival measure. The survival measures in the other studies are less directly comparable, but the direction is clearly the same. In Fawzy's research with melanoma patients the six-year death rate among intervention participants was one-third that of control subjects (9% compared with 29%), a statistically significant difference. He also noted a trend toward a lesser recurrence rate (21% and 38% in the intervention and control groups, respectively). In the Richardson trial of leukemia and lymphoma patients, participants in behavioral or educational interventions lived significantly longer than those who did not participate, in what amounted to a 39 percent reduction in the relative risk of death after controlling for possible confounding variables (Richardson et al. 1990).

It is certainly true that Taxol was tested and used in the clinic with thousands of patients before it was elevated to first-line therapy on the basis of the 1996 trial by McGuire and colleagues. Yet, in broad terms, much the same can be said about psychosocial interventions for cancer. Although early studies were methodologically flawed, they were remarkably consistent. Pioneers in the field, such as Lawrence LeShan (1977), Stephanie and O. Carl Simonton (Simonton et al. 1978), Ainslie Meares (1980), and Jeanne Achterberg and Frank Lawlis (Achterberg 1985; Achterberg et al. 1977) conducted uncontrolled studies from the 1960s through the 1980s confirming the psychological "safety and efficacy" of psychosocial interventions for cancer patients, while hinting at possible medical benefits. (Such studies are analogous, in many respects, to the early, uncontrolled phase I and phase II clinical trials conducted on agents such as Taxol.) Indeed, many of these investigators documented survival benefits (LeShan 1977, 1989; Meares 1980; Simonton et al. 1978), although their methods were imperfect. Nonetheless, all these investigations revealed the "cross-study consistency" referred to by Alistair Cunningham in his review of early psychosocial studies (Cunningham 1984). In other words, the consistency among the studies suggests that they tapped a meaningful dimension of efficacy, one that needed testing in better-designed clinical trials. As Michael Lerner of Commonweal has pointed out, the earlier studies presaged the significant survival benefits turned up in the methodologically tighter Spiegel and Fawzy studies of the 1990s (Lerner 1994).

The debate over numbers is relevant, but it presents a myopic view of the big picture. Also relevant is the statistical adjustment built into any well-designed randomized clinical trial. In a recent discussion, David Spiegel responded to this issue. "If you can prove an effect in a small sample, you really have to get a robust effect," he commented. "To the extent that there is no power inherent in the intervention to make a survival difference, the small 'n' [number of subjects] just makes it harder to show such a difference."

Spiegel elaborated that phase II and phase III chemotherapy trials (the former to test safety and efficacy, the latter to compare new agents with standard regimens) typically search for small differences among drug combinations that are roughly similar except for one minor change, such as a substitute agent or a new agent added to a multidrug regimen. In these instances the higher numbers are needed to detect such modest distinctions.

244 But with a trial of intervention versus no intervention a relatively small *N* is sufficient to reveal statistically significant differences that may be just as meaningful as those revealed in larger studies. Such has been the case with the Spiegel, Fawzy, and Richardson trials.

FROM STUDIES TO CLINICAL APPLICATION: IS THERE A
DOUBLE STANDARD?

There are countless examples of chemotherapy drugs that move rapidly into clinical use as soon as they demonstrate even marginal improvements in clinical outcomes. Some agents that are added to chemotherapy regimens have no appreciable survival benefit but simply improve response rates—the number of patients who experience tumor regression during treatment. Others carry only minimal benefits in terms of survival.

Consider one example from the annals of hematologic oncology. Acute myelogenous leukemia (AML) is an aggressive hematologic malignancy that often responds to first-line chemotherapy; unfortunately, the majority of patients relapse within three years. The standard treatment for AML has been cytarabine combined with an anthracycline agent. In the past few years idarubicin has largely replaced daunorubicin as the anthracycline of choice. The introduction of idarubicin has been based mainly on three clinical trials (Berman et al. 1991; Vogler et al. 1992; Wiernik et al. 1992). In these trials the differences in median survival between the two drug regimens were three months, six months, and twenty days, respectively. Idarubicin was introduced more for its significantly higher percentage of initial responses to treatment than for its survival advantage, which was fairly modest.

I have no problem with how such drugs are introduced; if they are even modestly better, why not? My problem, again, is that a nontoxic therapy that may confer greater survival benefits than some widely used chemotherapy drugs should continue to be overlooked on the pretext that more studies are needed. Only three studies were needed for idarubicin to supplant daunorubicin, even though the survival advantage was modest. Why aren't three sound studies showing survival benefits sufficient for adjunctive psychosocial interventions to become part of cancer medicine? One answer is that shifting an experimental drug into the cancer pharmacopeia requires no shift in paradigms or perspectives nor the effort required to fund and implement a challenging new program.

Then there is the recent FDA directive to streamline new chemotherapy drugs in the same manner as AIDS drugs. Specifically, the directive enables drug companies to shepherd drugs into use before they pass muster in phase III clinical trials. In other words, they no longer have to be proven more effective at producing clinical responses or survival advantages than other regimens; they must only be shown to produce tumor regressions. Of course, psychosocial interventions are not drugs and require no FDA approval. But other federal agencies, including the National Institutes of Health (NIH), could fast-track these interventions in comparable fashion by issuing a "clinical alert" regarding their effects.

Consider this parallel: One of the first drugs to qualify under the new FDA fast-track directive was irinotecan, used as second-line chemotherapy for colon cancer patients whose disease recurred after treatment with the standard regimen. Irinotecan was fast-tracked for a good reason: it can produce tumor regressions in patients who have no other medical options. (I am completely in favor of the directive for irinotecan and any other drug that is safe and shows such benefits.) However, it produces these regressions in only one-quarter of the patients, and the median survival of all patients is 10.4 months (Rothenberg et al. 1996). Compare these findings with Spiegel's metastatic breast cancer patients, who had nineteen months' life extension, and Fawzy's melanoma patients, who experienced a two-thirds reduction in death rates. Though head-to-head comparisons are difficult across studies of different cancers with somewhat different methodologies, by any yardstick the psychosocial interventions yield results every bit as clinically meaningful as this new drug, if not more so.

But the FDA fast track is for pharmaceutical vehicles only. Here again is evidence of a biomedical bias against nonpharmacologic therapies. If the FDA directive (or a similar directive from the NIH) made room for nonpharmacologic therapies, psychosocial interventions would qualify as safe adjunctive treatments with the *potential* to extend life, treatments that should be made available in every cancer treatment center and hospital. And *potential* is a litmus test no less stringent than that applied to drugs like irinotecan, which has no effect at all in three-quarters of the recipients.

In terms of broad application, psychosocial interventions for cancer should not even be held to the same standard as chemotherapy agents since they are safe, nontoxic "agents" with proven psychological and quality-of-life benefits. But when they are promoted specifically for their survival benefits, they *should* be held to the same standard. On that basis, I believe they are sufficiently close to meeting the chemotherapy criteria that potential survival benefits are a credible *additional* argument in favor of broad applicability.

To extend the medical analogy, here we have an inexpensive, nontoxic "pill" that is highly likely to make you feel and cope better, and by the way, methodologically solid evidence suggests that it may extend your life.

246 Should this "pill" be promulgated for widespread use by cancer patients? Of course, but with a simple caveat: the part about long survival needs more inquiry, so take your "pills" with hope but without illusions. That strikes me as an ethically and scientifically sound position.

Coping Patterns, Social Support, and Quality of Life: "Preclinical" Clues to Medical Benefits

In the field of oncology the development of a safe and efficacious chemotherapy is based not only on drug development and later clinical trials but on a series of intervening steps commonly referred to as *preclinical* research. Preclinical research includes in vitro laboratory studies that determine a drug's molecular mechanisms of action on cancer cells and identifies types of cancer cells responsive to the agent. It also includes in vivo animal studies that explore mechanisms of action and begin to characterize the safety and efficacy of the agent in different tumor models that are roughly comparable to human cancers. Preclinical studies provide rich information about how drugs work, how they might be applied, and how they might perform in the clinic. And this research usually does not end when a drug enters clinical use. It often continues so that a better understanding of the drug's actions can be gained, and its applications refined.

Analogous endeavors are carried out in the field of psychosocial oncology. Studies that explore psychological states and social factors associated with better medical outcomes provide a sound basis for answering the questions, What kinds of intervention heal? What components should be included in interventions that improve mind-body state and medical status? What are the "mechanisms of action" of effective psychosocial interventions for cancer? Such studies are surely comparable in purpose to the molecular biology and animal research that undergird chemotherapy trials.

One set of indices for effective psychosocial interventions in general are biological, and they include immunological and endocrine alterations associated with particular mind-states and the interventions that presumably cultivate them. Only one study to date suggests specific immune changes associated with a successful psychosocial intervention in cancer. Prior to the publication of his study showing survival benefits for a psychosocial intervention, Fawzy showed that patients participating in his intervention experienced a significant increase in natural killer cells, large granular lymphocytes, and the ability of interferon to augment natural killer cell activity (Fawzy et al. 1990). These cells and cell activities are considered by many cancer immunologists to be crucial to the immune system's capacity to control the metastatic spread of cancer (Temoshok and Dreher 1992).

In the current replication of his research with breast cancer patients, Spiegel is conducting a variety of immune measurements to determine *(a)* whether immune alterations are associated with his psychosocial intervention and *(b)* whether any such alterations are associated with medical outcomes, including longer survival. A few other upcoming psychosocial intervention trials (which I discuss below), one at the University of Massachusetts and a multicenter trial in Canada, will also include immune and endocrine measures in the search for mediating biological mechanisms relevant to cancer progression or control.

But by using the term *preclinical* research I do not mean to limit the analogy to studies of mediating biological mechanisms. Other forms of psychosocial research identify sources of the "anticancer activity," if you will, of psychosocial interventions. These studies evaluate whether naturally occurring psychosocial factors such as quality of life, social support, and various mind-states influence medical outcomes in cancer patients, and they tell us a lot about what might occur in psychosocial interventions to influence survival. The studies shed light on the dynamic psychosocial changes stimulated by participating in interventions, changes that presumably interact with mediating biological factors in ways just as complex as the molecular mechanisms of chemotherapeutic cell destruction. Put differently, there are many different kinds of preclinical studies in the mind-body field relevant to psychosocial intervention for cancer, and all fit together to help us understand what works, why it works, and how clinicians can optimize the chances that it will work.

For example, Lydia Temoshok and I have written about the psychological states and traits associated with better outcomes in cancer—fighting spirit, emotional expression, and active or assertive coping (Temoshok and Dreher 1992). These factors have been associated with various indices of favorable outcome, including immune enhancement, less aggressive tumors, and longer survival (Greer et al. 1990; Temoshok 1985). In terms of the interventions we are focusing on here, two of the factors, emotional expression and active or assertive coping, are central to Spiegel's Supportive/Expressive Therapy, which led to longer survival; active or assertive coping is also the explicit goal of Fawzy's cognitive-based group treatment, which led to better survival outcomes.

The data on two other "preclinical" factors—social support and quality of life—have received less attention than emotional expression and active coping, but existing studies show that they fit hand-in-glove with the

248   intervention trials. For instance, a neglected Canadian study published in 1995 in the journal *Cancer* dramatizes the survival effects of social support. Led by the epidemiologist Elizabeth Maunsell, the investigators followed 224 women with breast cancer that was either confined to the breast or had spread to regional lymph nodes (Maunsell et al. 1995). To measure social support, the researchers asked the patients whether they had confided in one or more people during the three months after surgery. The seven-year survival rate among women with no confidants was 56 percent. By contrast, the survival rate for those with one confidant was 66 percent, while those with two or more confidants was 76 percent. The researchers concluded that "social support appears to warrant serious consideration as a factor that may favorably affect breast cancer survival."

By any standard, the twenty-point difference between the survival rate of women who had no confidants and that of women who had two or more confidants is clinically important. No grand leap in the imagination is needed to suggest that group psychotherapy offers cancer patients more than two people in whom they can confide their fears, sadness, the everyday trials of therapy, their hopes for the present and future. Maunsell's epidemiological study captures a reality present in the fabric of people's lives; intervention studies evaluate the effects of an experimental process. But that experimental process can become part of the patients' real-life fabric, and although Maunsell's study does not prove the survival benefits of an intervention, it can be viewed as preclinical research elucidating the psychosocial mechanisms underlying the benefits of a group intervention.

The so-called quality-of-life studies, in which oncologists and epidemiologists have found often unexpected associations between patients' quality of life—primarily physical functioning, capacity to work, mood, pain, and energy—and survival, arguably represent the most overlooked body of research shedding light on factors that influence cancer survival. Not all quality-of-life studies show a relation between baseline measures and later survival (see, e.g., Ringdal et al. 1996; and Tross et al. 1996), but a review of the literature suggests that the positive studies greatly outnumber the negative ones.

Since 1948 the reigning measure of quality of life has been the Karnofsky Performance Status scale, a somewhat imprecise but nevertheless useful index of three dimensions of health status—activity, work, and self-care (Karnofsky et al. 1948). A 1992 editorial in the leading mainstream journal of cancer medicine, the *Journal of Clinical Oncology*, pointed out that "performance status has been shown repeatedly to be an extraordinarily powerful prognostic factor in a wide variety of malignancies, often functioning as an even better predictor of response and survival than stage

[of disease]" (Weeks 1992). The editorial elaborated that more sophisti-   249
cated quality-of-life measures had largely come to replace the Karnofsky
measure and went on to praise a New Zealand study published in the same
issue that used these measures in a population of advanced breast cancer
patients (Coates et al. 1992). The study showed that patient self-ratings of
physical well-being and their physician's ratings of overall quality of life
at the start of the study were powerful predictors of survival. In addition,
improvements over time in patient self-ratings of mood and pain were also
associated with longer survival. (These quality-of-life factors held firm
as independent predictors after adjustments were made for other biological risk factors.)

In methodologically sound studies quality-of-life measures have been
shown to predict survival in lung cancer (Buccheri et al. 1995; Degner and
Sloan 1995; Ganz et al. 1991; Ruckdeschel and Piantadosi 1989; Sorensen
and Badsberg 1990; Stanley 1980), lymphoma (Shipp et al. 1986), and
mixed tumor types (Tamburini et al. 1996). In the Ganz lung cancer study,
for example, patient-reported quality of life (on the Functional Living
Index—Cancer) and marital status were significant predictors of survival,
and those who rated themselves high on the Functional Living Index lived
twice as long as those who rated themselves low (Ganz et al. 1991).[*]

It is worth considering these preclinical studies in light of a recent
meta-analysis of forty-five psychosocial intervention trials involving cancer patients (Meyer and Mark 1995). The meta-analysis tested the efficacy
of psychosocial interventions to improve psychosocial functioning. The
researchers discovered that psychosocial interventions taken as a whole
yielded significant beneficial effects for all the key dependent measures—
emotional adjustment, functional adjustment, measures of treatment and
disease-related symptoms, and compound and global measures. "These
interventions have a consistent beneficial effect on all [these] areas," write
Meyer and Mark, who further suggest that "it would be an inefficient use of
research resources to conduct more studies in the United States" merely to
ask the simple question whether such interventions improve quality of life.

Since we know that psychosocial interventions improve quality of life,
and we know that quality of life can predict cancer survival, the puzzle
pieces begin to take shape in clear and undeniable form. Psychosocial can-

---

[*]A frequent criticism of quality-of-life measures is that they only reflect an early perception of disease
progression. But in patients with equal degrees of clinically measurable disease at the outset, it is hard
to understand how such an interpretation is possible. That is why I accept the New Zealand investigators' thesis that "our data are also compatible with an effect of some aspect of QL [quality of life] on the
disease process, in that the physical and psychological state reflected by more favorable QL scores may
be causally related to tumor progression" (Coates et al. 1992).

250   cer research into social support, quality of life, and coping patterns must be considered a legitimate and inextricable part of the scientific "preclinical" inquiry into the mystery of how a psychological treatment could possibly extend life for cancer patients.

Psychosocial Interventions for Cancer: Where We Stand Now

Having argued that there are enough data on both the psychosocial and medical end points to justify broad-based application of psychosocial interventions, the question arises, Where do we stand now? Although there is progress to report, overall the response from the medical establishment seems inadequate. However, a fine distinction can be made: the effort to expand research has been slightly more enterprising and substantial than the effort to expand applications.

PSYCHOSOCIAL INTERVENTION RESEARCH

In the area of research the NIH, its National Cancer Institute (NCI), and the American Cancer Society (ACS) have done a better job of supporting investigations into quality-of-life effects of psychosocial interventions than they have of supporting investigations into the medical effects of these interventions. The current director of the NCI, Richard Klausner, M.D., has opened an Office of Cancer Survivorship, headed by the pediatric oncologist Anna T. Meadows. Meadows, who reports that the office has been funded with "a few million dollars," will work with various centers within the NCI and will coordinate with other institutes and outside organizations to develop research on factors that influence the quality of life of cancer survivors. But there is no intention to test the relation between quality of life or psychosocial interventions and survival. "It is not our bailiwick," commented Meadows, currently the sole member of the office. Research on survival outcomes, she thought, would be the purview of other offices within the NCI.

But the only psychosocial intervention studies the NCI appears to be supporting on disease progression or survival outcomes are the two ongoing replications by Spiegel of his own study. Both are randomized, controlled clinical trials that will follow patients, chart their psychosocial well-being, assess mediating biological factors (including immune functions), and determine medical outcomes and survival. One study includes 450 early breast cancer patients; the other, 128 women with metastatic breast cancer.

A few psychosocial intervention trials have received support from other sectors of the biomedical establishment. The U.S. Army is sponsoring a trial at the University of Massachusetts Medical Center in Worcester led by Jon Kabat-Zinn, director of the Stress Reduction Program, and the epidemiologist James Hebert. Kabat-Zinn, Hebert, and their colleagues are tracking 180 early breast cancer patients randomized into three groups: an "individual choice" group, who receive usual supportive care; a group receiving Kabat-Zinn's eight-week stress management program (built around mindfulness meditation) plus six additional sessions tailored for the women with breast cancer; and an "intention control" group, who receive nutrition instruction for the same number of hours as the participants in the stress management and meditation program. Preliminary results show that women in the stress management group experienced significantly greater improvements in quality of life, as well as increases in melatonin excretion, which may have positive prognostic implications for women with breast cancer (Massion et al. 1995). Hebert says that his study was not conceived to follow disease progression or survival, but he may have an opportunity to track survival and will do so, if possible, for as long as twenty years.

The Army, along with the ACS and National Institute of Mental Health, has also funded an important study at Ohio State University led by psychologist Barbara Andersen. Andersen has randomized 234 cancer patients with disease stage II (small tumor with lymph node involvement, or large tumors without such involvement) or disease stage III (large tumors with lymph node involvement) into a control group and a psychosocial intervention group. The intervention includes relaxation techniques, cognitive-behavioral change, group support, and diet and exercise instruction. Andersen is tracking five-year survival; in addition, she is collaborating with the immunovirologist Ronald Glaser and other bioscientists from four labs at Ohio State to measure potential endocrine and immune mediators among subjects in her intervention trial. Andersen reported that the study, which is halfway completed and will cost $4 million, has been inordinately complex and difficult to coordinate and that no data would be available until 2003 or later.

The NIH's National Center for Complementary and Alternative Medicine has provided small grants for research on the effects of imagery and hypnosis on cancer patients, and it has also awarded a million-dollar grant to the University of Texas Health Science Center for cancer research emphasizing biopharmacologic and herbal therapies. The center is not currently supporting group psychosocial interventions for cancer patients.

There are also quite a number of ongoing clinical trials in the United States evaluating quality-of-life outcomes of psychosocial interventions, many of them supported by the NIH, the NCI, and the ACS. But over-

252 all, there is very little research on the disease-related outcomes of participation in psychosocial interventions. In the United States, then, the only
studies explicitly designed to evaluate survival are those directed by
Spiegel, Andersen, and perhaps Kabat-Zinn and Hebert.

Canada may be doing a better job. The medical oncologist Pamela
Goodwin, director of the Marvelle Koffler Breast Center at Mt. Sinai Hospital in Toronto, is conducting a rigorous replication of Spiegel's original
study. Unlike any past or present U.S. effort, Goodwin's trial is similar to
large-scale clinical investigations of new procedures or drugs in clinical
oncology; it is a multicenter trial involving treatment centers in six Canadian cities. The study will follow 254 patients with metastatic breast cancer and determine psychosocial outcomes, biological mediators, and survival after three years. The therapists have been trained in the particulars
of Spiegel's Supportive/Expressive Therapy, with oversight by Spiegel's
colleagues. Goodwin's multicenter trial has been supported by the Medical Research Council of Canada and the Canadian Breast Cancer Initiative to the sum of 1.5 million Canadian dollars. Results, including data on
psychosocial end points and survival, are also expected by 2002.

Alistair J. Cunningham, director of the Cancer Coping Skills Training
Program at the Ontario Cancer Institute, is conducting a randomized clinical trial of sixty-six cancer patients in a multifaceted psychosocial intervention he designed to stimulate psychological transformation and spiritual growth; he expects survival data in the near future. Cunningham is
also conducting a correlative study with thirty cancer patients, evaluating
the relationship between survival and the extent of psychological change
brought about by participation in his psychosocial intervention. Though
he awaits final data, he has produced an interim report on twelve patients.
In a telephone interview, Cunningham called the preliminary results
"quite striking." He went on to say that "there seems to be a relationship
between the amount of work and change people make psychologically and
survival" (see the last section of this chapter, "UPDATE 2002," for the
complete, published results of Cunningham's study, which expand upon
and confirm his preliminary findings).

While the Canadian studies are promising and single studies in both
France and Australia are reportedly under way, the scope of the worldwide
effort to study this question is nonetheless disappointing. Jessie C. Gruman, director of the Center for the Advancement of Health, a health policy group in Washington, D.C., agrees that more research with medical
end points is justified. But she makes the interesting case that biomedical
scientists are not the only naysayers: many psychosocial researchers are
themselves resistant. "There is a very strong feeling among psychosocial

researchers and clinicians that it delegitimizes research directed toward quality of life to imply that the only really important outcome is survival," commented Gruman, who sees some validity in this viewpoint but still supports research on survival. "Some feel that their commitment to their patients and their patients' experiences is in some way invalidated by trying to tie this to harder endpoints." These investigators worry not only about the fate of present-day efforts to improve quality of life but also about what survival research means for the future. When it comes to supporting psychosocial interventions, said Gruman in a telephone interview, "a large number of researchers feel that the medical community will be let off the hook if [research] finds that psychosocial interventions don't make a difference in morbidity and mortality."

The skittishness of the psychosocial researchers is understandable, and admittedly the issues at stake are complex. Certainly the validity of quality-of-life research must never be sacrificed at the altar of sexier survival data—findings more likely to galvanize media attention. At the same time, it seems shortsighted if not self-defeating to dichotomize these two goals, as if they can or should be set apart. The argument in favor of psychosocial interventions loses nothing in rationality or compassion by elevating both goals, one proven and one provisional. In fact, if psychosocial interventions became more widely available as a result of publicity about survival effects, their profound quality-of-life benefits might become more readily apparent to all concerned. The stance of some quality-of-life researchers also smacks of scientific timidity; to protect their area of concern, they disavow an inseparable area of research with major psychobiological ramifications and the potential to extend or even save some lives.

PSYCHOSOCIAL INTERVENTIONS: CURRENT IMPLEMENTATION

If the interest in studying the benefits of psychosocial interventions is thin, the interest in implementing such interventions is thinner. Leaving aside the survival studies, established research on the quality-of-life benefits (Meyer and Mark 1995) has yet to prompt a well-coordinated effort by the NIH, the NCI, and the ACS to implement psychosocial programs in cancer treatment centers and hospitals throughout the United States.

While psychosocial interventions are offered in some teaching hospitals in association with psychiatric-liaison or behavioral-medical departments—Memorial Sloan-Kettering Cancer Center and Johns Hopkins are two examples—there is no mandate and certainly no directive from any powerful group inside or outside government for interventions in the form of psychotherapy groups to be made available to cancer patients. Although

254   the NCI funds research and does not mandate clinical programs, both the NIH and the NCI, through their publications and influence on healthcare institutions, could take a much stronger position in favor of psychosocial interventions.

One academic society that strongly supports psychosocial interventions for cancer patients is the International Psycho-Oncology Society, headed by Memorial Sloan-Kettering's Jimmie Holland, a longtime ardent advocate of these programs. But the society is not a health policy group, and the only organization pushing for broad implementation of these programs in the political arena is the aforementioned Center for the Advancement of Health, headed by Jessie Gruman.

The center, funded by the MacArthur and Nathan Cummings Foundations, promotes a biopsychosocial view of health and its translation into programs of research and medical care that are fully integrated into the mainstream. One of their key projects is a "cancer initiative" to raise awareness among policymakers and the public of the need for psychosocial interventions for cancer patients and their families. Under Gruman's leadership the center has flooded the media with research findings supporting psychosocial interventions for cancer. It has also lobbied federal health institutes for broad-based applications, including applications in "under-served" areas of the country. The center recently published a position paper detailing essential elements that should be present in any psychosocial program for cancer patients and their families.

Gruman emphasizes that survival as an outcome is not taken very seriously as a goal of research or an argument for broad implementation. "The potential of psychosocial interventions to change medical endpoints—specifically morbidity and mortality—has simply not caught on."

The Opportunity and the Obligation

Why was there no sense of urgency to move on the findings of Spiegel, Fawzy, and Richardson? I attribute this lack to multiple factors: the myopia of biomedical scientists who have no paradigm to explain this effect, the anxiety of psychosocial researchers who fear eroding interest in quality of life, and the dichotomous thinking of both groups, who pit psychological against medical outcomes.

There is also another factor: the lack of profit motive for broad application of psychosocial programs. If huge multinational corporations had vested interests in these programs, as the pharmaceutical companies have in new chemotherapy and biological drugs, we would see action: massive funding for research, federal funds and clinical directives for psychosocial programs in hospitals and treatment centers, implementation by health maintenance organizations (HMOs) and managed care companies, position papers from mainstream medical societies, and far-flung programs of public awareness.

David Spiegel suggests that the lack of profit motive is a key factor. "There is no mediating industry," commented Spiegel in an interview with me. "Who is interested in promoting good therapy for cancer patients? People who sell chairs? There is nothing like the drug industry out there with their detail people and their advertising firms saying, 'Hey, use this.'" While the psychological and psychosomatic medicine societies have interests on behalf of professionals, they obviously cannot compare with the massive efforts of profit-driven corporations.

There is one available route for profits, however, and it possibly offers an alternative avenue for broad implementation. Consider the TV commercials being run by Cancer Treatment Centers of America, a for-profit concern with three treatment centers in the United States. The commercials tout their complementary treatments for "mind, body, and spirit." Patients at Cancer Treatment Centers have access to group programs run by psychologists, as well as to nutritional and "spiritual" counseling. Perhaps other profit-driven managed-care companies will pick up the mantle of psychosocial interventions once focus groups suggest that patients will select plans including such programs. But first the public must be fully aware of the benefits of psychosocial interventions.

Biomedical and biobehavioral researchers and clinicians should closely consider the chemotherapy analogy as a scientific and moral basis for action. Recently, according to a story reported by Spiegel, one mainstream oncologist showed a spark of common sense that cut through the collective layers of denial and obfuscation. Spiegel tells about I. Craig Henderson, of the University of California, San Francisco, widely known as one of the country's leading medical oncologists for breast cancer. After Spiegel had given a talk at a medical society meeting, Henderson spoke in support of research and application of psychosocial interventions for cancer patients. According to Spiegel, he got up and said, "If you proceed on the basis of the published literature, there is better evidence right now that group therapy extends survival time with breast cancer than there is similar evidence for bone marrow transplantation."

Henderson's comment is instructive, particularly in an era of managed care, when we agonize over the benefits, costs, and limitations of high-tech medicine. Perhaps we do not agonize enough. Bone marrow transplants are the most expensive—and dangerous—cancer treatment available, yet despite their mixed record of success in metastatic breast cancer, millions

256   of dollars were expended on their research and clinical usage. (Recent studies have proven that bone marrow transplantation is absolutely no better, in terms of survival, than standard chemotherapy for metastatic breast cancer.) Maybe bone marrow transplantation will someday live up to its promise, but how in good conscience can the nontoxic therapy of psychosocial support, with arguably a better record of clinical results, be pursued in such a halfhearted and disjunctive fashion?

    The bias against nonpharmacologic therapies has no basis in science or biomedical ethics. Indeed, this bias is blatantly unscientific and probably unethical. With evidence of quality-of-life benefits and of life-extending potential, biomedicine's lack of an initiative is nothing short of a scandal. If more studies weigh in with survival benefits, will the nationwide initiative begin? Or will there be a call for more randomized, controlled clinical trials? How much data will be enough? When will biomedicine finally recognize its obligation to provide cancer patients with therapies that build strength, hope, and physical resilience?

UPDATE 2002: New Data, New Questions

Since this chapter was first published in 1997, several new developments in research on psychosocial interventions for cancer have raised new questions about their role in cancer recovery or survival. Of most seeming significance, a major replication of David Spiegel's famous study of supportive-expressive group therapy for metastatic breast cancer patients, conducted by Pamela Goodwin, director of the Marvelle Koffler Breast Center at Mt. Sinai Hospital in Toronto, failed to show a survival benefit for patients in the intervention group (Goodwin et al. 2001). Goodwin and her colleagues randomly assigned 235 women into either weekly therapy groups ($N = 158$) or no intervention ($N = 77$). While patients in the treatment groups received some psychological benefits, there was no survival benefit: the treated patients had a median survival of 17.9 months, while those in the control group had a median survival of 17.6 months (Goodwin et al. 2001). Goodwin's findings were published in the *New England Journal of Medicine* and therefore received a great deal of press attention. In a 2001 article on the study in the *New York Times* by reporter Gina Kolata entitled "Cancer Study Finds Supports Groups Do Not Extend Life" the subtext was clear: the idea that psychological interventions might influence cancer survival has been proven false, once and for all.

    While the Goodwin study certainly casts some doubt on the thesis I presented in 1997—that psychosocial interventions may indeed prolong survival—it would be a scientific and even ethical mistake to declare this a settled issue. In my view the total body of existing evidence still leans clearly toward at least a modest survival benefit when the psychosocial intervention itself yields significant psychological benefits.

An important editorial by David Spiegel, "Mind Matters—Group Therapy and Survival in Breast Cancer," appeared in the same issue of the *New England Journal of Medicine* as Goodwin's study (Spiegel 2001). Spiegel noted that half of the studies published to date—five out of ten randomized clinical trials (Cunningham. 1998; Edelman et al. 1999; Fawzy et al. 1993; Goodwin et al. 2001; Ilnyckyj et al. 1994; Kogon et al. 1997; Kuchler et al. 1999; Linn et al. 1982; Peto et al. 2000; Ratcliffe et al. 1995; Richardson et al. 1990) —have reported that psychotherapy prolongs survival among cancer patients. Most importantly, Spiegel noted that three of the five negative studies provided only transient psychological benefits (Edelman et al. 1999) or no psychological benefit of any kind (Cunningham et al. 1998; Ilnyckyj et al. 1994). In his editorial Spiegel stated the obvious but salient point: "A psychological intervention that does not help emotionally is not likely to provide a physical benefit."

Spiegel's argument should be the reference point for analysis of this literature. The scientific theories behind survival benefits for psychological treatments for cancer patients depend primarily on mind-body interactions, which means that a treatment without psychological benefit would not be expected to have medical benefits. Thus, I would argue that the central question in this field should be restated. Instead of asking, Have psychosocial intervention trials shown survival benefits? we should ask, Have trials of psychosocial interventions *with proven psychological benefits* also shown survival benefits? If one sets aside studies of treatments that failed to produce significant psychological improvement, then 71 percent, or five of seven, of the trials to date have shown survival benefits. It is also important to consider that both of the studies showing psychological improvements but no survival benefits involved metastatic or end-stage cancer patients, which according to most analysts are those patients in whom survival benefits are least likely to result from psychosocial treatments that conceivably enhance host defenses. (The capacity of such defenses, including immunological ones, to overcome large tumors and widespread tumor growth is certainly constrained, to say the least.) Spiegel's 1989 result with metastatic breast cancer patients should not be considered a fluke, though in retrospect it is all the more remarkable that such a marked survival advantage was shown among women with advanced cancers that have spread to distant sites in the body.

In his editorial David Spiegel noted several other reasons why the Goodwin study, which he believed was well carried out and methodolog-

258 ically sound (he had acted as an advisor to Goodwin and to the study's clinicians), might not have shown a survival advantage for psychosocially treated patients. One was that psychosocial and emotional supports were far less well understood and available decades ago, when the first Spiegel study was carried out. Today, members of control groups in such studies are more likely to seek out such supports and perhaps to engage in a variety of supportive interventions on their own, thus limiting differences between control groups and psychosocial treatment groups (Spiegel 2001).

In a recent article in *Integrative Cancer Therapies*, aptly titled "Change is Complex: Rethinking Research on Psychosocial Interventions and Cancer," Lydia Temoshok and Rebecca Wald asked deeper questions about whether a psychosocial treatment is likely to produce medical benefits (Temoshok and Wald 2002). As I posited in chapter 4, the factors involved in cancer development and progression cannot be reduced to simplistic categories such as "distress," "negative emotion" or even "depression." The key variables are more likely longstanding coping strategies, including repression or nonexpression of emotions; a stoical or passive response style; and masked depression or hopelessness. Temoshok and Wald's point is that interventions might have to bring about shifts in such usually stable traits or chronic states in order to have an impact on survival. Thus, in order for such treatments to pass muster as therapies that might influence survival, measures are needed to determine whether they actually induce such significant changes in both stable coping styles and emotional states.

With regard to the Goodwin trial, Temoshok and Wald question whether the psychological measures were adequate to determine whether the psychosocial intervention produced such changes. They note that the primary psychological measure used, the Profile of Mood States (POMS), explicitly asks subjects to report on their moods "over the past week." Temoshok and Wald note that "what is more appropriately called for is not a measurement of ephemeral or transient states, but rather, a determination of whether the psychological intervention affected more stable (i.e., habitual, trait-like) psychosocial factors over the course of 6 months to a year . . . and thus, could be capable of having a effect on survival years later" (Temoshok and Wald 2002).

The Goodwin study produced a seemingly anomalous finding that may also be telling. Patients who at the outset of the study scored high on measures of distress and pain benefited psychologically from the treatment (with significantly lower distress scores at the study's end), while those who scored lower on measures of distress and pain from the outset did not benefit with regard to their psychological well-being (Goodwin et al. 2001). Temoshok and Wald (2002) present a trenchant hypothesis about this find-

The Scientific and Moral Imperative

ing. Referring to the substantial literature (reviewed in chapter 4) showing that open expression of distress and other negative emotions in the face
of a cancer diagnosis is not maladaptive and damaging to one's health but
rather is adaptive and promotes health, Temoshok and Wald hypothesize
that patients who benefited from the intervention—those in more evident
distress—were actually more expressive to begin with and therefore had
some of the skills that were needed to benefit from this supportive-expressive intervention. On the other hand, those who evidenced little distress may have been *less expressive* (more Type C, as explained in chapter
4) rather than more genuinely tranquil in response to their life-threatening diagnosis. (Indeed, most psychotherapists would investigate whether
a patient just diagnosed with metastatic breast cancer who reported "little
distress" was really protecting him- or herself from waves of negative emotion—fear, sorrow, or anger.) In theory, a supportive-expressive intervention should help less expressive individuals to open up more, but one won-
ders whether once-a-week group treatment of this kind is sufficiently deep
to cause a significant shift in longstanding traits or coping styles in most
people. Perhaps such an intervention would be more beneficial to those
who were already able to express emotion but would fall short in the case
of those who were not, an interpretation that is consistent with the findings in the Goodwin trial. The less expressive patients might need far more
focused and intensive help. Temoshok and Wald also note that Goodwin
failed to ask whether the more distressed patients who benefited psychologically from supportive-expressive therapy also lived longer. Here again,
more nuanced questions about psychological states and traits, a more penetrating analysis of measures and methods, and a more critical view of the
efficacy of interventions are all needed.

Another fascinating development in the field involves the work of the
psychologist Alistair Cunningham, Ph.D., a senior scientist in the Department of Epidemiology, Statistics and Behavioral Science, at the Ontario Cancer Institute in Toronto. In 1998 Cunningham published one of
the negative randomized trials of a psychosocial intervention for cancer
(Cunningham et al. 1998). Despite this disappointing result, Cunningham
observed that some of the intervention patients were far more committed
than others to the psychological work of change: they were more likely to
"take home" the principles of emotional and cognitive transformation and
to practice mind-body and other self-help methods learned in the group
settings. So he designed a correlative study, rather than a randomized one,
to determine by a sophisticated battery of measures whether participants
in the psychosocial intervention he designed were more or less committed
to the program. He then wanted to know whether patients more commit-

ted to change who experienced more benefits from the intervention were more likely to survive longer.

Though it involved a small number of metastatic cancer patients—twenty-two—Cunningham's correlative study fully supported his hypothesis. While controlling for disease severity, Cunningham found that the intervention patients who became more strongly involved in psychological and spiritual self-help work not only experienced more pronounced improvements in quality of life but also survived significantly longer (Cunningham et al. 2000). Cunningham's important work suggests that every intervention study should include measures of commitment and change, since patients less committed to processes of change would also be less likely to gain psychologically and physically from any psychosocial intervention. Perhaps his insight about psychotherapy for illness is comparable to a question that might be posed in a drug trial: Are the patients taking their pills when they get home?

Such subtle, nevertheless trenchant considerations must be brought into research designs and discourse surrounding this ongoing and persistently controversial question. But there is also a cultural aspect to the debate. Why are some mind-body clinicians and many patients and members of the public convinced of the survival benefits beyond evaluating a shred of data? And why do some in the biomedical community and public seem so averse to the idea of survival benefits? Why, for instance, did the Goodwin study get so much attention, while another recent study, that of Thomas Kuchler, Ph.D., a psychologist, of Christian-Albrechts University in Germany, has received no media attention at all? Kuchler and his colleagues randomly assigned 271 patients with gastrointestinal cancers to a group that received regular, one-on-one psychotherapy sessions or to a no-treatment control group (Kuchler et al. 1999). (The treatment, given both before and after hospitalization, was described as a highly individualized intervention, consisting of both emotional and cognitive support, designed to foster fighting spirit and to reduce feelings of helplessness and hopelessness.) After two years of follow-up the therapy participants lived significantly longer ($p = .002$) than those who did not receive treatment (Kuchler et al. 1999). (Cox regression models, statistical methods that can account for differences in disease stage and residual tumor classifications, showed that the results held up after controlling for disease severity.) Kuchler's study, published in *Hepatogastroenterology*, was even larger than Pamela Goodwin's, but it has received virtually no notice in the United States, though it was cited in Spiegel's editorial in the *New England Journal of Medicine*.

The superficial tug of war between conservative critics and true believers should be replaced by a cooperative investigation of the deeper questions, with a reasonable assumption, based on the 71 percent of positive findings in this still nascent field of inquiry, that "something is going on here." What is that something? What kind of changes will help cancer patients to not only feel better but also possibly live longer? What kind of interventions can be tailored to bring about such transformations? And what kind of research is best able to determine treatments that will help sustain people's emotional health, physical energy, and spiritual vitality as they engage in a critical encounter with illness?

REFERENCES

Achterberg J. 1985. *Imagery in Healing*. New Science Library. Boston & London: Shambhala.

Achterberg J, Lawlis GF, Simonton OC, Simonton S. 1977. Psychological factors and blood chemistries as disease outcome predictors for cancer patients. *Multivar Exper Clin Res.* 3:107–122.

Berman E, Heller G, Santorsa J, et al. 1991. Results of a randomized trial comparing idarubicin and cytosine arabinoside with daunorubicin and cytosine arabinoside in adult patients with newly diagnosed acute myelogenous leukemia. *Blood.* 77:1666–1674.

Buccheri GF, Ferrigno D, Tamburini M, Brunelli C. 1995. The patient's perception of his own quality of life might have an adjunctive prognostic significance in lung cancer. *Lung Cancer.* 12:45–58.

Coates A, Gebsk V, Signorini D, et al. 1992. Prognostic value of quality of life scores during chemotherapy for advanced breast cancer. *J Clin Oncol.* 10:1833–1838.

Cunningham AJ. 1984. Psychotherapy for cancer. *Advances.* 1:8–14.

Cunningham AJ, Edmonds CVI, Jenkins GP, et al. 1998. A randomized controlled trial of the effects of group psychological therapy on survival in women with metastatic breast cancer. *Psychooncology.* 7:508–517.

Cunningham AJ, Edmonds CVI, Phillips C, et al. 2000. A prospective, longitudinal study of the relationship of psychological work to duration of survival in patients with metastatic cancer. *Psychooncology.* 9:323–339.

Degner LF, Sloan JA. 1995. Symptom distress in newly diagnosed ambulatory cancer patients and as a predictor of survival in lung cancer. *J Pain Symptom Manage.* 10:423–431.

Dreher H. 1996. Can hypnosis rotate a breech baby before birth? *Adv Mind Body Med.* 12:46–50.

Edelman S, Lemon J, Bell DR, Kidman AD. 1999. Effects of group CBT on the survival time of patients with metastatic breast cancer. *Psychooncology.* 8:474–481.

Fawzy FI, Fawzy MO, Hyun CS, et al. 1993. Malignant melanoma: effects of an early structured psychiatric intervention, coping, and affective state on recurrence and survival six years later. *Arch Gen Psychiatry.* 50:681–689.

262   Fawzy FI, Fawzy NW, Amdt LA, Pasnau RO. 1995. Critical review of psychosocial interventions in cancer care. *Arch Gen Psychiatry.* 52:100–113.

Fawzy FI, Kemeny ME, Fawzy NW, et al. 1990. A structured psychiatric intervention for cancer patients. II. Changes over time in immunological measures. *Arch Gen Psychiatry.* 47:729–735.

Ganz PA, Kee JJ, Siau J. 1991. Quality of life assessment: an independent prognostic variable for survival in lung cancer. *Cancer.* 67:3131–3135.

Goodwin PJ, Leszcz M, Ennis M, et al. 2001. The effect of group psychosocial support on survival in metastatic breast cancer. *New Engl J Med.* 345:1719–1726.

Greer S, Morris T, Pettingale KW, Haybittle JL. 1990. Psychological response to breast cancer and fifteen-year outcome. *Lancet.* 335:49–50.

Ilnyckyj I, Farber J, Cheang M, Weinerman B. 1994. A randomized controlled trial of psychotherapeutic intervention in cancer patients. *Ann R Coll Physicians Surg Can.* 27:93–96.

Karnofsky DA, Abelman WH, Craver LF, et al. 1948. The use of nitrogen mustards in palliative treatment of carcinoma. *Cancer.* 1:634–656.

Kogon MM, Biswas A, Pearl D, Carlson RW, Spiegel D. 1997. Effects of medical and psychotherapeutic treatment on the survival of women with metastatic breast carcinoma. *Cancer.* 80:225–230.

Kolata G. 2001. Cancer study finds support groups do not extend life. *New York Times,* 13 December.

Kuchler T, Henne-Bruns D, Rappat S, et al. 1999. Impact of psychotherapeutic support on gastrointestinal cancer patients undergoing surgery: survival results of a trial. *Hepatogastroenterology.* 46:322–335.

Lerner M. 1994. *Choices in Healing: Integrating the Best of Conventional and Complementary Approaches to Cancer.* Cambridge, Mass: MIT Press.

LeShan L. 1977. *You Can Fight for Your Life.* New York: M. Evans & Co.

LeShan L. 1989. *Cancer as a Turning Point.* New York: E. P. Dutton.

Linn MW, Linn BS, Harris R. 1982. Effects of counseling for late stage cancer patients. *Cancer.* 9: 1048–1055.

Massion AO, Teas J, Hebert JR, et al. 1995. Meditation, melatonin, and breast/prostate cancer: hypothesis and preliminary data. *Med Hypotheses.* 44:39–46.

Maunsell E, Brisson J, Deschenes L. 1995. Social support and survival among women with breast cancer. *Cancer.* 76:631–637.

McGuire WP, Hoskins WJ, Brady MF, et al. 1996. Cyclophosphamide and cisplatin compared with paclitaxel and cisplatin in patients with stage III and stage IV ovarian cancer. *New Engl J Med.* 334:1–6.

Meares A. 1980. What can the cancer patient expect from intensive meditation? *Aust Fam Physician.* 9:322–325.

Meyer TJ, Mark MM. 1995. Effects of psychosocial interventions with adult cancer patients: a meta-analysis of randomized experiments. *Health Psychol.* 14:101–108.

Peto R, Boreham J, Clarke M, Davies C, Beral V. 2000. UK and USA breast cancer deaths down 25 percent in year 2000 at ages 20–69 years. *Lancet.* 355:1822.

Ratcliffe MA, Dawson AA, Walker LG. 1995. Eysenck Personality Inventory L-scores in patients with Hodgkin's disease and non-Hodgkin's lymphoma. *Psychooncology.* 4:39–45.

Richardson JL, Shelton DR, Krailo M, Levine AM. 1990. The effect of compliance with treatment on survival among patients with hematologic malignancies. *J Clin Oncol.* 8:356–364.

Ringdal GI, Gotestam KG, Kaasa S, et al. 1996. Prognostic factors and survival in a heterogeneous sample of cancer patients. *Br J Cancer.* 73:1594–1599.

Roath S. 1997. On psychosocial interventions for cancer (letter). *Adv Mind Body Med.* 13(3):2.

Rothenberg ML, Eckardt JR, Kuhn JG, et al. 1996. Phase II trial of irinotecan in patients With progressive or rapidly recurrent colorectal cancer. *J Clin Oncol.* 14:1128–1135.

Ruckdeschel JC, Piantadosi S. 1989. Assessment of quality-of-life by the Functional Living Index-Cancer (FLIC) is superior to performance status for prediction of survival in patients with lung cancer. *Proc Am Soc Clin Oncol.* 8:311.

Shipp MA, Harrington DP, Klatt MM, et al. 1986. Identification of major prognostic subgroups of patients with large-cell lymphoma treated with m-BACOD or M-BACOD. *Ann Intern Med.* 104:757–765.

Simonton OC, Matthews-Simonton S, Creighton J. 1978. *Getting Well Again.* Los Angeles: J. P. Tarcher.

Sorensen JB, Badsberg JH. 1990. Prognostic factors in resected stage I and II adenocarcinoma of the lung: a multivariate regression analysis of 137 consecutive patients. *J Thorac Cardiovasc Surgery.* 99:218–226.

Spiegel D. 1995. How do you feel about cancer now? Survival and psychosocial support. *Public Health Rep.* 110:298–300.

Spiegel D. 2001. Mind matters—group therapy and survival in breast cancer. *New Engl J Med.* 345:1767.

Spiegel D, Bloom J, Kraemer HC, Gottheil E. 1989. Effect of psychosocial treatment on survival of patients with metastatic breast cancer. *Lancet.* 2:888–891.

Stanley KE. 1980. Prognostic factors for survival in patients with inoperable lung cancer. *J Natl Cancer Inst.* 65:25–32.

Tamburini M, Brunelli C, Rosso S, Ventafridda V. 1996. Prognostic value of quality of life scores in terminal cancer patients. *J Pain Symptom Manage.* 11:32–41.

Temoshok L. 1985. Biopsychosocial studies on cutaneous malignant melanoma: psychosocial factors associated with prognostic indicators, progression, psychophysiology, and tumor-host response. *Soc Sci Med.* 20:833–840.

Temoshok L, Dreher H. 1992. *The Type C Connection: The Behavioral Links to Cancer and Your Health.* New York: Random House.

Temoshok L, Wald RL. 2002. Change is complex: rethinking research on psychosocial interventions and cancer. *Integrative Cancer Therapies.* 1:135–145.

Tross S, Herndon J II, Korzun A, et al. 1996. Psychological symptoms and disease-free and overall survival in women with stage II breast cancer: cancer and leukemia group B. *J Natl Cancer Inst.* 88:661–667.

Vogler WR, Velez-Garcia E, Weiner RS, et al. 1992. A phase III trial comparing idarubicin and daunorubicin in combination with cytarabine in acute Myeloge-

264   nous leukemia: a southeastern cancer study group study. *J Clin Oncol.*
10:1103–1111.

Weeks J. 1992. Quality-of-life assessment: performance status upstaged? *J Clin Oncol.* 10:1827–1829.

Wiernik PH, Banks PL, Case DC Jr, et al. 1992. Cytarabine plus idarubicin or daunorubicin as induction and consolidation therapy for previously untreated adult patients with acute myeloid leukemia. *Blood.* 79:313–319.

Chapter 7

Mind-Body Medicine for Women:

Gender-Specific Treatments

Fortunately, the assertion that women's health issues have gotten short shrift from biomedical researchers is no longer dismissed by the biomedical elite as so much feminist bluster. The evidence for this neglect is now viewed as incontestable, particularly with regard to the exclusion of women as research participants. The glaring example is heart disease, an area in which medicine's fundamental assumptions, such as the role of cholesterol and diet and the efficacy of certain treatments for heart attack patients, have been predicated solely on data from studies of men (Stanton 1995). For instance, the Physicians' Health Study, which informed us that a regular intake of aspirin could prevent heart attacks, cannot be the basis for recommendations for women, since all of the twenty-two thousand participants in the study were male (Steering Committee of the Physicians' Health Study Research Group 1988).

Because of this bias, mainstream biomedicine has hardly investigated gender differences in the aging process; evaluated the health issues surrounding menopause; sufficiently grappled with the autoimmune diseases so prevalent among women; or adequately funded breast cancer research. In 1990 the United States spent roughly ten times as much on AIDS research as it did on breast cancer even though breast cancer had claimed roughly six times as many lives (Altman 1996). The problem, of course, is not that too much is being spent on AIDS research, since AIDS is an infectious disease with disastrous human and public health consequences,

Reprinted by permission, with changes, from *Advances in Mind-Body Medicine* 13 (1997): 68–74.

266   but that too little is still being expended on breast cancer, considering its prevalence and mortality rate.

But meaningful change is on the horizon, due mainly to the obscene blatancy of these discrepancies, coupled with the strenuous efforts of women's health advocates. Since 1990 the Centers for Disease Control, the Food and Drug Administration, the National Institutes of Health, and the U.S. Public Health Service have opened offices focusing on women's health. A few large prospective studies on risk factors in women's health, including both gender-specific and gender-nonspecific diseases, have been launched, although women's health advocates continue to fight for funding levels for these trials commensurate with the problems they address. The $92.7 million spent on breast cancer in 1991 ballooned to $323.7 million in 1995, which was still not enough but obviously a vast improvement (Altman 1996).

So it is fair to report that mainstream biomedicine has made strides toward rectifying years of unjustifiable inequities. But what about mind–body medicine? Sadly, behavioral-medicine researchers have paid scant attention to women's health, in a manner that is uncomfortably similar to the neglect by mainstream biomedicine. A prime example is the lack of female subjects in biobehavioral research on heart disease. The renowned Western Collaborative Group Study, in which the cardiologists Meyer Friedman, M.D., and Ray Rosenman, M.D., established the Type A behavior pattern as an independent risk for heart disease, involved more than three thousand men and no women (Rosenman et al. 1975). Similarly, most early research on the association between hostility and heart disease relied on male subjects, with too few exceptions to allow researchers to generalize about the role of emotional factors in heart disease among women (Williams 1993).

Certainly, there are exceptions to the all-male rule in mind–body research. A fine example is the work of Margaret Chesney, M.D., of the University of California at San Francisco, on biobehavioral factors in heart disease among women, and Nancy Frasure-Smith, Ph.D., of McGill University in Montreal, has included a sizable proportion of women in her studies of depression and heart attack recovery and psychosocial interventions for heart patients (Frasure-Smith et al. 1993; Frasure-Smith et al. 1997). There has also been at least one federally sponsored effort to stimulate behavioral research into women's health, the daylong conference "Mind-Body Interactions in Health and Diseases," held in 1996 by the U.S. Public Health Service's Office on Women's Health as part of its annual Healthy Women 2000 program.

Although in the 1990s there has been a notable increase in biobehavioral investigations of heart disease in women, the stark reality is that women's health still does not receive its proportionate share of consideration by the mind-body research community. Just as mainstream researchers have lagged in explaining the physiological differences between women and men that are pertinent to their health, so too have mind-body researchers lagged in explaining how psychosocial factors may differ in their physiological influence on men and women. Too little basic research means too few clinical translations—mind-body treatments for women's health conditions, proven to work in clinical trials and made available in clinics and medical centers. And the few treatments proven effective in clinical trials are not being widely investigated or implemented for conditions—such as menopausal hot flashes, infertility, and certain autoimmune disorders—for which there are only partly (or in some cases minimally) successful medical treatments with numerous side effects.

In this chapter I briefly review basic research regarding sex differences in mind-immune interrelationships. But the greater part of the chapter covers clinical applications, specifically a body of promising research on mind-body treatments that complement, or in some cases supplant, mainstream therapies for severe premenstrual syndrome (PMS), menopausal hot flashes, and infertility.

Gender, Immunity, and Women's Conditions

The balance of sex hormones in men and women are obviously different, but the effects of the variations go well beyond reproductive and sexual functions. Sex hormones—estrogen, progesterone, testosterone, prolactin, and luteinizing hormone-releasing hormone (LHRH), to name the most prominent—have profound regulatory influences on the immune system. (Some also regulate the cardiovascular system in clinically important ways.) Here is another instance of mind-body unity: A biological subsystem, in this case gonadal hormones of the reproductive system, engages in extensive crosstalk with other biological systems that have no seeming connection to reproduction. The dialogue is so incessant that sex hormones can no longer be thought to "belong" exclusively to the reproductive system.

Broadly speaking, what is needed is a psychoneuroimmunological (PNI) perspective that gives full weight to hormonal activity, in other words, psychoneuro*endocrin*immunology. A small group of investigators have pursued the linkages among sex steroids and the nervous, cardiovascular, and immune systems and have turned up findings with great potential relevance for the treatment of women's conditions. Research on how sex hormones influence neural circuitry and neurotransmitters is gaining ground (McEwen 1998); it is no longer the province of a small coterie of investigators but a major subject of study by the National Institutes of Health. (Academic researchers are beginning to test and apply hormonal treatments for Alzheimer's disease and psychiatric disorders ranging from schizophrenia to clinical depression [Klaiber 2001].) The study of sex-hormone regulation of the immune system, however, is still poised on the outer boundaries of basic biomedical research even though it has already produced a treasure trove of discoveries, findings that will ultimately reshape our understanding of women's biology and women's diseases.

Why, from a teleological standpoint, might reproductive hormones have regulatory power over immunity? The first and foremost answer is the granting of "immune privilege" to an embryo in utero. Since sex hormones govern all reproductive processes, from mating to conception to fertilization to implantation to pregnancy, they are also partly responsible for shutting down immune responses against the embryo and developing fetus (McCruden and Stimson 1991). We now understand quite a bit about how this immune stoppage occurs. The hypothalamic-pituitary-gonadal (HPG) axis manages reproductive functions. Messenger molecules (specifically LHRH) produced by cells in the brain's hypothalamus prompt the pituitary gland to release its hormones, which in turn regulate the sex-hormone output of ovaries and testicles. With good reason this HPG axis intertwines, in many places, with the hypothalamic-pituitary-adrenal (HPA) axis, governor of the "stress response" that regulates the flow of adrenal stress hormones, themselves major players in immune modulation. In a chapter on HPG and the immune system Bianca Marchetti and her colleagues (2001) explain that "signals [of the HPG axis], generated within the brain and peripheral target organs, symbiotically interact to finely orchestrate every aspect of reproduction. Luteinizing hormone-releasing hormone (LHRH), a hypothalamic peptide, is defined classically as the neuroendocrine trigger and essential pacemaker of mammalian reproduction. LHRH acts not only at the level of the brain-pituitary-gonadal unit, but also is recognized now to directly influence immune organs and cells. As such, it finely regulates reproductive homeostasis."

By *reproductive homeostasis* Marchetti and colleagues mean that LHRH influences immunity so as to save the embryo and fetus—which contain genes from the father that signal "foreignness"—from being destroyed by the immune system. (LHRH is not the only gonadal hormone participating in this protection.) Beyond (or because of) this function, LHRH is directly or indirectly involved in an array of immune responses. It influences mast cells and their release of histamine. It shares messenger molecules and information with brain cells (astroglia) and immune cells. It acts as an immune modulator within the thymus gland, the "master gland" of immunity. Most tellingly, perhaps, some LHRH is produced by lymphocytes, and lymphocytes have receptors for LHRH that are molecularly indistinguishable from the ones found in the pituitary gland. "LHRH acts as an immunological response modifier in the brain-pituitary-lymphoid-gonadal axis," write Marchetti and colleagues. The braiding of reproductive/sexual, neuroendocrine, and immune systems is both intimate and elaborate, with several cascading networks of cells and signaling molecules, once thought to be discrete, meeting and twisting together at multiple points in their natural byways.

Androgens, estrogens, progestogens, and prolactin all modulate immune functions (McCruden and Stimson 1991). Estrogens have generally been shown to depress cell-mediated (T-cell) immunity, but they can stimulate antibody responses to foreign entities (antigens). At least one group of T cells have been shown to bear receptors for estrogen—the CD8 class, which can be cytotoxic (killers of foreign invaders) or suppressors (tamping down immune responses). The very presence of receptors on these immune cells means that sex hormones are among the orchestra leaders of their widespread activities. The thymus has estrogen receptors, and macrophages become highly active when estrogen is added to culture media. By exerting effects on a genetic level, estrogen, other sex hormones, and adrenal "stress" hormones collaborate to control the expression of corticosteroid receptors in the thymus, which turns out to be an important matter, since the thymus programs bodywide T-cell responses (Peiffer et al. 1994). And the action of these receptors for corticosteroids, the body's natural anti-inflammatories, is probably a key to women's abilities to maintain both normal pregnancy (without immune interference) and balanced immune responses throughout their life span. These are all instances in which sex hormones participate in the sprawling, complex activities of immune cells and substances in every corner of the body.

Progesterone too plays its part in immunity, mostly, though not exclusively, as an inhibitor (McCruden and Stimson 1991). Prolactin is a peptide hormone released by the pituitary gland that helps supervise the reproductive cycle. But it is yet another orchestrator of the immune symphony (Bernton et al. 1991). In rat studies, secretion of prolactin by the pituitary seems necessary for normal immune function, especially when stress or infection raises levels of immunosuppressive glucocorticoids. In a finding that would have shaken immunologists and reproductive endocrinologists a mere two decades ago, it has been shown that lymphocytes make a protein virtually identical to prolactin, which acts as a

270   self-regulator endowing these immune cells with the capacity to progress through the cell cycle (Bernton et al. 1991). Here is another example of immune cells getting regulatory signals from molecules, in this instance reproductive hormones, that immunobiologists thought had nothing to do with immunity.

What is the clinical relevance of the interplay between sex hormones and immune cells? The specifics remain cloudy, but the idea that these ubiquitous interactions influence health and disease, especially in women, can no longer be doubted. Understanding the congruence of the reproductive and immune systems is likely to illuminate pressing issues in women's health. For instance, why are autoimmune diseases so much more prevalent among women than among men? Rheumatoid arthritis (RA) is three times as common among women; multiple sclerosis (MS), two times; and lupus (SLE), nine times (Domar and Dreher 1996). Some specialists speculate that estrogen imbalances play a pivotal role in these diseases through their effects on immunity. But is stress also a factor? If so, does stress upset the balance of estrogens and other sex steroids in a manner that causes immune cells to react against the host's normal tissues, as they do in autoimmune disease? On these matters the evidence has been gradually building for thirty years.

It is certain that estrogen can influence autoimmune disease, because the high levels occurring during pregnancy often accompany dramatic remissions of RA, MS, and autoimmune thyroiditis (Wilder and Elenkov 2001). The same patients who experience remissions often find their diseases flaring up again during the postpartum period, when estrogen levels plummet. The finding makes sense since these disorders are caused largely by T-cell damage to normal tissues, and T-cell responses tend to be tamped down by estrogen. By contrast, an autoimmune disease caused by antibody damage—SLE—often develops or flares up during pregnancy, which also suits this theory: estrogen generally promotes humoral (antibody-based) immunity. Other mechanisms critical to the onset or worsening of autoimmune disease seem directly attributable to a destructive *pas de deux* of ovarian and adrenal hormones, acting individually and in concert, to cause the release of too many proinflammatory cytokines and too few anti-inflammatory cytokines. (A propitious *pas de deux* would keep them in proper balance and prevent autoimmunity.)

Meanwhile, both adrenal and ovarian hormones can fluctuate under stress. This situation underlies the contention of some mind-body investigators that psychological factors contribute to autoimmune disease via sex-steroid changes (such as a drop in estrogen) that switch on proinflammatory cells and substances, switch off anti-inflammatory forces, or both. While the mechanisms are not fully understood, the thesis is more than conjecture: over thirty years of research has correlated stress with exacerbation of RA, MS, SLE, and other autoimmune diseases (Rogers and Brooks 2001). It is also reasonable to theorize that stress-linked hormonal fluctuations are involved in inflammatory disorders with a proven stress component, such as temporomandibular joint (TMJ) syndrome and irritable bowel syndrome (IBS), although the role of sex steroids per se is not clear in either case. Considered as a whole, the lopsided prevalence among women of RA, MS, and SLE; the fact that stress can worsen each condition; and the influence of sex-steroid oscillations on the clinical course of each disease lead to a reasonable inference: mind-body treatments emphasizing stress management have untapped clinical potential for autoimmune diseases.

Other common women's conditions may also have a stress component, including infertility, menopausal hot flashes, and severe PMS. In these instances, stress-initiated imbalances of ovarian hormones have been variously implicated, and in the case of hot flashes a rush of adrenal hormones (catecholamines) could explain the oft-observed connection between stress and the frequency or intensity of hot flashes (Kronenberg 1984). While the mind-immune connection may not have a hand in hot flashes or PMS, in theory it could contribute to unexplained infertility. One hypothesis being considered is that after ovulation, cell-mediated immunity is suppressed so the embryo can implant in the uterine lining without being annihilated or otherwise hampered by an immune response (Marchetti et al. 2001). Sex hormones are likely responsible for this immune suppression; one avenue would be by regulating the flow of immune-dampening corticosteroids and their receptors in the thymus. If ovarian hormones do not do their job properly—due to a dearth or imbalance—immune cells and their messengers may interfere with implantation, arguably the most delicate biochemical moment for the evolving zygote on the path to a viable pregnancy.

What about breast cancer? Studies support links between maladaptive coping, neuroendocrine perturbations, hormonal factors, and immune deficits in the development and progression of the disease. But no one study (or series of them) puts this puzzle together, leaving strong inferences but no crystal-clear picture (Temoshok and Dreher 1992). And yet, despite grave skepticism the puzzle pieces are compelling, and they tend to cohere in a meaningful fashion. Research from the 1970s and 1980s suggests that emotional factors play a role in the progression of breast cancer (Greer et al. 1990; Levy et al. 1987; Levy et al. 1990). A recent replication of Steven Greer's British study from the 1970s failed to show that fighting spirit was associated with long survival, but it confirmed a statistical link between hopelessness and shorter survival (Watson et al. 1999) (see chapter 4, "Cancer and the Mind," for a full discussion of Greer's study, its replication, and emotional factors in cancer progression.) Sandra Levy, of the University of Pittsburgh, and colleagues correlated stress factors, poor social support, and deficits in natural killer cells with an unfavorable breast cancer prognosis (Levy et al. 1987; Levy et al. 1990).

Despite these advances, investigation of psychosocial-endrocrine-immune relationships in breast cancer is still in its early stages. But the questions are finally being asked with more committed intensity, in part due to the psychiatrist David Spiegel's finding that metastatic breast cancer patients who participated in supportive-expressive group psychotherapy lived twice as long (36 months) as patients who did not participate (18 months) (Spiegel et al. 1989). In his ongoing replication of this study and in a new randomized trial of psychosocial therapy for early breast cancer patients Spiegel is running extensive batteries of neuroendocrine and immune mediators to try to find out whether the mind-immune network explains any improvements in survival for patients in the treatment group.

Whether for autoimmune diseases, female cancers, PMS, menopausal symptoms, or infertility, basic mind-body research has more or less scratched the surface of putative causes and mechanisms. In some cases immunobiologists, endocrinologists, psychiatrists, psychologists, and neuroscientists have made sufficient progress to justify more intensive study, not to mention early clinical trials of mind-body treatments for conditions that are likely to respond.

Mind-Body Treatments for Women: What Works?

What mind-body treatments for women's disorders have been tested and proven useful? A review of the literature turns up few studies of targeted mind-body treatments for menopausal symptoms, PMS, gynecologic cancers, infertility, multiple miscarriages, endometriosis, or pelvic pain. By contrast, there is a sizable literature (albeit, much of it popular) on the applicability of *alternative* medicine for these women's health conditions, the most common modalities being Western and Chinese herbology, acupuncture, Ayur-Veda medicine, and homeopathy. Women searching outside the mainstream medical model for effective ways to prevent and treat their most common health concerns, then, are more likely to turn to these modalities than to mind-body medicine.

Having in the first part of this chapter sketched in both the promise of

mind-body medicine for women and the problem of neglect, I wish to
focus on the lack of attention paid to mind-body applications for women
that have *already* been established as effective. A prime example is the work
of Alice D. Domar, Ph.D., who directs the programs for women's health
at the Division of Behavioral Medicine at Harvard Medical School and is
director of the Center for Women's Health within the division. Domar has
developed and researched the women's health programs at the Beth Israel
Deaconess Hospital in Boston, under the auspices of the Division of Behavioral Medicine and the Mind/Body Medical Institute, both directed
by Herbert Benson, M.D. As I will detail, her mind-body interventions
for women have proven effective in the treatment of PMS, menopausal hot
flashes, and infertility. Yet the potential for broad clinical application remains untapped.

   In the interests of full disclosure I should note that I am the coauthor
of two books with Domar, *Healing Mind, Healthy Woman* (1996) and *Self-
Nurture* (2000). In *Healing Mind, Healthy Woman* we describe Domar's research, delineate her data, and offer clinical guidelines for the techniques
and practices she teaches to her patients. While I cannot disclaim my par-
tiality, I ask that readers place it in perspective and consider the value and
broad applicability of her work. Her findings need to be replicated, but
they clearly suggest that the integration of mind-body treatments into
mainstream gynecologic and medical practice could contain costs and ease
suffering for vast numbers of women.

PREMENSTRUAL SYNDROME

Premenstrual syndrome, PMS, is a complex of conditions that occur in
the late luteal phase of women's menstrual cycles. The symptoms, which
may be psychological (irritability, anxiety, and depression) or physical
(swelling and pain in breasts, joints, and genitals; headaches; fatigue; di-
arrhea; and weight gain), range from mild to severe. About one-third to
one-half of all adult women—some 10 million to 40 million—experience
mild to moderate PMS symptoms. Approximately 5 percent experience
symptoms so severe that they are incapacitating (Semler 1985). Biomedical researchers are not certain of the causes of PMS, although hormonal
fluctuations are generally implicated. Until recently pharmaceutical treatments were singularly ineffective; today, the serotonin-reuptake inhibitor
class of antidepressants, mainly Prozac (fluoxetine), is effective for a sizable percentage of women with severe PMS.

   In designing a mind-body intervention for PMS, Domar and her colleagues considered the role of stress in exacerbating the condition. A pos-

274   sible explanation for this stress-related worsening of symptoms is the increased sensitivity of women to adrenal stress hormones in the days prior to their periods (Collins et al. 1985). One such neurohormone, noradrenaline, may in particular be implicated because it has been associated with the emotional states common to PMS, namely, anxiety, anger, and irritability. Further, research has shown that sensitivity to noradrenaline can be reduced by the *relaxation response* (Hoffman et al. 1982), Herbert Benson's well-known term for our capacity, using certain meditative-like techniques, to becalm a wide range of physiological responses (including blood pressure, heart rate, brain wave activity, skin conductance, and muscle tension). Domar reasoned that the relaxation response, partly by reducing sensitivity to noradrenaline, might also alleviate the symptoms of PMS.

In collaboration with her late colleague Irene Goodale, Ph.D., Domar tested her hypothesis in a five-month study of forty-six women with diagnosed PMS (Goodale et al. 1990). The women were randomly assigned to three groups. All three groups carefully charted their symptoms throughout their menstrual cycle. One group did only that; a second group also read leisure materials twice a day; and the third group, the experimental subjects, used audiotapes to elicit the relaxation response twice a day.

Goodale and Domar found that women practicing relaxation showed significantly greater improvement in physical symptoms than did the women in the charting only and the reading groups. Women with severe PMS in the relaxation group also experienced marked improvement in psychological symptoms and became less socially withdrawn, while comparable changes did not occur among women with severe PMS in the two control groups. Women with severe PMS who practiced relaxation showed a 58 percent improvement in all PMS symptoms, compared with a 27 percent improvement in the reading group and a 17 percent improvement in the charting group.

Significantly, the 58 percent improvement among women practicing relaxation is as good as or better than the results seen in most studies of Prozac for serious PMS. A 1995 report in the *New England Journal of Medicine*, considered a watershed study, used three different measures of PMS symptoms and two different dosages of Prozac and concluded that patients with severe symptoms experienced, on average, a 39–52 percent reduction in symptoms with Prozac (Steiner et al. 1995).

It is hard to compare the results of Goodale and Domar's one study, which is avowedly rather small, to the many Prozac studies that have been published. (It should be noted that at least a few of the Prozac studies have produced results far less favorable than those reported in the *New England Journal of Medicine*.) But the methodology employed by Goodale and

Domar has not been questioned, and the positive results suggest that the inexpensive and completely safe treatment of eliciting the relaxation response can improve severe symptoms of a condition that disables countless women. PMS is often the source of jokes, but it is no laughing matter to women whose lives are disrupted. Goodale and Domar's work should be replicated because a safe and effective first-line therapy eliminates the problem of serious side effects that affect a subset of people on Prozac, and it would save millions, if not billions, in healthcare outlays.

Indeed, the current recommendation of physicians and gynecologists for women with severe PMS is to take Prozac *continuously,* not just during the late luteal phase, to avoid symptoms prior to their periods. This continuous regimen is necessary because it takes at least two weeks for Prozac to achieve a level of efficacy, yet the question remains, Does it make sense for women who are not otherwise depressed to live their lives on Prozac in order to treat symptoms that strike for less than a week each month? The answer may be yes for women with utterly incapacitating symptoms, but is it yes for *all* women with severe PMS, especially when a viable alternative exists?

For now it would seem prudent to recommend that women with mild to moderate symptoms practice relaxation twice each day as a first-line approach for PMS. Domar makes the same recommendation to women with severe PMS, with a commonsense caveat: if your symptoms do not abate, you can always start taking Prozac. This approach upholds the medical dictum found in the writings of Hippocrates, "First, do no harm."

MENOPAUSAL SYMPTOMS

Over the past decade there has been a shift in cultural attitudes toward menopause. No longer a silent passage, it has become one that invites expression; it is talked about, analyzed, alternately feared and embraced. Although the negative attitudes about menopause are waning, the cultural outbreak of talk and media stories has yet to exorcise fully our view of "the change" as a time of energetic, emotional, and sexual decline. Such cultural attitudes and the psychosocial stress they create may also have medical consequences, exacerbating the symptoms associated with menopause.

Perhaps the most vexing menopausal symptoms are hot flashes, intermittent sensations of roiling heat. Approximately 75 percent of postmenopausal women are beset by hot flashes, which can hamper quality of life by causing social embarrassment, sleeplessness, and depression. (The depression is sometimes the result of sleeplessness rather than estrogen loss.) Stress is so often cited as a trigger for hot flashes that even main-

276   stream gynecologists seem to accept that daily pressures, hassles, intense emotions, or psychological traumas contribute to the frequency and intensity of these episodes. At least one study supports this long-held belief (Swartzman et al. 1990).

The usual conventional treatment for hot flashes (and other menopausal symptoms) is the introduction of oral or transdermal estrogen and progesterone after the onset of menopause—hormone replacement therapy, or HRT. (Natural therapies, including some herbs, may also be of some benefit for hot flashes.) The publication of numerous studies in the past several years has cast serious doubts on the safety of HRT, so the search for viable alternatives has intensified.

Several years after studying the use of the relaxation response in alleviating PMS, Domar joined with Judy Irvin, Ph.D., to test the possible benefits of the response for women with severe menopausal hot flashes (Irvin et al. 1996). Thirty-three women, aged forty-four to sixty-six, were placed into one of three groups: the first group practiced relaxation using audiotapes every day for seven weeks; the second read leisure materials; and the third simply recorded their hot flashes. All three groups kept careful records of their symptoms. Women practicing relaxation experienced a statistically significant (28%) decrease in the intensity of their hot flashes, while no such decrease occurred in women in the two control groups. The women in the relaxation group also experienced a significant decline in depression and feelings of dejection, a decline that again was not observed in the control groups. Finally, the frequency of hot flashes dropped among women practicing relaxation and not among women in the control groups, but not at a statistically significant level. Three other studies, however, have shown a significant drop in frequency using the relaxation response. A study at Wayne State University in Detroit showed a 70 percent reduction in hot flash frequency (Germaine and Freedman 1984); a study at the Lafayette Clinic, also in Detroit, showed a 40 percent drop (Freedman and Woodward 1992); and a study at Eastern Michigan State University showed a 70 percent reduction (Stevenson and Delprato 1983).

Domar has further observed in her group and in individual practice that women who not only practice relaxation but also follow a comprehensive mind-body program, including cognitive restructuring, emotional expression, and social support, experience even better results, with a reduction in both intensity and frequency of hot flashes and a marked improvement in mood (Domar and Dreher 1996). (Irvin and Domar limited their study to relaxation because of the age-old methodological problem in intervention studies: when you include too many treatments in a "package," it becomes impossible to differentiate the healing properties of each component.)

Domar and Irvin's findings, then, strongly suggest a viable, reasonably effective, and safe alternative to HRT as the exclusive treatment for hot flashes (and other menopausal symptoms). The emphasis here is on *safe.* The questions and controversies regarding the suitability and safety of HRT for all women are beyond the scope of this chapter, but there is no doubt that significant numbers of women cannot or should not take supplemental estrogen to control menopausal symptoms, primarily because HRT may increase the risk for breast cancer after approximately five years of use. The data on the risks of HRT are now overwhelming; its efficacy in preventing heart disease is uncertain, and physicians and gynecologists are becoming increasingly cautious about recommending HRT for all women, not just those with a family history of breast cancer.

Thus, women with known genetic or other risk factors for breast cancer and many others concerned about risks may be left to suffer with debilitating psychological and physical symptoms when they choose to avoid HRT and its potential pitfalls. But there is no risk with relaxation techniques. The techniques also yield benefits that may not occur with HRT, such as a renewed sense of control over one's physiological and emotional states during a time of profound psychophysical transformation.

Relaxation and the other mind–body methods that Domar uses (which have not been studied in controlled trials) are not merely alternatives to HRT. They also can be used in conjunction with HRT to improve symptomatic relief and to enhance coping since estrogen replacement alone is not effective for all women and is not always fully effective. Domar has found that cognitive restructuring enables women to ward off the inimical cultural mind-set of menopause as a time of decline, a mind-set that causes anxiety and depression regardless of whether hormonal fluctuations are severe. Emotional expression and coping skills are also needed to help women adapt to the social upheaval so common during this stage of life, as children leave the home, aging parents require caretaking, and grief attends inevitable losses at midlife.

INFERTILITY

Today one in six couples—15 percent—are infertile. And among many of these couples infertility reaps an enormous toll. They suffer not only from childlessness but also from an emotional roller-coaster ride of high-tech medical treatments. It is a ride of rising expectations and dashed hopes, and it often leaves couples financially depleted and emotionally ex-

278   hausted. In a study conducted with Patricia Zuttermeister, M.A., and
Robert Friedman, Ph.D., Alice Domar showed that infertile women had
depression scores that were indistinguishable from those of patients with
cancer, heart disease, hypertension, or HIV (Domar et al. 1993). The only
group of medical patients with significantly higher depression scores were
those with chronic pain.

A small but intriguing body of research has linked stress and depression with tubal spasms or hormonal fluctuations that can cause infertility
(Domar and Dreher 1996). (There is also the putative relationship, mentioned above, between psychological factors, hormonal imbalances, and a
glitch in the immune privilege "granted" to the embryo, a glitch that allows the immune system to interfere with implantation [Marchetti et al.
2001].) In the past decade depression has eclipsed stress or anxiety as a factor likely to contribute to disruptions in reproductive processes. In one
study, women with a history of depression were nearly twice as likely to
report a subsequent history of infertility (Lapane et al. 1995), and two
studies have shown that depressed women undergoing in vitro fertilization had significantly lower pregnancy rates (Demyttenaere et al. 1998;
Thiering et al. 1993). Based on this work, as well as a few small intervention studies with positive outcomes, in 1987 Domar developed a ten-week
Mind-Body Program for Infertility, which included relaxation techniques,
cognitive therapy, emotional-expression exercises, self-nurturance, couples' communication, and group support, with a special emphasis on em-
bracing the potential for joy and meaning in daily life (Domar et al. 1990).
To achieve this end, Domar encouraged her patients to let the groups become a refuge from painful preoccupations with getting pregnant, to view
the mind-body skills not as a new way to get pregnant but as a way off the
emotional roller coaster of high hopes and grave disappointments. Domar
did not discourage patients from continuing medical treatments for fertility; rather, she encouraged them to restructure their cognitive and emotional responses to the ongoing experience of treatment.

In two separate studies with a total population of 106 women with unexplained infertility, Domar demonstrated that this ten-week program significantly reduced depression, anxiety, and distress among infertile women
(Domar et al. 1990; Domar et al. 1992). On average, the women had been
struggling with infertility, including the rigors of high-tech medical treatments, for 3.5 years. The primary purpose of the two studies was to see
whether the intervention reduced distress, and both studies showed that
patients experienced meaningful reductions in depression and anxiety. But
Domar also found that one-third of the women had become pregnant
within six months of completing the program (Domar et al. 1990; Domar

et al. 1992). Domar has now tabulated results from 284 participants in her program, who have averaged three years of struggle with infertility (Domar and Dreher 1996; Domar et al. 1999). Overall, 42 percent of the women became pregnant within six months, and a total of 36 percent went on to give birth. Those who conceived had not used significantly more medical fertility treatments than those who did not.

Without a control group, these findings could not carry the claim that mind-body medicine definitely improves the odds of conception for infertile women. However, Domar's hunch that the pregnancy rate was unusually high was supported by a study conducted at McMaster University, in Hamilton, Ontario, and at the University of British Columbia in Vancouver (Collins and Rowe 1989). Among a similar group of infertile women who did not participate in a mind-body program only 18 percent conceived within a six-month period. Based on this comparison and on her clinical instincts, Domar suspected that her psychological treatment was having a biological effect, which seemed to support the controversial notion that emotional states were involved in many cases of unexplained infertility.

Searching for clues about the stress-infertility connection and the seeming benefits of her treatment, Domar reviewed her data and found what at first glance appeared counterintuitive. Women with higher depression scores at the start of the Mind-Body Program were significantly more likely to get pregnant after the program than women with low depression scores at the start. Among 132 women who initially scored high on the Beck Depression Inventory, a sensitive measure of depression, a remarkably high 60 percent became pregnant within 6 months, compared with a 24 percent viable pregnancy rate in women who were not depressed when they began the program ($p < .035$) (Domar et al. 1999).

Why would women who were *more* depressed at the outset be more likely to conceive? To Domar the finding suggested that depression, through an influence on reproductive hormone balance, may indeed have contributed to infertility through psychobiological mechanisms (including those mentioned above). The depressed women were most likely to conceive, in her view, because they were most likely to benefit from the program, which she repeatedly demonstrated could *reduce* depression dramatically among participants. Put differently, these depressed women, unable to conceive and becoming increasingly depressed as a result, entered the Mind-Body Program and reclaimed their sense of control and their capacity for relaxation and pleasure, and a sizable majority became pregnant within a short time span. Many still needed medical treatment, but such treatment had previously failed to reverse their infertility.

280   Domar's first two published studies, in which a third of the women in her program became pregnant within six months, spurred interest in a randomized clinical trial that would provide a more definitive answer to the question, Can mind–body treatments improve the odds that infertile women will bear children? In the mid-1990s Domar received a five-year grant from the National Institute of Mental Health to compare the psychological results and pregnancy rates among women in her Mind–Body Program for Infertility, in a standard support group, and in a control group. The final results were published in 2000 in the leading journal in the field, *Fertility and Sterility* (Domar et al. 2000).

Participants in the study were 184 women who had been trying to conceive for one to two years; they were randomized into one of three groups: (1) Domar's 10–week, multimodal Mind–Body Program; (2) a standard support group for infertility patients; and (3) a routine-care control group. Sixty-four women dropped out, the majority from the control groups because they wished to be part of a psychosocial intervention. The final analysis included 47 women in the mind–body program, 48 in the support group, and 25 in the control group. At the end of the year-long study, 55 percent of the Mind–Body Program participants and 54 percent of the support group participants experienced a viable pregnancy, compared with only 20 percent of the controls (Domar et al. 2000). The pregnancy rate among the mind–body participants was significantly higher than the rate among the controls ($p = .001$); the same held true for the support group participants ($p = .0146$). There was no significant difference between the pregnancy rates for the mind–body and support group participants.

Domar and her colleagues presented evidence that the number of dropouts did not compromise the validity of their data (Domar et al. 2000). They also showed no differences between the groups with regard to medical therapy for infertility; the intervention groups did not use more high-tech fertility treatments than the controls. In fact, Domar compared the percentage of patients in each group who got pregnant spontaneously, without any medical therapy. Her finding was not statistically significant, but it was intriguing: among the mind–body participants, 42 percent of the pregnancies resulted from spontaneous conception, compared with 11 percent and 20 percent in the support and control groups, respectively.

The overall findings validated Domar's hypothesis that patients in psychosocial intervention programs would do better than controls, though she had also theorized that mind–body participants would do better than the support group members. She believes that women dealing with infertility for a longer time frame—like the subjects in her earlier studies, who had been struggling with infertility for more than three years—would display more depression, and since the mind-body program is tailored to relieve depression, she surmises that a study of this population might favor her program over support groups with regard to pregnancy rates.

Domar's study suggests that psychosocial interventions, whether of the mind-body or support-group variety, can improve pregnancy rates among infertile women. If her finding can be repeated, the ramifications for fertility medicine, the healthcare system, and suffering patients would be momentous: they would include a humanization of this branch of medicine, incalculable cost savings, and less prolonged misery for countless couples.

Domar's work at Harvard Medical School's Division of Behavioral Medicine underscores the potential of mind-body medicine for women. The mind and the reproductive system are as intertwined as the mind and the immune system, which is why targeted psychosocial interventions appear to have salutary physical effects on women with PMS, menopausal symptoms, and infertility. Replications of Domar's work are badly needed, but I cannot help pondering the response of the biomedical establishment if early clinical trials of a pharmaceutical agent had produced results similar to Domar's. How long would it take for the corporate funding gears to be set in motion? How lavish would the expenditures be for research and development?

While the benign neglect of behavioral-medicine treatments for women is no conspiracy, it may be related to the fact that there is no private-sector advantage to broad-scale applications. If anything, effective mind-body treatments could mean reduced reliance on pharmaceutical solutions for a range of conditions. Fewer women might have to depend on Prozac to treat PMS and HRT to treat hot flashes, and fewer cycles of hormonal drugs and exorbitantly expensive in vitro technologies might be needed for infertile couples. All of these pharmaceutical and high-tech strategies are marvelous for women who genuinely need them, but what if many fewer women genuinely needed them? These are not questions that the biomedical establishment or even the mind-body research community is facing head-on. And the same questions apply to other conditions that affect women in ways that are different from men, such as heart disease, breast cancer, and autoimmune diseases, to name only the most conspicuous examples.

A clear strategy is hard to map out, but the responsibility for change should be shared equally by public and private biomedical funding institutions that have been overly skeptical about mind-body treatments, as well as the mind-body medicine community itself, which has also given short shrift to women's health. One place to start would be the replication

282 and expansion of studies that have already hinted at the vast promise of mind-body medicine for women.

REFERENCES

Altman R. 1996. *The Politics of Breast Cancer.* New York: Little, Brown.

Bernton EW, Bryant HU, Holaday JW. 1991. Prolactin and immune function. In: Ader R, Felton DL, Cohen N, eds. *Psychoneuroimmunology II.* New York: Academic Press.

Collins A, Enroth P, Landren B. 1985. Psychoneuroendocrine stress responses and mood as related to the menstrual cycle. *Psychosom Med.* 47:512–527.

Collins J, Rowe T. 1989. Age of the female partner is a prognostic factor in prolonged unexplained infertility: a multicancer study. *Fertil Steril.* 52:15–20.

Demyttenaere K, Bonte L, Ghelof M, et al. 1998. Coping style and depression level influence outcome in in vitro fertilization. *Fertil Steril.* 69:1026–1033.

Domar AD, Seibel M, Benson H. 1990. The mind-body program for infertility: a new behavioral treatment approach for women with infertility. *Fertil Steril.* 53:246–249.

Domar AD, Zuttermeister P, Friedman R. 1993. The psychological impact of infertility: a comparison with patients With other medical conditions. *J Psychosom Obstet Gynaecol.* 14:45–52.

Domar AD, Zuttermeister P, Seibel M, Benson H. 1992. Psychological improvement in infertile women following behavioral treatment: a replication. *Fertil Steril.* 58:144–147.

Domar AD, Clapp D, Slawsby EA, Dusek J, Kessel B, Freizinger M. 2000. Impact of group psychological interventions on pregnancy rates in infertile women. *Fertil Steril.* 73:805–811.

Domar AD, Dreher H. 1996. *Healing Mind, Healthy Woman.* New York: Henry Holt & Co.

Domar AD, Dreher H. 2000. *Self-Nurture: Learning to Care for Yourself As Effectively As You Care for Everyone Else.* New York: Viking Press.

Domar AD, Friedman R, Zuttermeister PC. 1999. Distress and conception in infertile women: a complementary approach. *J Am Med Womens Assoc.* 54:196–198.

Frasure-Smith N, Lesperance F, Prince RH, et al. 1997. Randomised trial of home-based psychosocial nursing intervention for patients recovering from myocardial infarction. *Lancet.* 350:473–479.

Frasure-Smith N, Lesperance F, Talajic M. 1993. Depression following myocardial infaction: impact on six-month survival. *JAMA.* 270:1819–1825.

Freedman RR, Woodward S. 1992. Behavioral treatment of menopausal hot flashes: evaluation by ambulatory monitoring. *Am J Obstet Gynecol.* 167:436–439.

Germaine LM, Freedman RR. 1984. Behavioral treatment of menopausal hot flashes: evaluation by objective methods. *J Consult Clin Psychol.* 52:1072–1079.

Goodale, I, Domar AD, Benson H. 1990. Alleviation of premenstrual symptoms with the relaxation response. *Obstet Gynecol.* 75:649–655.

Greer S, Morris T, Pettingale KW, Haybrittle J. 1990. Psychological response to breast cancer and fifteen-year outcome. *Lancet.* 1:49–50.

Hoffman JW, Benson H, Arns PA, et al. 1982. Reduced sympathetic nervous system responsivity associated with the relaxation response. *Science.* 215:190–192.

Irvin JH, Domar AD, Clark C, Zuttermeister PC, Friedman R. 1996. The effects of relaxation response training on menopausal symptoms. *J Psychosom Obstet Gynaecol.* 17:202–207.

Klaiber EL. 2001. *Hormones and the Mind: A Woman's Guide to Mood, Mental Sharpness, and Sexual Vitality.* New York: HarperCollins.

Kronenberg F, Cote LJ, Linkie DM, Dyrenfurth I, Downey JA. 1984. Menopausal hot flashes: thermoregulatory, cardiovascular, and circulating catecholamine and LH changes. *Maturitas.* 6:31–43.

Lapane KL, Zierler S, Lasater TM, et al. 1995. Is a history of depressive symptoms associated with an increased risk of infertility in women? *Psychosom Med.* 57:509–513.

Levy SM, Herberman RB, Lipman M, D'Angelo T. 1987. Correlation of stress factors with sustained depression of natural killer cell activity with predicted prognosis in patients with breast cancer. *J Clin Oncol.* 5:348–353.

Levy SM, Herberman RB, Whiteside T, et al. 1990. Perceived social support and tumor estrogen/progesterone receptor status as predictors of natural killer cell activity in breast cancer patients. *Psychosom Med.* 52:78–85.

Marchetti B, Morake MC, Gallo F, et al. 2001. The hypothalamo-pituitary-gonadal axis and the immune system. In: Ader R, Felten DL, Cohen N, eds. *Psychoneuroimmunology.* 3rd ed. Vol. 1. San Diego, Calif: Academic Press; 363–390.

McCruden AB, Stimson WH. 1991. Sex hormones and immune function. In: Ader R, Felten DL, Cohen N, eds. *Psychoneuroimmunology,* 2nd ed. New York: Academic Press; 475–488.

McEwen BS. 1998. Multiple ovarian hormone effects on brain structure and function. *J Gend Specif Med.* 1:33–41.

Peiffer A, Morale MC, Barden N, Marchetti B. 1994. Modulation of glucocorticoid receptor gene expression in the thymus by the sex steroid hormone milieu and correlation with sexual dimorphism of immune response. *Endocrine J.* 2:181–191.

Rogers MP, Brooks EB. 2001. Psychosocial influences, immune function, and the progression of autoimmune disease. In: Ader R, Felten DL, Cohen N, eds. *Psychoneuroimmunology.* 3rd ed. Vol. 2. San Diego, Calif: Academic Press; 399–419.

Rosenman RH, Brand RJ, Jenkins CD, et al. 1975. Coronary heart disease in the Western Collaborative Group Study: final follow-up experience of eight-and-one-half years. *JAMA.* 223:872–877.

Semler TC. 1985. *The Complete Guide to Women's Health and Well-Being.* New York: HarperCollins.

Spiegel D, Bloom J, Kraemer HC, Gottheil E. 1989. Effect of psychosocial treatment on survival of patients with metastatic breast cancer. *Lancet.* 2:888–891.

Stanton AL. 1995. Psychology of women's health: barriers and pathways to knowl-

284   edge. In: Stanton AL, Gallant SJ, eds. *The Psychology of Women's Health.* Washington, D.C.: American Psychological Association.

Steering Committee of the Physicians' Health Study Research Group. 1988. Preliminary report: findings from the aspirin component on the ongoing physician's health study. *New Engl J Med.* 316:262–264.

Steiner M et al. 1995. Fluoxetine in the treatment of premenstrual dysphoria. *New Engl J. Med.* 332:1529–1534.

Stevenson DW, Delprato DJ. 1983. Multiple component self-control program for menopausal hot flashes. *J Behav Ther Exper Psychiatry.* 14:137–140.

Swartzman LC, Edelberg CR, Kemmann E. 1990. Impact of stress on objectivity recorded menopausal hot flashes on flush report bias. *Health Psychol.* 9:529–545.

Temoshok L, Dreher H. 1992. *The Type C Connection: The Behavioral Links to Cancer and Your Health.* New York: Random House.

Thiering P, Beaurepaire J, Jones M, et al. 1993. Mood state as a predictor of treatment outcome after in vitro fertilization/embryo transfer technology (IVF/ET). *J Psychosom Res.* 37:481–491.

Watson M, Haviland JS, Greer S, Davidson J, Bliss JM. 1999. Influence of psychological response on survival in breast cancer: a population-based cohort study. *Lancet.* 354:1331–1336.

Wilder RL, Elenkov IJ. 2001. Ovarian and sympathoadrenal hormones, pregnancy, and autoimmune diseases. In: Ader R, Felten DL, Cohen N, eds. *Psychoneuroimmunology.* 3rd ed. Vol. 2. San Diego, Calif: Academic Press; 421–431.

Williams R. 1993. Hostility and the heart. In: Goleman D, Gurin J, eds. *Mind–Body Medicine: How to Use Your Mind for Better Health.* Yonkers, NY: Consumer Report Books.

Chapter 8

Somatization:

Secrets Disclosed to the Body

The syndrome is all too familiar: patients who present physical complaints or disorders for which there are no clear causes, leaving them and their physicians in a state of confusion and even helplessness. When initial tests reveal no organic disease or overt pathophysiology, the frustrated doctor and patient begin a high-tech fishing expedition. Further tests are no more fruitful, except that they rule out a list of possible organic causes. What is left? A clinical entity called *somatization disorder*, which is considered one of the *somatoform disorders*, also known as psychosomatic illness. These terms refer to physical conditions that are not imagined (as in hypochondriasis) but are clearly caused or exacerbated by psychosocial factors.

Theories about somatization depend on who is doing the theorizing. Freudians and neo-Freudians believe that somatizers transduce repressed ideas or emotions into bodily symptoms, a process also know as *conversion disorder*. Behaviorists believe that somatizers' illness behaviors are learned in childhood or later. Cognitive psychologists blame anxiety disorders caused by distorted thought processes. But the different schools share a broad definition: somatization disorders are characterized by numerous physical complaints without an evident organic basis. Physical pathologies may underlie the symptoms, but they are not easily traced or readily perceived. Psychological factors are taken to be the fundamental cause, but how to establish this in a given case and how to then treat the disorder are problems that seem beyond the ken of physiological biomedicine.

By several estimates, somatization accounts for at least 50 percent of

Reprinted by permission, with changes, from *Advances in Mind-Body Medicine* 12 (1996): 50–57.

286   patients seen in primary care medicine (DeGruy et al. 1987; Roberts 1994).
Family medicine researchers have identified somatization disorder as the
fourth most common diagnosis encountered in primary care, placing it
ahead of ischemic heart disease, diabetes, obesity, urinary tract infections,
and the common middle-ear disease of childhood, otitis media (DeGruy
et al. 1987). Nearly two decades ago an article in the *Journal of the American Medical Association* described somatization as "one of medicine's blind
spots" (Quill 1985). About the same time, an editorial in *Psychosomatics*
described it as "medicine's unsolved problem" (Lipowski 1987). While
mainstream medicine appears to recognize the scope of the problem, clinicians still get caught in the bind of ordering tests and treatments that
usually fail to identify or address the condition's underlying causes.

The costs of such disorders can hardly be calculated. Consider the bills
accumulated for the increasingly expensive medical tests that fruitlessly
search for organic causes. How many patients with chronic headaches, for
example, are given magnetic resonance imagery (MRI) tests to rule out
brain tumors when psychosocial factors are the real (and sometimes fairly
evident) root causes? Consider also that a variety of conditions that can
have organic origins are, more typically, the result of somatization. These
conditions include irritable bowel syndrome, primary hypertension,
chronic pain, Raynaud's disease, and food allergies, to name a few (Wickramasekera et al. 1996). Other disorders with organic components or infectious origins may also have psychosomatic contributors, such as ulcers,
asthma, and autoimmune disorders. Finally, life-threatening diseases such
as cancer or ischemic heart disease may not be directly caused by somatization, but their progression may be influenced by psychosocial factors
(Temoshok and Dreher 1992; Williams 1989).

A concerted effort to understand, diagnose, and treat somatization disorder would certainly reap copious benefits in improved patient care and
reduced healthcare costs. Yet most biomedical practitioners remain so ignorant of (or resistant to) psychosocial diagnosis and intervention that little
is being done to rectify this situation. Of course, the biomedical model itself does not lend itself to a psychosocial approach, and efforts in behavioral-medicine research, psychophysiology, and psychoneuroimmunology
have yet to be sufficiently integrated into the mainstream to make a major
impact on attitudes and practices. Malpractice jitters also account for part
of the problem. If doctors began actively searching for psychosocial causes
without ruling out every organic possibility, the occasional instances of undetected organic disease would trigger lawsuits—and further erode the respectability of biopsychosocial investigations.

What is needed is a rigorous and reproducible procedure for diagnosing and treating somatization disorder. If at a relatively early stage in the course of doctor-patient interaction, somatization could be ruled *in* rather than left as a grab-bag diagnosis of last resort, doctors could save time, the healthcare system could save money, and patients could save themselves from undue, chronic suffering. With due respect for the realistic possibilities of organic disease and the concurrent use of needed diagnostic procedures, tragic mistakes could be avoided. More to the point, successful early psychosocial intervention would prevent the costly high-tech fishing expeditions that often leaves patients floundering in deeper and deeper waters.

Ian Wickramasekera's High Risk Model

For more than two decades the psychologist Ian Wickramasekera, currently a visiting professor at both the Saybrook Institute and Stanford University Medical School, has been developing a psychosocial method and a model to diagnose and treat somatic disorders. He has devised a series of tests that, according to his model, identify somatizers, and he has constructed a clinical method custom-tailored to their conditions. Although Wickramasekera's clinical approach is given the familiar tag *applied psychophysiology*, commonly used to describe mind-body treatments involving biofeedback, aspects of his therapy go well beyond standard biofeedback and are uniquely designed to address the underlying causes of somatization.

Wickramasekera described his approach in an article written with two family practitioners, Terence E. Davies and S. Margaret Davies, "Applied Psychophysiology: A Bridge between the Biomedical Model and the Biopsychosocial Model in Family Medicine" (Wickramasekera et al. 1996), published in an issue of *Professional Psychology: Research and Practice* that had a special section on applied psychophysiology. (Other articles highlighted the efficacy of applied psychophysiology, including biofeedback as well as cognitive-behavioral therapies, in the treatment of disorders such as irritable bowel syndrome [Whitehead and Drossman 1996] and several disorders of elimination [Blanchard and Malamood 1996].) Wickramasekera's work is notable for two reasons. Firstly, if his diagnostic approach proves reliable and replicable, he will have solved the riddle of how to expeditiously ferret out somatizers from people with organic disease or outright mental illness. Secondly, he has developed a mind-body treatment method for somatization, which he calls *psychophysiologic psychotherapy*, that is arguably more targeted and more refined than previous efforts. If further studies confirm that it is both effective and teachable, he will have contributed a therapy that can simultaneously ease the suffering of countless patients with chronic ailments and save billions of healthcare dollars. Psychophysiologic psychotherapy, which Wickramasekera first developed as a professor in the Departments of Psychiatry and Family Medicine at Eastern Virginia Medical School, is designed to overcome the somatizers' typical resistance to psychotherapy. It is a resistance that is normally stiffened by doctors or therapists who reinforce the invidious message that somatizers' symptoms are either "all in their heads" or proof of mental illness.

In Wickramasekera's view, somatizers are people who tend to block from consciousness any perception of emotional threat or, put differently, who repress distressing emotional states and memories until they are utterly unaware of them. (These are common psychic defenses and personality traits, not mental illnesses per se.) The perception of threat, whether past or present, and the associated thoughts, memories, and emotions (such as fear, grief, and anger) become sequestered from consciousness. But these banished thoughts and feelings drive bodily symptoms through mind-body channels, causing perturbations in the autonomic nervous system and the networks it helps regulate, including the cardiovascular and immune systems. According to his theory, when people block the perception of threat, they are susceptible, on the physical level, to "autonomic dysregulation." The threatening thoughts and emotions are "secrets kept from the mind but not from the body" (Wickramasekera 1999).

That is why special tests are needed to identify somatizers. It has long been noted by a number of experts in emotion and consciousness that a subset of individuals who appear "normal," even on standardized psychological tests, are in fact distressed. These individuals, who employ so-called repressive coping as a habitual mode of handling stress or trauma, can be detected only when standardized tests are combined in tricky ways to unmask their veiled, unconscious tendency to squelch authentic emotions (Schwartz 1990; Weinberger et al. 1979). These individuals can also be identified through psychophysiological testing. In this procedure the person's vital signs (like blood pressure, heart rate, and skin conductance) spike upwards (indicating physiological arousal) when he or she is exposed to upsetting emotional stimuli, even though he or she simultaneously reports feeling no pain, anxiety, or sadness and claims to be imperturbably calm (Kneier and Tomoshok 1984; Schwartz 1990).

Wickramasekera approaches this "unmasking" process from a somewhat different perspective. He claims, first of all, that people who score either very high or very low in "hypnotizability" have a higher than usual risk for somatization. (He measures a person's ability to respond to hypnotic induction with the Harvard Group Scale of Hypnotic Ability [Shor and Orne 1962].) He goes on to argue that the highest risk for somatization occurs in highly hypnotizable people who also score high in a category he calls *negative affectivity* (Wickramasekera 1999).

What is the import of hypnotizability and so-called negative affectivity to the understanding of somatizers and their suffering? People who are hypnotizable are highly suggestible but also creative and exquisitely sensitive, Wickramasekera said in a recent interview with me (May 1996). He likens such people to the princess in the Hans Christian Andersen tale *The Princess and the Pea,* who can feel the pea in her bed no matter how many mattresses it is buried under. But this very sensitivity—a talent in many circumstances—prompts and enables many of the people who possess it to adeptly "keep secrets from themselves." They are so sensitive to discomfort that they have learned to shift states of consciousness to quickly blot out unpleasant sensations and feelings. Wickramasekera points to evidence that highly hypnotizable people often report feeling no pain during surgery even though physiological monitors demonstrate levels of activation commensurate with the experience of pain. "They unconsciously use their abilities to exclude or block things from consciousness," said Wickramasekera. This makes the somatizer something of a paradox: he is so intrinsically open to painful stimuli that he has developed the ability to slam shut his emotional and sensory window.

But not all highly hypnotizable people are repressors who also somatize. According to Wickramasekera, the ones to be concerned about are those who demonstrate high negative affectivity, a tendency to chronically experience negative emotions such as fear, anxiety, anger, or jealousy even when there is no real-world trigger for such intense feelings. "The important point is that such individuals don't need anything stressful to happen to them to be in that negative state."

Put simply, the person with high hypnotic ability will not be a repressor or a somatizer unless beset by disturbing and persistent negative emotions that he or she needs to shunt into bodily symptoms. In the absence of so-called negative affectivity, the hypnotizable person may simply be open, creative, suggestible, empathic, and capable of shifts in consciousness. Indeed, he or she may be healthy in mind and body. However, with high levels of negative affectivity, such people have reasons to use their ability to "block things from consciousness," Wickramasekera told me.

Negative affectivity can take many forms, and Wickramasekera measures this tendency with tests of *overt* or *covert neuroticism* (Wickramasekera 1999). *Overt neuroticism* generally refers to consciously experienced negative affect that is not well integrated, expressed, or resolved; while *covert neuroticism* is another term for repression, or the presence of nega-

290   tive affect that has been pushed underground. (Wickramasekera uses the Eysenck Personality Inventory [Eysenck and Eysenck 1968] to detect overt and covert neuroticism, and the Marlowe-Crowne Social Desirability Scale, which taps the tendency to maintain a socially desirable front at all costs, as a further test of covert neuroticism.) Wickramasekera claims that in a person with high hypnotic ability, neuroticism, whether overt or covert, is a prescription for somatic complaints that cannot be cured until the person comes to grips with subterranean states of mind.

In a different way, low hypnotizability and negative affect are also major risks for somatization. People with these traits are individuals whose lack of suggestibility may be associated with less sensitivity, a blunting of intuitive and emotional awareness. Such individuals, says Wickramasekera, tend to be skeptics, critics, analytic thinkers. They are not likely to accept the notion that emotions or psychosocial factors have anything to do with their symptoms. In an unpublished study now under review, Wickramasekera evaluated a group of eighty individuals suffering from morbid obesity who were seeking medical management for their condition—restrictive diets, medications, or surgery. He predicted that a higher than normal percentage would not be hypnotizable, and his hypothesis was borne out. In a general population, roughly 10 percent would score very low in hypnotizability; in this obese population 68 percent scored very low. Wickramasekera reached his conclusion because these individuals were not seeking psychotherapy or support; instead, they were seeking medical treatments to solve a problem that is frequently associated with emotional factors. In other words, they displayed a limited emotional awareness, which is consistent, in his view, with low hypnotizability.

The Nine Key Factors in Somatization

Although the tests for hypnotizability and overt and covert neuroticism represent the core of Wickramasekera's "unmasking" procedure for diagnosis, he also evaluates six additional risk factors. Together these nine factors, all of which he measures with standardized tests, constitute the High Risk Model of Threat Perception (Wickramasekera 1995; Wickramasekera et al. 1996). He groups the nine factors into three subcategories: predisposers, triggers, and buffers. The predisposers include hypnotic ability; both overt and covert neuroticism; and a propensity for catastrophizing, the tendency to see the world through the gloomiest possible glasses. These personality tendencies, which Wickramasekera believes are partly genetic and partly psychosocial in origin, set the person up for somatization. The triggers are factors common in stress research (Sternbach

1986; Weinberger et al. 1987): major life changes and minor hassles. The buffers—which may prevent symptoms in people disposed to somatizing—are good social support, high satisfaction with social support, and well-developed coping skills (House et al. 1988; Lazarus and Folkman 1984). Thus, Wickramasekera has constructed a multidimensional model of somatization and, more broadly, health and disease. Somatizers—which to some degree include many of us—are not simply disease-prone personalities, nor are they abject victims of stress, loneliness, or lack of education. They are complex people whose personalities, inner lives, upbringings, genetics, relationships, social opportunities, and social environments all interact to help determine whether they are likely to somatize distressing emotions into bodily symptoms.

A high score on all nine factors is not necessary to pose a risk for somatization disorder. Wickramasekera does not suggest that his model be applied in a mechanistic fashion, like the yardstick approaches in psychiatry's *Diagnostic and Statistical Manual,* with fairly arbitrary cut-off points that determines risk versus no risk. Rather, clinicians may be alerted to the possibility of somatization when a person scores high in hypnotizability and high negative affectivity. The other tests then provide useful additional data to refine risk profiles—a predisposed person who also has many triggers and few buffers will be that much more likely to somatize. According to Wickramasekera, such an individual will also be at a high risk for somatic symptoms to develop into true organic disease. In a study of seventy-eight people complaining of chronic chest pain, a colleague of Wickramasekera's found a consistent pattern of covert neuroticism along with low hypnotizability in those who developed frank cardiovascular disease (Saxon 1996).

In another study Wickramasekera (1995) provided strong evidence that his model is indeed a useful tool for identifying people at risk for somatization disorder. Eighty-three patients with previously noted chronic somatic complaints were tested on the nine factors in the High Risk Model. Thirty-two percent scored very high and 28 percent scored very low on hypnotic ability, figures that were significantly higher ($p < .05$) than those for a community control sample matched for age and sex. In addition, the patients scored significantly higher than control subjects on all of the risk factors in Wickramasekera's multidimensional model (see table 8.1).

Critics of Wickramasekera's model might argue that certain psychosocial factors would likely increase as a result of a recalcitrant symptom— that the mind-states and traits came after the symptom, not before. For example, a person struggling with severe back pain might begin to catastrophize, experience more life hassles, and lose social support. But would

TABLE 8.1

Comparison of Somatizers and Normal Subjects on High-Risk Variables for Somatization Disorder

	N	MEAN	SD	T*	DF	P
Hypnotic ability						
Patients	83	6.60	3.60			
Normals	78	4.80	3.40	2.597	119	.05
Catastrophizing						
Patients	83	37.00	12.80	—	—	—
Normals	78	31.56	8.34	9.456	118	.001
Neuroticism (NA†)						
Patients	83	18.40	5.50			
Normals	78	9.00	4.80	11.65	201	.001
Lie scale (covert NA)						
Patients	83	4.10	1.10			
Normals	78	2.10	1.20	11.00	159	.001
Major life changes						
Patients	83	668.30	70.80			
Normals	78	362.90	230.90	11.19	159	.001
Minor hassles						
Patients	83					
Number		29.30	18.60			
Intensity		1.60	.43			
Normative group	78					
Number		20.60	15.10	3.24	159	.001
Intensity		1.47	.28	2.25	157	.025
Social support						
Patients	83					
Number‡		3.40	1.60			
Satisfaction‡		5.10	.78			
Normative group	78					
Number		4.48	1.96	−3.84	159	.0001
Satisfaction		5.38	.73	−2.34	159	.020
Coping skills						
Patients	83	19.00	28.60			
Normative group	78	31.30	23.20	−2.98	159	.003

Source: Adapted from Wickramasekera 1995.
Note: Comparative results on standardized tests for Wickramasekera's nine risk factors among somatizers ($N = 83$) and normal subjects ($N = 78$). The risk for somatizers was greater on all nine factors. (For the first six factors, higher scores indicate greater risk; for the last three factors, lower scores indicate greater risk.) In the last column, the p-values of .05 or less indicate significant between-group differences in the expected direction (higher risk for somatizers) for each variable.
* Independent t-test for differences in means
† Negative affectivity
‡ Number of social support episodes and satisfaction with social support count as separate factors.

his or her scores on hypnotizability or repression change drastically? The literature of personality and psychodynamics suggests that they would not, since these traits are fairly stable over time. Moreover, the extent to which psychosocial factors *cause* a particular symptom may be of minor consequence when that condition simply cannot be traced to organic causes, is utterly recalcitrant, and is clearly *exacerbated* by psychosocial factors. (Beyond this, at a certain point ignoring emotional and social factors in the crossfire of a chicken-and-egg debate results in a denial of the needs of patients and the potential of mind-body therapies.)

One virtue of Wickramasekera's model is that it overcomes the limitations of the typical one-dimensional tests that have been used to determine whether feelings of intense stress or distress are present in people with chronic illness, usually whether negative emotions or stressful life events can be associated with the illness. As often as not, no correlation is found, and this result is taken as confirmation that the mind does not contribute to the condition. Wickramasekera and others (notably Daniel Weinberger, Gary Schwartz, and Lydia Temoshok) rightly argue that such tests are insufficiently sensitive and multidimensional to identify people whose negative affectivity is covert and who have little or no awareness of their own psychic defenses. Indeed, the "illusion of mental health" has been documented among many subjects who "pass" standard psychological tests but who are shown, through further (and more probing) psychophysical tests, to employ maladaptive defenses and harbor repressed negative emotions (Dreher 1995).

Still, for some, Wickramasekera's model might seem too complex. Are all those factors really necessary? In the mainstream medical world, we now understand that cholesterol levels are helpful, but doctors must also know the levels of HDL and LDL (high- and low-density lipoproteins), not to mention HDL-LDL ratios, homocysteine levels, and C-reactive protein tests, to fine-tune a patient's risk profile for cardiovascular disease. Nowadays, cholesterol alone is considered a crude measure of heart disease risk. If it is widely acknowledged that blood workups for cardiovascular risk must include multiple measures and that a proper panel of immune tests must include a wide variety of differential cell counts and measures of cell function, why should a comparable degree of complexity be unnecessary in tests of psychosocial factors involved in chronic illness? Are not our personalities and emotional states as layered and complex as our blood systems?

The Trojan Horse Procedure

Once Wickramasekera has evidence of somatization, he turns to another procedure that is valuable both to confirm the diagnosis of somatization and as a first phase of treatment. This procedure is called the Psychophysiologic Stress Profile, in which Wickramasekera (or another trainer) hooks the patient up to biofeedback instrumentation that measures physiological arousal by measuring skin conductance, temperature, blood volume pulse, heart rate, forehead muscle tension. The clinician keeps an eye on these channels while speaking with the patient and in various ways applying emotional pressure, for example, by conducting a mental arithmetic stress test and asking questions about upsetting subjects. When the instruments indicate that the person is physiologically aroused but the person reports little or no distress, the clinician has further evidence of repression (blocking awareness of emotional distress) and a high risk for somatization.

Wickramasekera then uses the discrepancy as a teaching tool. He shows the person the telltale graphs, which prove that the person's physiology has been drastically altered under conditions of stress even though he or she has not been aware of it.

Describing the effect of this procedure, Wickramasekera says, "That's how I get my foot in their heads," conjuring the image of the mind of the somatizer as a door that he has managed to crack open. Somatizing patients often resist psychotherapy as a sign of characterological weakness, hypochondria, or the last resort for people with severe mental illness. These attitudes may be culturally ingrained, but they are also defenses the person uses to sidestep investigation into the quarantined contents of the unconscious. It frequently takes both Wickramasekera's medical instruments and the graphic evidence they provide to convince an individual that his or her health may depend on states of mind that directly influence states of body.

Wickramasekera calls this approach his "Trojan Horse" method since he creates an elaborate procedure, practically a ruse, to convince patients to open their minds to the possibility that their conditions are largely psychosocial in origin even though they have a real biological component (Wickramasekera 1992). Wickramasekera relies on as many psychophysiological demonstrations as needed to encourage receptivity in patients, all the while developing a therapeutic alliance with them. If this alliance is rooted in empathy, Wickramasekera (or any other clinician employing his method) can present the patient with "objective" evidence of his psychological "split" in a way that gradually overcomes his reflexive defenses.

This psychophysiologic psychotherapy continues through three broad phases: (1) an educational phase, in which the person learns about mind-body connections; (2) a "coinvestigator" phase, in which the patient and the doctor search for further understanding of psychosocial contributors to the patient's condition; and (3) a psychotherapy phase, in which the cat comes out of the bag and the patient acknowledges the need for, and accepts, deeper investigations of his or her anxiety, depression, anger, or grief. As in any sound form of psychodynamic psychotherapy, these investigations go wherever they must—to family dynamics of the past or present, long-held emotional distress, traumatic memories, or conflicts and creative blocks in the present. Each phase is guided by biofeedback, which offers physiological information and hard evidence that mind and body are unified.

Clinical Success: A Woman with Multiple Somatic Complaints

In their recent paper in *Professional Psychology: Research and Practice* Wickramasekera and his colleagues (1996) offer a compelling case example of the High Risk Model and Wickramasekera's clinical methods. Susan, a forty-three-year-old married woman, came to her family physician, Terence Davies, with complaints of severe respiratory allergies, sinus infections, and terrible chronic headaches. The headaches were persistent despite treatment with narcotics. Prescription antihistamines and desensitization had not effectively controlled her food allergies, which her allergist called "the worst I had ever encountered." Davies referred her to Wickramasekera after she suffered "a classic anaphylactic reaction" to an injection of allergens, in which she developed "hives in waves from head to toe."

In her initial interview Susan was "pleasant and cooperative," and there was no evidence of psychopathology based on the standards of the *Diagnostic and Statistical Manual of Mental Disorders.* Wickramasekera tested her with the High Risk Model and found that she scored high on only two of the nine risk factors, but they were two pivotal variables: high hypnotizability and high covert neuroticism (or repression). Wickramasekera writes that these are "two of the . . . most potent mechanisms for blocking the perception of threat (negative affect) from consciousness and appeared relevant to the psychodynamics of this case." He goes on to say that "these potent cognitive blocking mechanisms may account for why all of Susan's prior clinical interviews and verbal report psychological tests . . . were free of psychopathology, producing an 'illusion of mental health.'"

Psychophysiological tests confirmed Wickramasekera's suspicions. Despite her overtly calm presentation, she had high mean levels across such parameters as skin conductance, heart rate, and forehead muscle tension,

296   all of which indicated high physiological arousal. Her temperature and blood volume pulse levels were low, which is common among tense individuals with classic psychosomatic symptoms such as functional headaches. Also relevant was her report that her hands and feet were "always cold and wet." Here was someone who exemplified Wickramasekera's clinical concept of the somatizer, a person who "hadn't the foggiest idea" that she was in a constant state of fight or flight. "Her implicit or unconscious suffering was clearly evidenced in her body by her cold and wet hands and by her multiple chronic somatic symptoms."

Although a bit of role-playing was involved in the early, Trojan Horse part of therapy, Wickramasekera moved quickly to form a therapeutic alliance with Susan based on truth-telling and trust. He explained that the test results had revealed "two cognitive mechanisms" by which she "kept secrets from herself but not from her body." He then moved to his therapeutic strategy, which could be summed up by his own phrase, "First we put out the fires, then we find the matches."

To "put out the fires," he taught Susan self-hypnosis and temperature biofeedback skills to temporarily becalm body and mind. "As she acquired an ability to physiologically self-soothe and to be less fearful, the previously unconscious, metaphorical dragons that were driving her body's red alert status stepped into consciousness," writes Wickramasekera. "As she identified her dragons and learned to deal with them more effectively, she learned not only how to put out her symptomatic fires, but also how to locate and diffuse the matches."

As Susan was able to calm herself, anxiety and anger about her troubled marriage rose to the surface. "Several suppressed or repressed traumatic marital incidents . . . emerged into consciousness. These incidents were independently documented by public record and her employer." She came to realize that her husband had control over key areas of her life, including her finances and social life. He treated her alternately "like a child" and like his mother, and there had been no intimacy between them for years. In the course of therapy she not only became aware of her anger but also developed greater self-assertion at home and at work. But it was not an easy transformation. "As her rage at her husband surfaced, she became very depressed about her marital situation." Susan was experiencing the well-known psychotherapeutic truism that things often get much worse before they can possibly get better.

"As this strong negative affect came to consciousness, her headache pain reduced," writes Wickramasekera. "Cognitive-behavioral therapy was used to treat her depression and to encourage self-care. She began to allocate more of her time and money to self-care. She became less concerned about the disapproval of her husband and coworkers. Both her allergic reactions to multiple food and environmental substances and her pain reports were reduced, in spite of the withdrawal of all allergic and analgesic medications."

Efforts to get her husband to participate in marital therapy failed, but Susan continued her own therapy process and continued to make improvements. At a follow-up seven months later psychological tests demonstrated that she "is not aware of mental distress but has less somatic stress." Two years later she reported 100 percent remission of all her allergies and somatic symptoms, increased self-confidence, and sustained high self-assertion. Wickramasekera also notes that "under further serious stress, the marriage may require professional attention."

Perhaps most intriguing, her physiological parameters at the seven-month follow-up showed marked transformations. Her skin conductance, heart rate, and forehead muscle tension dropped precipitously, while her temperature and blood volume pulse rose considerably.

The case of Susan is a good illustration of what can be accomplished in mind-body therapy with due regard for the complexities of experience and the layeredness of personality. If one accepts Wickramasekera's precepts, self-soothing alone, whether in the form of biofeedback, hypnosis, meditation, or yoga, would not have been enough to bring about such sustained changes in physiology and symptomatic improvements. Indeed, Wickramasekera strongly believes that clinical behavioral medicine has concentrated far too much on dousing fires and far too little on searching for matches.

According to Wickramasekera, one of several factors that prevent recognition of the need for sophisticated mind-body diagnosis and therapy is the "stigma of mental illness in the medical sector, which inflates the psychological distance between the primary care physician's office [and mind-body therapy] from several miles to several light years." His hope is that the empirical evidence for his model, along with his therapeutic successes, will persuade family physicians and primary care doctors to adopt at least some of his methods; to have the necessary instruments in their clinics, or in close proximity; and to utilize psychophysiological procedures to help patients accept psychosocial therapies they might otherwise avoid.

Of course, before this can happen, mainstream medicine must be willing to take a serious look at Wickramasekera's model and his data. This may take some time. To date, medicine has been afflicted by its own blinkered vision of somatization disorder—hypnotizing itself into believing that vast numbers of its patients are somehow helped by tests and treatments that all too often are as ineffective as they are shortsighted.

REFERENCES

Blanchard EB, Malamood HS. 1996. Psychological treatment of irritable bowel syndrome. *Prof Psych Res Practice.* 27:241–244.

DeGruy F, Columbia L, Dickenson P. 1987. Somatization disorder in family practice. *J Fam Pract.* 25:445–515.

Dreher H. 1995. *The Immune Power Personality: Seven Traits You Can Develop to Stay Healthy.* New York: Dutton/Signet.

Eysenck SB, Eysenck HJ. 1968. The measurement of psychoticism: a study of factor stability and reliability. *Br J Soc Clin Psychol.* 7:286–294.

House JS, Landis KR, Umberson D. 1988. Social relationships and health. *Science.* 241:540–545.

Kneier AW, Temoshok L. 1984. Repressive coping reactions in patients with malignant melanoma as compared to cardiovascular disease patients. *J Psychosom Res.* 28:145–155.

Lazarus RS, Folkman S. 1984. *Stress, Appraisal, and Coping.* New York: Springer.

Lipowski ZJ. 1987. Somatization: medicine's unsolved problem [editorial]. *Psychosomatics.* 28:294–297.

Quill TE. 1985. Somatization disorder: one of medicine's blind spots. *JAMA.* 254:3075–3079.

Roberts SJ. 1994. Somatization in primary care: the common presentation of psychosocial problems through physical complaints. *Nurse Pract.* 19:50–56.

Saxon J. 1996. Discriminating patients with organic disease from somatizers among patients with chest discomfort using factors from the high risk model of threat perception. Ph.D. diss., Virginia Consortium for Professional Psychology.

Schwartz GE. 1990. Psychobiology of repression and health: a systems approach. In: Singer JL, ed. *Repression and Dissociation: Implications for Personality Theory, Psychopathology, and Health.* Chicago: University of Chicago Press.

Shor RE, Orne EC. 1962. *Harvard Group Scale of Hypnotic Susceptibility, Form A.* Palo Alto, Calif: Consulting Psychologists Press.

Sternbach RA. 1986. Pain and "hassles" in the United States: findings of the nuprin pain report." *Pain.* 26:69–80.

Temoshok L, Dreher H. 1992. *The Type C Connection: The Behavioral Links to Cancer and Your Health.* New York: Random House.

Weinberger DA, Schwartz GE, Davidson RJ. 1979. Low-anxious high-anxious, and repressive coping styles: psychometric patterns and behavioral and physiological responses to stress. *J Abnorm Psychol.* 88:369–380.

Weinberger M, Hiner SL, Tierney WM. 1987. In support of hassles as a measure of stress in predicting health outcomes. *J Behav Med.* 19:19–32.

Whitehead WE, Drossman DA. 1996. Biofeedback and disorders of elimination: fecal incontinence and pelvic floor dyssynergia. *Prof Psych Res Practice.* 27:230–240.

Wickramasekera I. 1992. Diagnosis by inclusion: the perspective of a behavioral medicine practitioner. *Advances.* 8:17–30.

Wickramasekera I. 1995. Somatization: concepts, data, and predictions from the high risk model of threat perception. *J Nerv Ment Dis.* 183:15–23.

Wickramasekera I. 1999. Secrets kept from the mind but not the body. *Adv Mind Body Med.* 15(1)75–77.

Wickramasekera I, Davies TE, Davies SM. 1996. Applied psychophysiology: a bridge between the biomedical model and the biopsychosocial model in family medicine. *Prof Psych Res Practice.* 27:221–233.

Williams R. 1989. *The Trusting Heart.* New York: Times Books.

Chapter 9

Mind–Body Interventions for Surgery:
Evidence and Exigency

The techniques of mind-body medicine are reasonably well accepted for
certain chronic and hard-to-treat medical conditions, from pain syndromes to hypertension. In well-designed studies, relaxation, guided imagery, biofeedback, hypnosis, and related strategies have proven workable,
and mainstream medical institutions are taking baby steps toward implementing them—here and there, in small pockets within departments of
psychology, psychiatry, neurology, and rehabilitation. Although progress
is arguably insufficient, there is at least some sense of movement on these
fronts. By contrast, one proven indication for mind-body intervention—
preparation for surgery—has received little attention and scant implementation.

The precepts of mind-body unity underlie the use of psychological or
behavioral interventions before, during, or after surgery. One of these precepts is that patients are not passive receptacles for medical treatments but
are participants, since their own healing systems, which involve mind-body
interactions, are engaged in the process at many levels. This might seem
far-fetched in the surgical arena, since the patient is unconscious when
he or she is being operated upon. The archetypal image of surgery is of
the active physician fixing the patient's pathology as he or she lies prone,
passive, and unaware on the operating table. But this image belies the fact
that the mind is consciously engaged before and after surgery, when
thoughts and feelings about the experience may influence physiology, and
the fact that the mind may even be engaged during surgery, though below

Reprinted by permission, with changes, from *Advances in Mind-Body Medicine* 14 (1996): 207–222.

the level of consciousness, in ways that affect physiological responses to the manipulation and incision of skin, muscle, and organs. How well patients respond to surgery—how anxious they are beforehand, how rapidly they heal afterwards, whether they suffer complications, how much pain they subsequently experience—may be affected by states of mind and emotion.

Although mind-body interventions are used before, during, and after surgery, most studies involve preoperative applications because they are the most widely employed. Therefore, in this chapter I focus primarily on preoperative interventions.

By any standard the field of behavioral anesthesia, as it was named by the psychologist Henry L. Bennett, a pioneer and leading figure in the field, has produced an impressive body of evidence. Several hundred studies involving thousands of patients confirm that relatively simple behavioral interventions prior to surgery can demonstrably improve postoperative outcomes. Patients undergoing a wide range of different surgeries need less pain medication after their operations, lose less blood, and have fewer surgical complications and shorter hospital stays (Devine 1992a, 1992b). In most interventions a practitioner (or less frequently, an audiotape) prepares the patient with *comforting* words, *information* about the surgical procedure, and *instructions* on coping. In some cases the clinician presents hypnotic suggestions or guided imagery to the patient with the aim of priming the patient to produce specific outcomes, such as faster healing of wounds, the movement of blood away from the surgical site to prevent excess blood loss, the timely return of bowel motility, and swifter overall recovery.

The methods employed in these "instructional interventions" vary greatly from one study to the next. One purpose of this chapter is to analyze the elements that seem to work best, and why. One finding I discuss is something of a surprise: while methods for inducing relaxation are currently the cornerstone of much of behavioral (mind-body) medicine, in the literature on preparation for surgery the effects of garden-variety relaxation techniques are inconsistent and may be limited. One theory about this anomaly is that surgery is unlike many other stressors, and the most effective preparatory interventions are those that best address the actuality—and the meaning—of the experience.

In examining the field of behavioral anesthesia I first report on several meta-analyses of the literature. Given the wealth of literature, pooled data with proper statistical interpretations, as in meta-analysis, make it easier to generalize about the efficacy of these mind-body methods. I then turn to a more detailed consideration of research that has begun to sort out

302 which interventions are most effective. My aim is to show that the benefits of these interventions are large—both for patients and for the balance sheets of the healthcare system. Yet, distressingly, even though mind-body approaches have been shown not only to save money but also to make operations less traumatic, more manageable, and safer for patients undergoing virtually any kind of surgery, the literature remains largely unknown.

Mind-Body Interventions for Surgery: What Is the Evidence?

A broad scope of the studies prove the effectiveness of mind-body interventions that prepare patients for surgery. Significant psychological and medical benefits have been documented in hundreds of studies involving thousands of surgical patients. In the largest meta-analysis to date, preoperative "psychoeducational" interventions were found to be effective in improving outcomes in surgery across 191 studies involving more than 8,600 patients (Devine 1992, personal communication). The interventions have been shown to work for virtually every imaginable kind of surgery, from back surgery to coronary-bypass operations to cancer resections. They are effective for men, women, the young, the elderly, and people from different geographic locations. Similar effects have been found in published and unpublished studies; in research conducted in the 1960s, 1970s, and 1980s; in every kind of hospital (teaching, general, HMO-affiliated); and with a wide range of interventions, whether administered by nurses, psychologists, doctors, or pastoral counselors.

The most compelling evidence for these assertions come from meta-analyses of clinical trials of psychological or behavioral interventions for surgical patients. In the early 1980s Emily Mumford and her colleagues at the University of Colorado reviewed thirty-four controlled studies, evaluating the effects of providing psychosocial intervention as an adjunct to medically required care for 3,254 patients facing surgery or recovering from heart surgery or a heart attack (Mumford et al. 1982). On average, the surgical and coronary patients provided with informational or supportive interventions experienced smoother and more rapid postsurgical recovery than those in control groups.

The statistical measure used in meta-analyses to quantify the effectiveness of an intervention is the *effect size,* which, generally speaking, represents the standardized mean difference between treatment and control groups measured in units of standard deviation. Based on the conventions of these forms of analysis, an effect size of 0.20 is considered a reliable though small effect, 0.50 is considered moderate, and 0.80 or greater is considered large. In the Mumford meta-analyses the effect sizes for

210 outcome measures in the thirty-four studies averaged +0.49 (the large numbers of outcome measures included a range of psychological and physical indices of surgical success), and the intervention groups did better than the control groups by about .5 standard deviation. As a rough guide to the practical meaning for patients of a moderate effect size, a value of +0.50 implies that the score of the average person in a treatment group is better than the scores of 69 percent of the individuals in the control group.

More impressively, in terms of the key outcome of speedy recovery, the effect size is +0.80, a "large" effect. In their analysis of thirteen students that used days in a hospital after surgery or heart attack as an outcome indicator, Mumford and colleagues showed that psychological interventions reduced hospitalization by an average of 2.4 days, a finding with immense ramifications for both quality of care and cost savings.

In 1986 Donna Hathaway, an assistant professor in the School of Nursing at the University of Tennessee, published a meta-analysis of sixty-eight studies of the effect of preoperative instructional interventions on postoperative outcomes (Hathaway 1986). (Hathaway's analysis included some of the same studies used by Mumford but consisted mostly of other studies.) The total number of treated subjects was 2,413, and there were 1,605 control group subjects, for a total of 4,018. The mean effect size was again moderate (+0.44), indicating that the average patient receiving any form of preoperative instruction had more favorable psychological, physiological, and psychophysiological outcomes than a similar group who did not receive instruction.

Using a formula to translate the meaning of such an effect size (Rosenthal and Rubin 1982), Hathaway demonstrated a 20 percent higher success rate for two-thirds of the experimental subjects. "So not only do 67 percent of the patients receiving preoperative instruction have more favorable outcomes," writes Hathaway, "but their outcomes are 20 percent better than those not receiving preoperative instruction." By any litmus, a 20 percent improvement in such indices as speed of recovery, length of hospital stay, and reliance on pain medication will translate into a meaningful increase in the cost-effectiveness of surgical treatments.

The most comprehensive meta-analyses of mind-body interventions for surgery have been spearheaded by Elizabeth C. Devine, professor of nursing at the University of Wisconsin School of Nursing (Devine 1992a, 1992b; Devine and Cook 1986, 1986). The vast majority of the studies involve what she calls "psychoeducational" interventions, most administered by nurses, although some were administered by psychologists or doctors. Devine identified three themes in these interventions: providing patients

304 with health-related *information* about their condition and surgical procedure; *teaching patient skills, exercises, or activities* likely to reduce pain, discomfort, or complications; and providing *psychosocial support*. A modest
13 percent of the studies involve techniques that can fairly be characterized as "mind-body medicine" (relaxation, hypnosis, cognitive reappraisal,
etc.), although the vast majority included some elements of behavior
change and psychosocial support. These preoperative interventions take
an average of 30–45 minutes for nurses or other healthcare personnel to
administer.

In her 1986 analysis involving 102 studies (including most, though not
all, of the 68 studies in Hathaway's analysis), Devine (with Cook) examined how psychoeducational interventions influenced four outcomes—recovery, pain, psychological well-being, and satisfaction with care—among
hospitalized adult surgery patients. Five broad groupings of surgical patients were identified: abdominal, thoracic, orthopedic, gynecologic, and
others (including those undergoing early cancer surgery and eye, ear, nose,
and throat surgery). "Statistically reliable and positive effects were found
on each of these four classes of outcomes," wrote Devine. "Based on the
research reviewed, psychoeducational interventions reliably facilitate the
recovery of surgical patients." Some specifics:

- The average effect size value for all measures of surgical recovery was
  +0.50, a moderate but statistically meaningful result that led Devine to
  conclude that psychoeducational interventions are effective.
- The most robust recovery effects were found in the ability of the interventions to reduce medical complications (+0.87) and to lessen the number of days after discharge until the person resumed normal activities
  (+0.68).
- More moderately, the interventions reliably reduced the patients' pain
  (+0.39) and increased their psychological well-being (+0.40).

Devine continued to collect the data through the mid- to late 1980s, and
in 1992 she published the largest meta-analysis of studies of psychoeducational care for surgery (Devine 1992b), covering 191 studies, including
the 102 studies from the earlier analysis. As I noted at the outset, the studies comprised more than 8,600 patients (Devine, personal communication). The overall results include the following:

- Based on the sample of studies, the average effect size values are +0.43 for
  recovery, +0.38 for pain reduction, and +0.36 for reduction of psychological distress.

- For these same outcomes, the percentage of studies indicating beneficial effects ranged from 70 percent to 84 percent, significantly larger than the 50 percent one would expect if there were no treatment effect.
- Devine evaluated whether the interventions influenced the length of hospital stay, a key index of both recovery and cost savings. Length of stay was measured in 118 comparisons between treatment and control groups from 76 studies. A shorter average length of stay for experimental subjects was found in 76 percent of the comparisons and in 79 percent of the studies. (In the other comparisons and studies there was no difference.)
- Across the 76 studies, length of hospital stay was decreased an average of 1.5 days, a figure with sizable implications for potential cost savings.

Devine noted a slight decrease in efficacy from her previous analysis, which she attributed to the advent of a managed-care "environment" in which many surgical patients are admitted the same day of the procedure and there is less time for preoperative psychosocial treatment. However, she viewed the glass as half full: "The overall efficacy of psychoeducational care provided to adult surgical patients has been reconfirmed with this larger sample of studies," she wrote. "It is particularly noteworthy that these findings are of more than strictly historical interest. Despite changes in healthcare delivery, small to moderate-sized beneficial effects continue even in the most recent studies" (Devine 1992b).

Devine also pointed to a limitation in her analysis. "For all we know," she said in a conversation with me in January 1998, "the control groups may have been getting some psychoeducational care or support." She pointed out that relaxation techniques, audiotapes, and guided imagery approaches have become more "available" in the broader culture and that studies through the late 1970s and 1980s may have included sizable numbers of control patients who were either privately practicing or being taught these techniques. But this limitation suggests potentially stronger rather than weaker effects for psychosocial interventions; that is, despite possible use of behavioral medicine or psychosocial support among control patients, the interventions still had a reliably moderate effect when compared with these controls.

Can Surgical Patients Influence Physiological Healing?

As Devine has carefully cataloged, the scores of studies in her meta-analyses include a range of psychosocial and behavioral interventions that tend to involve at least one and typically all of three elements: preparatory information, rehabilitation and coping skills, and psychosocial support. In some instances techniques explicitly referred to as "mind-body"—relaxation, hypnotic suggestion, and imagery—were used, but these techniques were not always designed to assist patients in producing specific physiological outcomes.

In recent years the field of behavioral anesthesia as elaborated by Henry Bennett and others has begun to focus more on manifest mind-body techniques to improve the already impressive results from preoperative "preparatory" psychosocial interventions.

Consider this approach, developed by Bennett, to mind-body preparation for surgery. On the evening before a patient is scheduled to undergo spinal-cord surgery a psychologist enters the patient's room. One aspect of spinal-cord surgery is that it often leads to profuse blood loss, although there is wide variability in the amount of blood lost from one patient to the next. The psychologist engages the patient in a discussion of how it might be possible for the patient to exert some control over the amount of blood loss that will occur. He or she starts with an illustrative example: blushing. How is it that a few words spoken by another person, whether they signal embarrassment or arousal, can cause blood to move rapidly up to the head, causing a rush of warmth and a reddening of the face? The mind must be able to influence the movement of blood, says the psychologist, suggesting that the patient may be able to exploit that facility during surgery.

The psychologist next offers these implicit specific suggestions: "Blood vessels are made of smooth muscle, and like any muscle, they contract or relax in localized areas to alter blood volume to the area. To make sure you will have very little blood loss in your surgery, it is very important that the blood move away from the area of the spine and out to other parts of your body during the operation. Therefore [*spoken slowly*], the blood will move away from the spinal cord during the operation. Then, after the operation, it will return to that area to bring nutrients to heal your body quickly and completely." The patient takes the implicit suggestions, and after the operation the patient is found to have lost 500 cubic centimeters of blood during the surgery, which is roughly 400 cubic centimeters less than is commonly observed in patients undergoing this form of spinal-cord operation.

This example illustrates Bennett's method of applying behavioral anesthesiology to patients undergoing surgery that can cause extensive blood loss. It also mirrors the techniques and results of an impressive study published by Bennett and his colleagues (1986) when Bennett was in the Department of Anesthesiology of the University of California, Davis, Medical Center. They randomly assigned ninety-four spinal-surgery patients into three groups, all of whom received a fifteen-minute preoperative visit from a psychologist trained to perform such interventions. The first group received only information about neural monitoring of spinal-cord function, a procedure that patients in each group would undergo. The second group served as the relaxation group; in addition to being given the information also provided to the first group, its members were also taught to relax their muscles during the administration of anesthesia and during their emergence from unconsciousness. The third group, referred to as the "blood-shunting group," received the information and directions given the first two groups but was also given specific instructions, as in the example above, for moving blood first toward and then away from the site of surgery.

Bennett believes that the blood-shunting approach, like his other presurgical interventions meant to enhance the recovery process, may call upon principles of hypnotic induction, but the procedures involve no explicit effort to put patients into a trance state. What is more, "I never use the word hypnosis," Bennett told me in an interview in January 1998. "I do not want to mystify this process for the patient."

The findings of the study supported Bennett's hypothesis that patients could exert mental control over the extent of their blood loss during surgery. As mentioned, patients in the blood-shunting group lost significantly less blood—a median of 500 cubic centimeters—than those assigned to either the control group or the relaxation group, where the median blood loss was almost a full liter—900 cubic centimeters. These results held firm after controlling for such potential confounding factors as time under anesthesia and length of incision. The amount of blood loss in all three groups was within the normal range, but patients in the blood-shunting group were at the low end of the continuum.

Over the past decade Bennett has contributed to our understanding that relatively simple interventions can influence surgical variables other than blood loss. He has shown, for example, that they can influence the most notable side effect of gastrointestinal surgery, the complete cessation of the peristaltic action of the stomach and intestines, known as ileus. After surgery patients are unable to take food by mouth until they recover motility in the gastrointestinal system. Until then patients receive intravenous feeding and cannot be discharged from the hospital. Thus, the entire recovery process is influenced by the return of peristalsis.

In a study in 1993 Bennett and his colleagues randomized forty patients undergoing gastrointestinal surgery to two groups. One was the "suggestion" group, which received specific instructions from a psychologist for the early return of gastrointestinal motility (Disbrow et al. 1993). Patients were told, "Your stomach will churn and growl, your intestines will pump and gurgle, and you will be hungry soon after your surgery." Patients were

308   also told to identify their favorite foods, thoughts of which could lead to stomach growling. They were then given the suggestion, "So you can get back to eating [your favorite food] as soon as possible, your stomach and intestines will start moving and churning and gurgling soon after surgery." This entire intervention took about five minutes. The second group, the control subjects, received an intervention of equal length in which they were given information and instructions on clearing the lungs after surgery.

The results again supported Bennett's view that surgical patients can use their thoughts to affect their physiology. The suggestion group had a significantly shorter time to the return of gastrointestinal motility, 2.6 days compared with 4.1 days. As a result, the suggestion patients were also in the hospital for a significantly shorter time, 6.5 days compared with 8.1 days. The researchers calculated that this reduction of 1.5 days in the hospital translated into an average cost savings of $1,200.

Postoperative pain is another parameter that can be influenced by preoperative behavioral interventions. This area of research was pioneered in the 1960s by the anesthesiologist Larry Egbert of Massachusetts General Hospital. In a classic study the anesthesiologist gave presurgical instructions to forty-six patients on how to prevent and relieve postoperative pain by relaxing the muscles surrounding the site of incision (Egbert et al. 1964). These patients required significantly less narcotic pain medication, and they returned home sooner than a control group of similar patients who received no such instruction.

One of the more intriguing studies of the benefits of preoperative mind-body intervention was carried out by Carole Holden-Lund at the University of Texas. Holden-Lund gave surgical patients instruction in relaxation and in guided-imagery exercises based on the specific physiological processes involved in healing wounds (Holden-Lund 1988). She found that patients in her experimental group had lower postsurgical levels of cortisol, the stress hormone that can suppress antibody production and lymphocyte and natural killer cell activity, all of which are needed for the proper healing of wounds (Holden-Lund 1988). Whether for this reason or not, she found that the intervention patients did indeed experience more rapid healing of wounds.

Mixed Results

It may seem that the results of behavioral or mind-body interventions are all straightforward, that the intervention leads to the positive effect that the study anticipated. But some studies have led to mixed findings, and these results prompt deeper questions about preoperative interventions— what works and why?

Consider the research of Bjorn Enqvist of the Eastman and Karolinska Institutes in Sweden. An orthodontist and hypnotherapist, Enqvist and colleagues have carried out several trials of presurgical hypnosis. In one trial, Enqvist and his colleagues (Enqvist et al. 1995) provided hypnotherapy tapes to three randomized groups of patients who would undergo maxillofacial surgery in three weeks. The surgery is performed under general anesthesia, it involves a loss of blood that sometimes approaches 1,000 cubic centimeters, and it leads to extensive postoperative edema. Those in the first group ($N = 18$) were given hypnotherapy tapes containing preoperative suggestions for improved healing, less bleeding, lower blood pressure, relaxation, and faster recovery. They were instructed to listen to these taped inductions once or twice daily. Those in a second group ($N = 18$) received the same tape and instructions but were also given a tape with similar instructions to be played *during* the surgery while under anesthesia. Those in the third group ($N = 24$) were given only a hypnosis tape, to be played only during the surgery. Each of the three groups was matched by demographics and type of surgery to a group of control patients being treated presurgically at other institutions.

I focus here on the measure of blood loss. The patients who received preoperative suggestions exhibited a 30 percent reduction in blood loss, those who received suggestions before and during surgery showed a 26 percent reduction, and those who received suggestions only during surgery demonstrated a mere 9 percent reduction in blood loss. The extent to which the intervention stemmed blood loss was significant only in the first preoperative group. In theorizing why the group that also received "intraoperative" (during surgery) suggestions did not do as well, the investigators noted that the surgical procedures in this group were more complicated. The results of the third group also suggested that the intraoperative tape had little value, which raised at least two possibilities: that hypnotic induction during surgery is not effective or that the tape used in the study was not adequate. In any event, Enqvist and colleagues found in this study that a mind-body intervention could reduce blood loss.

However, in a repeat of the study with nineteen facial surgery patients and matched controls Enqvist was not able to reproduce the blood-loss findings. In the repeat study there was one experimental group, the nineteen subjects who received hypnotherapy tapes both before and during surgery. Compared with the controls, the hypnotherapy subjects experienced significantly less postsurgical edema, fever, and consumption of

310   antianxiety drugs, but their blood loss was not significantly different than that of the controls (Enqvist 1995). In searching for an explanation of why these patients did not lose less blood, Enqvist realized that in the prior study the patients in the hypnotherapy groups had had ongoing contact with an orthodontist-hypnotherapist (not identified, but presumably Enqvist himself), who "might have given these patients direct positive influence in comparison with patients in the control group. Thus, the 'wish to please' could explain some of the differences between groups." Enqvist went on to suggest that in his replication this potential "bias" was minimized, since most patients were treated by other orthodontists who were not aware of the study. He also noted that the techniques of maxillofacial surgery had been refined by the time of the replication, resulting in considerably reduced blood loss in all patients. (A larger group of forty-five patients did show a difference in blood loss, but Enqvist regarded this finding as "only tentative," since the patients were matched to controls by surgical type but not by gender, as had been done in the smaller sample.) As I will suggest later, the very attempt to minimize the "bias" of a personal relationship may explain why the findings on blood loss in the second study failed to reproduce the benefit achieved in the first study. The "personal touch" may matter a great deal in such interventions.

   Another study with mixed results was conducted by one of the country's leading cardiothoracic surgeons, Dr. Mehmet Oz of Columbia-Presbyterian Medical Center, who has received much attention for using complementary medical approaches in his surgical practice. In a recent study Oz and his colleagues randomized thirty-two patients about to undergo coronary-bypass surgery to two groups: one group received instructions on self-hypnotic relaxation techniques to use prior to surgery, while the other group received no such instructions (Ashton et a1. 1997). Psychological testing revealed that patients practicing preoperative self-hypnosis were significantly more relaxed than the control group in the days following surgery. Further, the patients who said they practiced the self-hypnosis techniques needed markedly less pain medication than did those who had not practiced the techniques. However, when the researchers also measured requirements for anesthesia, hospital stay, and postoperative morbidity and mortality, they found no significant differences between the two groups.

   How can the mixed results of the Columbia-Presbyterian study be explained? The investigators speculated that their results may have been limited because there was only a brief time to teach the patients self-hypnosis—on the eve of their surgery—because heart bypass patients are now admitted the day before the operation. "Effects may have been greater if patients were able to be taught self-hypnosis several days prior to surgery,

so they could practice the relaxation techniques for a longer period," wrote
Oz and colleagues.

Research by Bennett suggests another perspective. In his study on gastrointestinal motility (Disbrow et al. 1993) he found that certain presurgical approaches appeared to be more effective than others in reducing
postoperative pain and requirements for pain medication. Providing basic
educational information and teaching simple coping skills appeared to be
effective, but presurgical group therapy, specific information about the
surgical process, reassurance, and methods to redirect attention away from
the pain were not. Likewise, a presurgical program of self-hypnosis with
nonspecific suggestions for relaxation was also ineffective.

The techniques taught in the Columbia-Presbyterian study included
both relaxation and hypnotic suggestions about reduced bleeding and stable blood pressure. From the perspective of Henry Bennett, the emphasis
on instruction may have been the key to the benefits that were found, while
the relaxation components may have been less helpful. I will shortly take
a broader look at the issue of relaxation and behavioral anesthesia.

Taken together, these several studies indicate that not all preoperative
mind-body interventions are alike. Some work better than others. Nor do
all do the same things. What makes the difference? Recent studies have
begun to examine this issue, and the results are refining knowledge of how
to shape preoperative interventions.

Recent Intervention Data: Disappointment and Surprise

Although literature reviews broadly help to distinguish preoperative mind-
body methods that work from those that do not, for many years few well-
designed efforts attempted to compare clinical applications. The leading
researcher in this area (again) has been Bennett in several studies he conducted between 1993 and 1996 in the Department of Anesthesia of Pennsylvania State College of Medicine. (He has now formed his own company,
Patient Comfort, Inc.)

I have already referred to Bennett's 1993 study with Disbrow, in which
he distinguished between the ability of different preoperative verbal approaches to reduce pain and the need for pain medication after surgery.
His most interesting findings on this subject come from a recently reported
randomized, placebo-controlled, double-blind clinical trial of 335 surgical patients in which he compared four surgical-preparation audiotape
programs for their possible effect on three medical outcomes: intraoperative blood loss, length of hospital stay, and use of postoperative pain medication (Bennett 1996).

312   The patients, who were undergoing one of four different surgical procedures—spinal surgery, radical neck dissection, joint replacement, or abdominal cancer resection—were randomly assigned to five groups. There
were four experimental groups, each with a different tape, and a placebo
group with a tape whose "whooshing" noise had no meaningful physiological effect. (A second control group, identified just prior to the operations, comprised patients who reported that they had not listened to their
tapes.) A statistician later confirmed that each of the groups contained a
similar distribution of patients undergoing the four types of surgeries. The
four audiotape programs were

1. Bennett's own informational instruction with specific suggestions for physiological outcomes (as in the gastrointestinal study), taped by him.
2. A relaxation tape, largely of composed music designed to soothe, with a
   voice-over introduction about the rigors of surgery and the healing potential of relaxation, prepared by Linda Rodgers (Rodgers 1995).
3. A "hemi-sync" relaxation tape, which includes the delivery of tones in both
   ears at slightly different frequencies, producing what sounds to the listener
   like a "wah-wah" sound, prepared by Robert Monroe. (The differing frequencies are supposed to "drive" the brain toward greater relaxation, presumably by influencing brain wave patterns.) As the "wah-wah" becomes
   slower and deeper, a voice-over by Monroe prompts the listener to drop
   more deeply into a relaxed state.
4. A guided-imagery tape, a lushly produced visualization exercise prepared
   and read by Belleruth Naparstek, scored with specially composed music
   designed to highlight and accompany each image. The images are meant
   to take the listener to a "nonordinary state," with an emphasis on spiritual
   connectedness. Also included are lush or metaphoric visualizations of positive outcomes—faster wound healing, less pain, no nausea, and so on. (A
   highly regarded therapist and imagery practitioner, Naparstek has also created the Health Journeys series of guided-imagery audiotapes, each one designed to help people resolve a specific medical, emotional, or addictive
   conditions.)

Several days prior to surgery, the patients were told to take the tapes
home and listen to them through headphones as often as they wished. In
his analysis, Bennett found that most patients took this instruction seriously, averaging four listenings per patient in each of the four study groups,
though among these groups there were patients who did not listen to the
tapes, whom Bennett thus treated as a second control group. All subjects
also listened to tapes during surgery; the content of these tapes was mostly

similar to that of the presurgical tapes. The subjects in the two control groups listened to tapes of whooshing noises during their surgeries.

In many respects the results surprised Bennett. When the outcomes of patients in the experimental groups were compared with those of patients in the no-treatment control group, they revealed that three of the four tapes—those by Rodgers, Monroe, and Bennett himself—produced no significant benefits with regard to any of the three medical outcomes he was examining (blood loss during surgery, length of hospital stay, and use of postoperative pain medication). By contrast, the Naparstek imagery tape produced highly significant results with regard to two outcomes: the patients experienced far less blood loss and spent less time in the hospital. Specifically, the median blood loss for patients listening to the Naparstek imagery tape was 200 cubic centimeters, the least lost by any group, compared with 350 cubic centimeters in the placebo control group. And members of the Naparstek group were in the hospital one full day less than members of the placebo control. Table 9.1 reports the comparative results in each group, with p values of statistical significance.

Bennett also used the Profile of Mood States to evaluate emotional states before and after surgery. With regard to *state* anxiety (the experience of anxiety in response to particular stresses), those listening to the Naparstek imagery tape experienced a smaller before-to-after increase than did the patients listening to the other tapes. More unexpectedly, this group of patients was the only one to experience a *drop* in the Profile of Mood States measure of *trait* anxiety, the general tendency to experience anxiety, presumably a relatively unchanging facet of personality. Somehow, listening to the Naparstek tapes appeared to alter a person's characteristic emotional responses, at least for a short period of time after surgery.

A further unexpected, even startling finding was that the "did not listen" subjects had better outcomes for several variables than did many who listened to the audiotape interventions. Next to the patients in the Naparstek group, the "did not listen" subjects had the least blood loss and the shortest hospital stays, though neither of the figures was significant when compared with the placebo control group. Bennett showed that these patients were relatively less anxious and depressed from the outset, one possible reason why they did not bother to listen to the tapes preoperatively. Another anomalous finding is harder to explain: the placebo controls, as well as the "did not listen" group, used (nonsignificantly) less morphine to treat their pain in the first three days after surgery.

Yet there were aspects of the results that fit Bennett's expectations. He found that the patients who listened to the two relaxation tapes did worse than the placebo group on the three major medical outcome measures,

TABLE 9.1

Comparative Effects of Audiotaped Preparations for Surgery

PART A

VARIABLE	CONTROL	ROGERS	BENNETT	MONROE	NAPARSTEK	DID NOT LISTEN	P VALUE BASED ON ANOVA (OR KRUSKAL–WALLIS)
Intraoperative blood loss (in cubic centimeters)	350	375	300	500	200	300	0.0421‡
Length of stay (in hours after surgery)	121	144.12	121.14	117.5	92.5	93.2	.0129
Change in state anxiety	3.56	3.02	4.35	6.96	2.28	8.06	.3413
Preoperative state anxiety	40.98	40.10	42.79	42.63	42.1	41.22	.8600
Change in trait anxiety	0.59	2.05	2.79	4.04	−0.58	1.06	.4737
Preoperative trait anxiety	37.14	38.20	37.21	37.91	37.96	33.58	.4199
Total morphine use 3 days postoperative (in milligrams of morphine equivalence)*	62.1	92	70	125	90.33	65.3	.0285‡

PART B

VARIABLE	P VALUES				
	ROGERS	BENNETT	MONROE	NAPARSTEK	DID NOT LISTEN
Intraoperative blood loss (in cubic centimeters)	.97	.34	.39	.03†	.12
Length of stay (hours after surgery)	.40	.43	.83	.02‡	.08
Total morphine use 3 days postoperative	.26	.87	.006†	.09	.77

Source: Adapted from Bennett 1996.

Note: Part A lists significant differences between controls and the five experimental groups; Part B lists significant differences between controls and specific experimental groups. The p value based on ANOVA reflects the presence of statistically significant differences ($p < .05$) between the control group and at least one of the other groups. Such differences occurred in three areas: intraoperative blood loss, length of stay, and total morphine use. Part B shows the p values (statistically significant for $p < .05$) for comparisons between the control group and each of the other five groups for those three areas. In other words, the second analysis determined which treatment groups experienced significant difference from controls. The table indicates two such differences for patients using the Naparstek tape—significantly less blood loss and briefer length of stay—and one such difference for patients using the Monroe tape—significantly more total morphine use.

* Results in these rows are medians; all others are mean averages.

† Psychological measurements from the Profile of Mood States (POMS).

‡ Statistically significant difference at $p \le .05$.

confirming his view, based on previous studies and on his own theoretical beliefs, that tapes emphasizing relaxation, no matter how novel their methods or how soothing their veneer, do not necessarily produce the desired benefits. Lacking in these programs, he believes, are specific instructions to produce a salutary physiological change—moving blood, activating the bowel, healing wounds.

As for his own tape, Bennett was disappointed and mildly perplexed that it did not produce better results, though he points to a statistical trend toward reduced blood loss in patients listening to his instructions. Next to the Naparstek group, the Bennett and "did not listen" groups had the least blood loss—300 cubic centimeters. More to the point, Bennett does not view the findings as reason to reject the results of many previous studies confirming the benefits of instructional intervention as a whole, both because the most successful tape, by Naparstek, included specific instructions for physiological benefits and because his own instructional tape yielded relatively better results than the two relaxation-oriented tapes.

But the Naparstek findings have caused Bennett to rethink some of his assumptions. "I would modify my view to say that it appears that the integration and sophistication of the [tape] intervention makes a difference," he commented in an interview with me. "That sophistication probably will involve, for lack of a better term, 'guided imagery,' yet it probably cannot be guided imagery about rose gardens. It probably has to be [imagery] specific to the surgical process the patient is going through. Belleruth Naparstek's tape is an active intervention—she mentions blood loss, she mentions wound healing. But she also had someone compose music . . . that supports the words and their message of meaning. This may have added a synergistic element."

I mentioned another possible factor to Bennett. His intervention is brief, simple, informational, and to the point. When imparted in person by a human being who meets a patient eye to eye, it may have a considerably more powerful effect than when a patient listens to an audiotaped version of the same words. Belleruth Naparstek may have overcome this theoretical deficit with lush images, evocative words, warm vocal tones, and comforting music composed to deliver mind-pictures and suggestions with emotional punch. Bennett agreed that the human factor may have made a difference in his study and that it might explain why his intervention, which had repeatedly produced statistically significant results when delivered in person, failed to do so when delivered via a tape.

If the human factor is indeed the explanation, then the import of behavioral anesthesiology and other clinical applications of behavioral medicine must not be ignored. Administrators and practitioners in hospitals

316   and managed-care settings should think twice before they turn behavioral
medicine into a tape-dispensary business. While tapes can be valuable ad-
juncts, and in some cases effective interventions (as the Naparstek tape
seems to demonstrate), they may not always replace the human practitioner who spends even fifteen minutes with a frightened patient.

Naparstek Revisited

Were the results of the Naparstek tape a fluke? As I have indicated, the
question is critical to the development of behavioral anesthesia. Is it essential that a person deliver the interventions? Or can a tape, albeit a tape
that meets many criteria, do it?

A recently published study of surgical outcomes using the same Naparstek tape did in fact replicate the efficacy of her program. Diane Tusek
and colleagues at the Cleveland Clinic, in Cleveland, Ohio, conducted a
prospective, randomized trial of pre- and postoperative guided-imagery
interventions for patients undergoing elective intestinal surgery for diver-
ticulitis (Tusek et al. 1997). One hundred thirty patients were randomly assigned to a control or study group. The study group listened to Naparstek's
"guided imagery for surgery" tape on the three days prior to the procedure.
They then listened to a tape of soothing music in the preoperative holding
hour and in the operating rooms, and for six days postoperatively they listened to imagery tapes with positive suggestions about outcome. The control subjects received only standard preoperative instructions.

The data analysis revealed that among patients using guided imagery
the average length of hospital stay was 1.5 days less than the stay of the
control patients, for a total of 6.4 days rather than 7.9. The imagery patients used one-third less pain medication, and their bowel functions returned to normal 1.2 days sooner. Furthermore, both pre- and intraoperative anxiety was decreased in the study group, and these patients also
reported steadily declining postsurgical anxiety for five successive days,
while the control subjects' anxiety remained constant. One arguable flaw
in this study is the lack of a placebo for the control group, such as a tape
with white noise or whooshing sounds. But the fact that Naparstek's imagery tape proved far superior to a placebo in Bennett's larger study suggests that the findings of the Cleveland Clinic are reliable.

What makes Naparstek's guided imagery tape for surgery effective? As
I have suggested, there may be multiple features: the use of imagery, which
itself has a well-documented capacity to influence involuntary physiological processes; the warmth of Naparstek's voice; the somatosensory effects
of the accompanying music; and—critical from Bennett's perspective—

Naparstek's inclusion of suggestions for specific physical changes during the program. In a telephone interview I asked Naparstek what she thought made her tape so efficacious. She had an unequivocal response: "What works best is taking people beyond ordinary time into a different state of consciousness, preferably where they drop into their hearts. The tape is putting them in a place of love and power where they feel safe."

According to Naparstek, after providing an "induction," in which the person is transported to that place of safety, the tape uses images to suggest physical outcomes: the body will knit together bone and skin to heal faster; the blood will deliver what is needed to the surgical site; the body will send nutrients to the area, allowing cells to rebuild. In a calm, resonant voice she suggests to the listener that he or she will not bleed much and prompts the listener to imagine the surgical staff commenting, "Look, she [or he] is hardly bleeding at all." Naparstek places the patient in an operating room transmogrified into a hallowed space, filled with the faces of loved ones. "I encourage patients to have whole cheering sections—family, best friends, the dearly departed, guardian angels, power animals—anyone who had ever wished them well." (Naparstek's intraoperative tape is not so lavish. With headphones strapped on during surgery, patients listen to a tape of the same soothing, evocative music used in the preoperative tapes.)

Naparstek summarized the qualities of her tape that she feels have healing effects: "It is the kind of imagery—heart focused, schmaltzy, emotional, spirit-oriented. I want to take the person on a sort of shamanistic journey, one that moves them deeply into a nonordinary state. The music, language, and specific images are all designed to evoke spirit, to generate love and gratitude." Clearly, some would wave aside her content as "New Agey." But Naparstek has an earthbound quality that comes through in her voice, moderating syrupy or "flaky" connotations that some of her images might conjure up among more skeptical minds.

The efficacy of Naparstek's tape seems real, indicating that a tape can successfully transmit a preoperative behavioral intervention. But this efficacy seems to demand an elaborate format—a critical component, apparently—which seems to be less crucial when a human being presents the intervention in person. Put simply, the schmaltziness on her tape has a heartfelt rather than a forced quality, and her images speak to an honest desire to feel cared for and protected when one is about to lose control of the conscious mind and have one's bodily boundaries invaded. Further, granting Bennett's thesis about the central importance of instruction in preoperative interventions, one can make a case that the varied elements of Naparstek's tape serve to deliver its suggestive instruction—reducing

318 blood loss, healing wounds, and so on—in the most effective possible way. The mellifluous sounds and the reassuring images of a "safe place" filled with loved ones seem to steady the mind, perhaps by reducing fear and instilling calm confidence in one's ability to exert control over seemingly involuntary physiological processes.

Why Is Information Important? What's Wrong with Relaxation?

The majority of preoperative behavioral interventions are built around the information and instructions that a thoughtful physician, nurse, or anesthesiologist might make to a patient the night before surgery. The effort to focus the preoperative interventions on relaxation is a more recent development—and, it would seem, a less successful approach.

Bennett has given much thought to the issue of instruction versus relaxation. "Surgery is exertional," he asserted in our interview. "It takes a lot of work to go through surgery." A person would not prepare for a psychologically and physically demanding event, he maintained, as if he or she were about to lapse into slumber.

Bennett offered a helpful analogy: "What should I say to you if you were about to run steeple chase for the first time? You know it's rigorous, you know it takes long, but you don't know a damn thing about a steeple chase. Do I tell you to just go home and relax? Your life may depend on how you run, but is 'take it easy' all I say? Or should I tell you the history of the steeple chase; the fact that it has been run for centuries and is very hazardous. Is that helpful? What if I say instead, OK, when you hit the first bend you will see a water hazard in front of you. Make sure you go through the right-hand side of that hazard because there are snakes and vipers on the left, and it's shallow on the right. Next you come to a big hedge, and whatever you do, jump through the middle of that hedge. With this approach, I clearly am giving you useful instructions on how to negotiate a strenuous course successfully."

The steeplechase comparison—or any athletic analogy—does not suggest that the surgical patient should be *anxious*, Bennett argued. People about to enter competitive sporting events are said to do best when they exhibit calm confidence, a relaxed form of readiness. Similarly, some activation of catecholamine and corticosteroid stress hormones may be appropriate for presurgical preparation, though overactivation would be counterproductive, producing immune deficits, hypertension, and other untoward physical effects. Should a tennis player about to enter the biggest match of his or her life be unperturbed to the point of lethargy? Or should the person be so pumped up that he or she shakes with tension? Obviously, the answer lies in between—relaxed readiness—and the same applies to surgical patients.

First, Do No Harm

As the meta-analyses illustrate, the sweep of studies on behavioral anesthesia show regular, consistent benefits. However, several investigators believe that a small subset of patients may actually be harmed by these interventions. According to a review in the early 1980s by John F. Wilson of the University of Kentucky College of Medicine, these investigators theorize that patients who use denial as a coping style may become increasingly anxious when confronted with any information about surgery and its outcome, even if the information is presented in a nonthreatening manner (Wilson 1981). In a few reports, patients classified as deniers have responded to preparatory information about either their surgery or diagnostic procedures with increased use of pain medication (Andrew 1970), more frequent complaints (DeLong 1970), and higher heart rates (Shipley et al. 1978; Shipley et al. 1979).

Could such patients be harmed by a psychosocial intervention? Wilson sought to answer that question with a study of seventy patients undergoing elective cholecystectomy and abdominal hysterectomy. He prepared them for surgery with relaxation training and with information about sensations they would experience. He found that while personality variables such as denial, fear, and aggressiveness did influence outcomes, patients using denial were not harmed by the preparatory intervention, which reduced hospital stay, pain, and pain medication and increased indices of strength and energy. Wilson concluded that behavioral preparation for surgery benefits even frightened patients, aggressive ones, or those using denial as they confront elective surgery.

Although Wilson's study is reassuring, it nonetheless seems possible that patients employing denial as a rigid coping strategy might be negatively affected by straightforward facts about possible surgical outcomes, including information about pain, how long it will take to heal, and potential complications. Ian Wickramasekera, a psychotherapist whose work focuses on identification and treatment of somatizers (Wickramasekera 1998), suggests that the subgroup of patients who are repressors—who would score low on measures of hypnotizability—might respond to presurgical interventions, whether informational or suggestive or hypnotic, with more rather than less distress (Wickramasekera, personal communication, January 1998). The lesson here is that clinical common sense dictates that these interventions should be tailored to personality types.

320 For instance, some people cannot absorb much information and instruction and mainly need support, while others will experience a greater sense of control when they hear, in a supportive context, specifics of what they are about to experience.

For his part, Bennett grants that interventions with frank information but no instruction—without empowering guidance that gives patients a sense that they can do specific things to influence their recovery—could conceivably cause more harm than good for some people. And he believes that interventions relying *solely* on relaxation techniques are likely to be at best inadequate and at worst possibly even deleterious.

Elizabeth Devine, pointing to her meta-analyses, argues that there will always be "outliers" in such studies, individuals who do worse than expected. But in her statistical reviews she has not seen the large spread in standard deviations that would hint at a clear subset of people doing worse as a result of preoperative psychosocial interventions, whatever those interventions might be. Indeed, she told me in a telephone interview that based on her extensive research, she doubts "that there are any consistent groups of patients who are either not benefiting or doing worse" as a result of psychosocial interventions.

In sum, the data so far strongly indicate that interventions providing information, reassurance, *and* specific instructions on controlling various psychological and physical outcomes are broadly effective and largely without risk, as well as relatively easy to administer.

The Neglect of Behavioral Anesthesia

As a highly involved participant, Bennett has closely followed the use of behavioral anesthesia in surgical medicine. His progress report was not encouraging. "I think that we have come about two percent of the way toward where we need to be," he maintained in his interview with me, referring to an ideal situation in which psychosocial and mind–body interventions are delivered to every surgical patient. Most of Bennett's "two percent" of progress consists of consumers' use of such commercially available products as audiotapes and the presurgical support and mind–body instructions offered by private psychotherapists or mind–body practitioners. Hospital systems and the managed-care industry have shown virtually no interest.

But Bennett was optimistic that the atmosphere might be changing.

Thirty years ago the childbirth movement moved childbirth from the realm of disease to being a family bonding experience. It was the consumer who drove that. Of course, childbirth is something you have nine months to prepare for, and it's something you look forward to. With surgery, you often don't have time to prepare for it, and often there isn't much to look forward to. There is frequently an element of fear and even shame—something is wrong with you or you wouldn't need surgical intervention. But our society is moving forward in becoming aware of these matters. The population is aging, they are hitting life crises and wondering what they can do to help themselves. At the same time, HMOs and hospital systems are highly competitive, and it behooves both institutions to recognize that [behavioral] interventions for surgery, when done in a sophisticated manner, are highly efficacious—a win-win-win situation. Patients win because they are more satisfied and feel they have participated in their recovery. The surgeon wins because the patients do better, and they are happier consumers. The economic providers win because it costs less.

Bennett has spent years attempting to convince hospitals, HMOs, and other medical institutions to adopt behavioral-intervention programs. "I have yet to be successful in implementing any kind of program despite my offers to do it essentially for free." He told me several depressing stories about offering his program to various hospitals. In one case he proposed conducting a large-scale study at virtually no cost with miniscule outlays of time from healthcare professionals. There was no interest. In another instance a large, brand-name HMO was enthusiastic about Bennett's research and purchased two hundred sets of both his instructional tapes and Belleruth Naparstek's imagery tapes. But implementation hit a wall once the tapes entered the managed care-bureaucracy, and they have been sitting on a shelf for over two years.

One roadblock here might be the confusion among managed-care and hospital administrators about preoperative and intraoperative interventions. Preoperative interventions, as I have detailed, have a clear, virtually unqualified record of effectiveness. Intraoperative interventions, in which taped suggestions, instructions, or music are played through headphones during an operation, have a mixed record of success. Three detailed overviews of intraoperative research have shown positive results in some studies but not in others (Ghoneim and Block 1992, 1997; Merikle and Daneman 1996). The initial Enqvist study on blood loss is illustrative: patients undergoing preoperative suggestion experienced a marked reduction in blood loss, while those undergoing intraoperative suggestion alone did not (Enqvist 1995). The evidence suggests that the degree of unconsciousness achieved with varying anesthetic medications and dosages

322   may be pivotal in determining whether suggestive or relaxing tape content is integrated by the mind during surgery (Schwender et al. 1996). While learning appears to be possible during surgery, the surgical conditions, the anesthesia, and the nature of the intraoperative intervention will determine whether positive outcomes can be achieved. Conceivably, the equivocal results of *intra*operative studies may have tainted a story that should be clear-cut: when properly designed, *pre*operative mind-body interventions work.

    This said, one would still think that cost-effectiveness arguments would push the medical establishment to a careful consideration of preoperative interventions. The meta-analyses prove that hospital stay is shortened by anywhere from 1.5 days (Devine 1992a) to 2.4 days (Mumford et al. 1982). As Bennett's study of abdominal surgery indicated, the reduced 1.5 days of hospital stay achieved by the intervention translated into a $1,200 savings per patient (Disbrow et al. 1993). Clearly, just in terms of reduced hospital stays the savings for large HMOs and hospital systems could arguably be millions of dollars per institution and would far surpass the costs of brief interventions by single healthcare professionals.

    In their 1986 analysis of 102 studies Devine and Cook examined the cost benefits of psychoeducational care for surgical patients. Based on the assumption that nurses would administer the interventions, which would typically require forty-five to sixty minutes per patient, Devine and Cook, using 1986 healthcare salary figures, estimated that the cost would be approximately twenty dollars per hospitalization. Against this cost Devine and Cook put savings in reduced hospital stay, medical complications, medications for pain, anxiety, and nausea and offered this provisional prediction: "Since there are several million surgical procedures performed each year that are similar to the ones included in the research reviewed, the potential impact of increasing psychoeducational care on healthcare costs is large. If the actual cost saving is only $100 per patient . . . the cost savings to the nation would be hundreds of millions of dollars, and would justify the modest cost to increase levels of psychoeducational care" (Devine and Cook 1986).

    What, then, accounts for the disinterest? Is it simply insufficient cost-benefit data? The evidence on actual patient benefits is formidable. As with so many mind-body interventions, the problem may have most to do with the closed-mindedness of those who cannot accept any data, no matter how convincing, from a paradigm they do not accept or understand. As Bennett put it in his interview with me, "Viewing the patient as anything other than a warm set of organs raises the anxiety of the healthcare profession."

    The knee-jerk reaction of medical administrators and many scientists seems to be, "Why have a healthcare provider spend one costly moment on something we can't quite believe?" The implicit thought is "data be damned," and the unintended consequence is unneeded patient discomfort and worse—prolonged suffering and surgical complications.

Bennett nonetheless suggested that the bottom-line mentality of managed-care institutions is so "value-neutral" that it will eventually seize on these data in the relentless search for savings. (This implies that biomedical professionals, with their paradigmatic myopia, are greater impediments to this kind of change than bureaucrats.) I hope he is correct, but I worry that managed-care administrators are as implicitly skeptical of new medical models as are mechanistic doctors. Perhaps common sense will rule when doctors, hospitals, and HMOs are pressured by consumers— the patients—who intuitively believe they need support and preparation for surgery and who vigorously assert that need. Then the competitive dynamics of the marketplace will press institutions to provide such services.

Research findings and common sense should also continue to drive progress in behavioral anesthesia. In Bennett's words, "My assumption is that a patient who is moribund, upset, and exhausted is a more expensive patient than one who feels that he or she has actively participated in his or her surgery. The active participant who's had motivational instructions will know what to do physiologically to be able to get up and out of the hospital bed. Such a patient will feel part of the healing process rather than a passive body containing the work of the surgeon."

REFERENCES

Andrew JM. 1970. Recovery from surgery, with and without preparatory instruction, for three coping styles. *J Pers Soc Psychol.* 15:223–226.

Ashton C, Whitworth GC, Selomridge JA, et al. 1997. Self-hypnosis reduces anxiety following coronary artery bypass surgery: a prospective, randomized trial. *J Cardiovasc Surg (Torino).* 38:69–75.

Bennett HL. 1996. A comparison of audiotaped preparations for surgery: evaluation and outcomes. Paper presented at the annual meeting of the Society for Clinical and Experimental Hypnosis, Tampa, Fla.

Bennett HL, Benson DR, Kuiken DA. 1986. Preoperative instruction for decreased bleeding during spine surgery. *Anesthesiology.* 65:A245.

Bennett HL, Disbrow E. 1993. Preparation for surgery and medical procedures. In: Goleman D, Gurin J, eds. *Mind-Body Medicine: How to Use Your Mind for Better Health.* Yonkers, NY: Consumer Reports Books.

DeLong DR. 1970. Individual differences in patterns of anxiety arousal, stress-

324   relevant information, and recovery from surgery. Ph.D. diss., University of California, Los Angeles.

Devine EC 1992a. Effect of psychoeducational care for adult surgical patients: a meta-analysis of 191 studies. *Patient Educ Couns.* 19:129–142.

Devine EC. 1992b. Effect of psychoeducational care for adult surgical patients: a theory-probing meta-analysis of intervention studies. In: Cook ID, Cooper H, Coudray DS, eds. *Meta-Analysis for Explanation: A Casebook.* New York: Russell Sage Foundation.

Devine EC, Cook TD. 1986. Clinical and cost-savings effects of psychoeducational interventions with surgical patients: a meta-analysis. *Res Nurs Health.* 9:89–105.

Disbrow EA, Bennett HL, Owings JT. 1993. Preoperative suggestion hastens the return of gastrointestinal motility. *Western J Med.* 158:488–492.

Egbert LD, Battit GE, Welch CE, Bartlett MK. 1964. Reduction of postoperative pain by encouragement and instruction of patients. *New Engl J Med.* 270:825–827.

Enqvist E. 1995. Stress reduction, preoperative hypnosis and perioperative suggestion in maxillofacial surgery: somatic responses and recovery. *Stress Med.* 11:229–233.

Enqvist E, von Konow L, Bystedt H. 1995. Pre- and perioperative suggestion in maxillofacial surgery: effects on blood loss and recovery. *Int J Clin Exp Hypn.* 18:284–294.

Ghoneim MM, Block RI. 1992. Learning and consciousness during general anesthesia. *Anesthesiology.* 76:279–305.

Ghoneim MM, Block RI. 1997. Learning and memory during general anesthesia: an update. *Anesthesiology.* 87:387–410.

Hathaway D. 1986. Effect of preoperative instruction on postoperative outcomes: a meta-analysis. *Nursing Research.* 35:269–275.

Holden-Lund C. 1988. Effects of relaxation with guided imagery on surgical stress and wound healing. *Res Nurs Health.* 11:235–244.

Merikle PM, Daneman M. 1996. Memory for unconsciously perceived events: evidence from anesthetized patients. *Consciousness Cogn.* 5:525–541.

Mumford E, Schlesinger HJ, Glass GV. 1982. The effects of psychological intervention on recovery from surgery and heart attacks: an analysis of the literature. *Am J Public Health.* 72:141–151.

Rodgers L. 1995. Music for surgery. *Advances.* 11:49–57.

Schwender D, Klasing S, Konzen P, et al. 1996. Midlatency auditory evoked potentials during anaesthesia with increasing endexpiratory concentrations of desflurane. *Acta Anaesthesiol Scand.* 40:171–176.

Shipley RH, Butt JH, Horwitz B, Farbry JE. 1978. Preparation for a stressful medical procedure: effect of amount of stimulus pre-exposure and coping style. *J Consult Clin Psychol.* 46:499–507.

Shipley RH, Butt JH, Horowitz EA. 1979. Preparation to reexperience a stressful medical examination: effect of repetitious videotape exposure and coping style. *J Consult Clin Psychol.* 47:485–492.

Tusek DL, Church JM, Fazio VW. 1997. Guided imagery: a significant advance in

the care of patients undergoing elective colorectal surgery. *Dis Colon Rectum.* 325
40:172–178.

Wickramasekera I. 1998. Secrets kept from the mind but not the body or behavior.
Adv Mind Body Med. 14:81–132.

Wilson JF. 1981. Behavioral preparation for surgery: benefit or harm? *J Behav Med.*
4:79–102.

Index